DENTAL CARIES

Dental Caries
Aetiology, Pathology and Prevention

L. M. SILVERSTONE
N. W. JOHNSON
J. M. HARDIE
R. A. D. WILLIAMS

First published 1981 by
THE MACMILLAN PRESS LTD
London and Basingstoke
Associated companies in Delhi Dublin
Hong Kong Johannesburg Lagos Melbourne
New York Singapore and Tokyo

ISBN 0 333 21178 2 (hard cover)
ISBN 0 333 21179 0 (paper cover)

Printed in Hong Kong

Contents

Preface

This book is based on the 'Topic Course in Dental Caries', which was designed in 1972 for undergraduate dental students at The London Hospital Medical College and is now conducted annually. The objectives of the course are to provide the student with an understanding of dental caries as a disease process so that he can appreciate its impact on the orofacial tissues of his patients, on their general welfare, and on the community at large. Additional objectives are the provision of a sound biological basis for the treatment of carious teeth and of a scientific basis for the design and evaluation of preventive methods.

The book is thus aimed primarily at dental undergraduates at all levels; junior clinical students should be in a position to assimilate much of the scientific content because of their proximity to dental anatomy, biochemistry, microbiology and immunology. The practical implications of many of the concepts discussed will, however, be better appreciated by more senior students because of their greater clinical experience, and we hope that undergraduates will turn to the book at intervals throughout their education. Other professional groups should also find it a useful source of reference.

Because of the comprehensive treatment of most topics the book should be of value to graduate students in many specialities, and is deliberately aimed at them also. Some material, for example chapter 8 on the kinetics of enamel dissolution, is complex and will not be readily appreciated by the average clinical student. However, this has been deliberately included since it is part of the broad scientific base of cariology on which further progress in prevention and treatment depends. It is hoped that such detail will not inhibit the average reader from grasping the important principles involved, and we have therefore provided frequent summaries of the present state of knowledge.

All chapters describe the research findings upon which our current understanding is based. This makes the treatment lengthy at times, but it is in our view the proper approach to teaching in a university context.

L. M. S.
N. W. J.
J. M. H.
R. A. D. W.

Acknowledgements

We are grateful to numerous colleagues for helpful discussion and for providing tables and illustrations of their own original research. Mr George Walters and Ms Lindsay Hitchcock produced most of the photographs and Ms Jennifer Abrahams carried the major secretarial burden. Without them our task would have been impossible.

Part I
The Disease Process

Chapter 1

The Nature and Problem of Dental Caries in Man

1.1   Introduction

Dental caries and periodontal disease are the two most common oral diseases and study of them naturally dominates the teaching and practice of dentistry. To some extent they have a common cause and, frequently, a common end-point, namely loss of the affected teeth. As a generalisation, dental caries probably results in more pain and discomfort and periodontal disease in more tooth loss.

This book deals with dental caries in its broadest sense, a subject which is beginning to be defined as cariology in many countries. Cariology is a discrete subject because of the unique structure of the dental hard tissues and their response to environmental influences; it represents an application to a particular health problem of many other scientific disciplines such as epidemiology, pathology, microbiology, immunology, physical chemistry, biochemistry and biophysics. The fact that so many disciplines are involved in understanding caries is sufficient justification for the existence of cariology as a subject and for this book. However, in concentrating our attention on caries we should never lose sight of the equal importance of periodontal disease to the oral and general health of our patients.

Dental caries (*caries*—from the Latin, decay) simply means decay or rotting of the teeth (figure 1.1). It is a form of progressive destruction of enamel, dentine and cementum initiated by microbial activity at the tooth surface. Loss of tooth substance is characteristically preceded by a softening of these tissues, brought about by partial dissolution of mineral ahead of the total destruction of the tissue. Because of this, caries can be distinguished from other destructive processes of the crowns of teeth such as *abrasion* due to mechanical wear and *erosion* due to acid fluids which remove totally thin portions of the surface which they contact, layer by layer.

The purpose of this introductory chapter is to describe the problems that this widespread disease creates for the individual and for society as a whole, to explain, briefly, modern concepts of

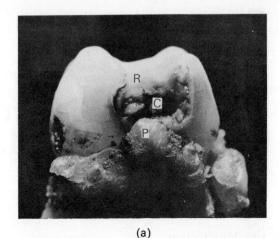

(a)

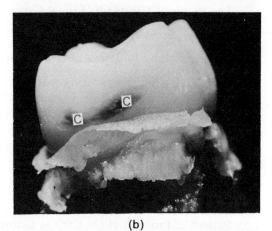

(b)

Figure 1.1   (a) Molar tooth extracted with the gingival soft tissues still attached to the cervical margin. This tooth has a large carious cavity (C) on the approximal surface which extends from just below the crest of the interdental papilla (P) upwards to undermine the occlusal marginal ridge (R). This is an advanced lesion which has taken many months to reach this stage, and represents a failure of caries control measures in this patient. (b) Molar tooth extracted with the gingival soft tissues attached to the cervical margin, showing an initial carious lesion (C) on the approximal surface. No cavity has yet formed but subsurface decalcification has occurred over a large area between the gingival crest and the area of contact with the adjacent tooth. This is the area in which plaque can grow relatively undisturbed. Lesions at this stage can be arrested or can be encouraged to regress if proper preventive measures are applied.

the cause and mechanisms of dental caries in man, and of how attempts can be made to reduce the ravages of the disease by preventive measures. All of these aspects are analysed in greater detail in subsequent chapters.

1.2 The Problems Created by Dental Caries

The need to restore carious teeth or to replace teeth lost due to caries obviously presents the individual with problems of time, discomfort, inconvenience and expense. Unless satisfactory prosthetic treatment is received, tooth loss may result in aesthetic deterioration and impairment of speech and masticatory function. Although rarely of life-threatening significance with modern processed diets, this latter problem can become an important consideration in aged individuals, and the impact on the quality of life of difficulty with chewing should not be underestimated. Loss of teeth leads inevitably to atrophy of the supporting alveolar bone and this may be accelerated by the provision of inadequate dentures. Following tooth loss there is a progressive alteration of the whole of the facial skeleton and associated musculature, and disease of oral soft tissues and of the temperomandibular joint may supervene (figure 1.2).

The pain and distress caused by inflammation of the pulp due to the progression of caries is all too familiar, and it has been estimated that one million nights of sleep are lost, and 5 million days disturbed by toothache each year in England alone[46]. As this condition is caused by bacteria, the possibility of spread of infection to surrounding bone, to and through contiguous soft tissues, and to more distant sites via the blood stream and lymphatic system must constantly be borne in mind. Today, caries rarely leads to fatal infection, but a few deaths each year are recorded by the Registrar General[1] as due to dental disease and a visit to any dental emergency clinic will confirm the extent of personal suffering which arises from dental infections. Oral infections in patients with rheumatic or congenital heart disease are particularly dangerous because of the risk of provoking infective endocarditis[2].

In addition to personal suffering, the almost universal presence of caries in Western com-

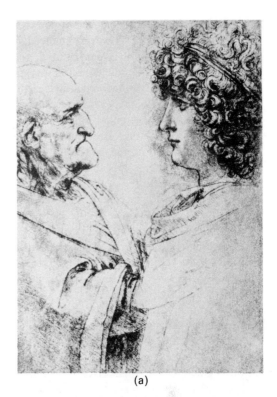

(a)

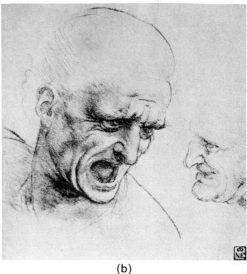

(b)

Figure 1.2 Two drawings by Leonardo da Vinci which illustrate poignantly the collapse of the face which follows tooth loss in old age. (a) 'Old Man and Youth' Red Chalk, about 1495, Uffizi Gallery, Florence. (b) 'Heads of Warriors' (Study for the battle of Anghiari) Black Chalk 1503–5, Museum of Fine Arts, Budapest. Reproduced by courtesy of The Phaidon Press Ltd., Oxford and London.

munities presents society as a whole with a considerable problem. However financed, the cost to the community is large. In the financial year 1977, approximately £250 million was spent in England and Wales alone on dental treatment within the General Dental Services section of the National Health Service and a little over half of this was required for the restoration of carious teeth[3]. This sum, by no means the total cost of oral disease, represents less than 4 per cent of total NHS expenditure[4, 5], although at one time dentistry received 10 per cent; it is exceeded as a single disease 'entity' only by the cost of the mental health services. The total cost of dental care is estimated to be £7.1 per head per annum, perhaps a modest figure when compared to what many individuals are prepared to spend on social and cosmetic activities.

Approximately 12 million working days are lost annually in Britain from dental disease and its complications. At the present time only approximately 40 per cent of the British population regularly avail themselves of the dental care services[10]. If all were to do, so, the cost would clearly rise steeply and the manpower resources, at present 20 000 dentists, 1050 hygienists and 500 operating auxiliaries[17, 46] would be unable to satisfy the demand.

It is clear, therefore, that much greater emphasis is necessary on the prevention of dental caries, as well as periodontal disease and other forms of oral disease. Only in this way will individual suffering be reduced while the cost to society is kept within practicable limits. Later in this chapter our present knowledge of the nature of the caries process is outlined, in order to point out those places in this complex series of events where the process may be interrupted by preventive methods. Each of these theoretical approaches to prevention are considered in detail in part II of the book.

1.3 The High Prevalence of Dental Caries

Although dental caries was known to ancient man, decay in his teeth usually began in dentine which had become exposed due to excessive wear associated with abrasive diets, and on root surfaces and cervical portions of the crowns[6, 7]. In modern communities, caries commences most often at the enamel surface in the pits and fissures of the crown, beneath the contact areas of approximal surfaces of teeth in contact, and in the cervical third of the crown between the gingival margins and the point of maximum convexity of the crown (figures 1.3 and 1.4). This is because it is in these areas that bacteria, in the form of dental plaque, adhere to the teeth, and are relatively protected from becoming scraped off. Root surface caries is still, however, common in primitive and developing societies and, on a global scale, may be the most prevalent form of the disease[8].

The prevalence of caries has increased steadily with the advance of civilisation; for example, studies of ancient Greek skulls show that at about the time of the birth of Christ 10 per cent of that population were affected[9]. By AD 1000 this had risen to 20 per cent and today, in most of the so-called advanced Western civilisations, the figure approaches 100 per cent.

Dental caries and periodontal disease are the most common diseases affecting Western man. In England and Wales the prevalence of caries in adults is 98 per cent, and a National Survey conducted in 1968 found that only 3 people in 1000 had 28 or more teeth present and free from decay[10]. In all the major industrialised nations the extent of disease increases with age, most rapidly during childhood and adolescence, but still steadily to middle age. In Britain, 25 per cent of all teeth erupted in children up to 12 years of age have been affected by caries; by the age of 15 years this has risen to 33 per cent and by age 30, to 67 per cent. By the age of 45 years caries is much less active, although many teeth continue to be lost from periodontal disease.

Apart from age and the advance of civilisation, many other factors influence the prevalence and incidence of dental caries in populations. These include dietary habits, race, geographical location, sex, familial patterns and the influence of treatment. The complex interrelationship of

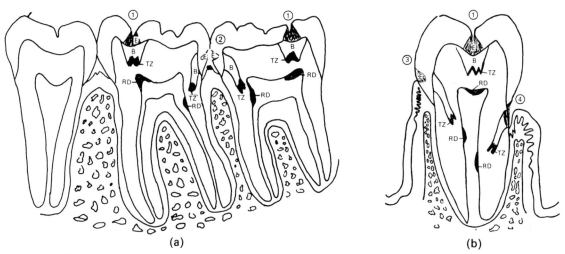

(a) (b)

Figure 1.3 Diagram of sites on the surfaces of teeth where plaque accumulates and carious lesions preferentially develop. (a) Mesio-distal section through a premolar and two molar teeth. (b) Bucco-lingual section through a premolar tooth. Lesions are labelled:

    (1) Class I caries, commencing in pits or fissures
    (2) Class II caries, interproximal lesions
    (3) Class V caries, gingival third lesions and (4) root surface caries arising on exposed cementum or root dentine following gingival recession.

The pattern of progress through tooth substance is also indicated: The lesion within enamel is labelled E. B represents the body of the dentine lesion, TZ the translucent zone defence reaction in dentine and RD the reactionary dentine formed in response to the early enamel and dentine lesions.

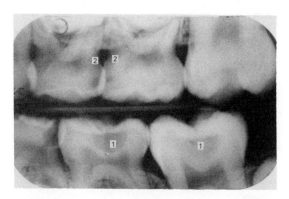

Figure 1.4 'Bite-wing' radiograph showing a child with deciduous molars and first permanent molars in function. Prominent occlusal pit and fissure lesions (1) and approximal (2) lesions are visible because of the marked radiolucency in the dentine. (Courtesy of Professor A. H. Brook)

these factors is analysed in detail in chapter 2, but the serious state of affairs in the whole of the Western world can be emphasised here by considering the extent of tooth loss. Complete tooth loss—a state indicating total failure of both past preventive dentistry and past dental treatment—

has been reached by approximately 25 per cent of the population of England and Wales at the age of 40 years, and this figure is 75 per cent at the age of 60; 37 per cent of the population over 16 years of age have no natural teeth[10].

1.4 The Causes and Initiation of Dental Caries

An oversimplified but essentially accurate concept of the aetiology and pathogenesis of dental caries has existed for a century and has come to be known as the chemicoparasitic or acidogenic theory. This holds that bacteria present in the mouth interact with retained food particles to produce substances capable of dissolving enamel. The three essential components of the caries process are thus immediately appreciated, namely the presence of a susceptible tooth, the presence of microorganisms and dietary factors.

An enormous amount of subsequent research has confirmed this concept and provided detail concerning those features of the structure and

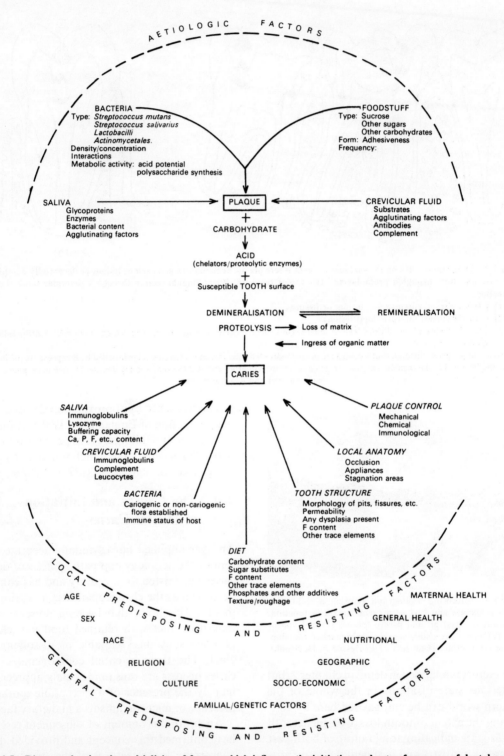

Figure 1.5 Diagram showing the multiplicity of factors which influence the initiation and rate of progress of dental caries.

composition of teeth which affect their susceptibility to caries, detail on which bacteria are most likely to be involved, and detail on those components of the diet which are particularly dangerous.

Many other factors, both local and systemic, influence the likelihood of caries developing and its speed of progression, so that caries is truly a multifactorial disease. These factors and their interactions are presented schematically in figure 1.5, the object of which is to indicate areas to be discussed in detail in subsequent chapters. It may be helpful to return to this diagram from time to time during the reading of subsequent chapters, and to use it as a structure for revision.

As might be expected from such a highly complex situation, the caries process is dynamic, with periods of attack alternating with periods of stasis or with regression of the lesion. This fact has an important bearing on any clinical approach to the management of patients, the prime objective of which should be to tip the balance towards arrest or regression; that is, to control the cariogenicity of the patient's mouth and to encourage remineralisation of damaged tooth structure.

1.4.1 The acidogenic (chemicoparasitic) theory of caries

A number of theories of caries aetiology exist but, as stated above, most of the available evidence supports the 'acidogenic theory', or 'chemicoparasitic theory', propounded in some detail as long ago as 1890 by an American, W. D. Miller[11]. Miller based his ideas on a series of experiments conducted in the laboratories of the famous German microbiologist, Robert Koch. He drew heavily on the new knowledge of bacteriology emerging in Europe at that time, principally from the laboratories of Koch and of his great rival Louis Pasteur in France. Of particular significance was the observation that many organisms could produce acid from the fermentation of sugar. Miller showed that a number of oral microorganisms had this property, that lactic acid was one of the major acids formed, and that extracted teeth could be de-

mineralised by incubating them in mixtures of sugar or bread with saliva. At about the same time, Williams[12] recognised the fact that bacteria adhered firmly to enamel surfaces, producing a gelatinous film which he considered might localise the acid to its most dangerous site, in contact with the tooth.

In essence, therefore, the chemicoparasitic theory postulates that acids are produced at or near the tooth surface by bacterial fermentation of dietary carbohydrates and that these acids dissolve the apatite crystals which make up some 95 per cent of the mass of the enamel. Washing away of the acid is reduced by the presence of dental plaque, which also serves to hold the products of dissolution close to the tooth surface (figure 1.6). We now know that many different kinds of bacteria aggregate in protected portions of the tooth surface to form dental plaque (chapter 4), and that if the kinds of organism we now recognise as cariogenic (chapter 3) are present in substantial numbers, damaging amounts of acid can be formed.

Following the ingestion of readily fermentable carbohydrates, particularly those with a low molecular weight such as the sugars glucose and sucrose, the pH in plaque falls to 4.5 or 5 within 1–3 minutes and takes 10–30 minutes to return to neutrality. Subsequent intakes of carbohydrate may depress the pH even further. This characteristic graph (figure 1.7), known as a Stephan curve after the dental scientist who first brought it into prominence[13], is further discussed in chapter 5. Such levels of acidity are dangerous because, whereas at neutrality human saliva and dental plaque are supersaturated with calcium and phosphate, at about pH 5 this saturation is overcome and enamel solubility increases markedly.

There is ample evidence that a direct correlation exists between type and frequency of carbohydrate ingestion and the lowering of intra-oral pH, and a similar correlation between dietary carbohydrate levels and caries incidence. The acids involved can be identified easily in the test tube in sugar–saliva mixtures, after incubation of various other foodstuffs with saliva

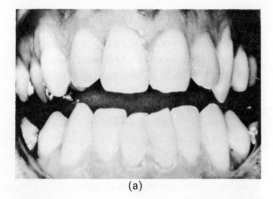

(a)

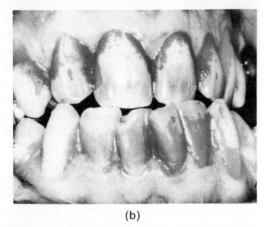

(b)

Figure 1.6   (a) Anterior view of adult dentition. Extensive plaque deposits are present but cannot easily be seen in this photograph. (b) Some subject as in (a) immediately after staining plaque deposits with disclosing solution. Plaque is particularly heavy interproximally and near to the gingival margin.

or dental plaque microorganisms[14a, 14b], and with more difficulty in the dental plaque[15] and in carious enamel itself. These are all organic acids, principally lactic acid, and are produced as end products of the Embden–Meyerhoff glycolytic pathway and of the Krebs tricarboxylic acid cycle, or of other pathways which these bacteria use in the catabolism of carbohydrate (see chapter 5). Lactic acid is capable of producing exact histological replicas of the early natural carious lesion when sound extracted teeth are placed in sterile artificial systems containing the acid and a gelatinous medium, such as gelatin, which apparently acts by providing a diffusion barrier for the products of enamel dissolution[16].

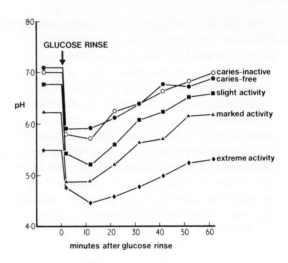

Figure 1.7   The 'Stephan' curve. This shows the rapid fall in pH following a glucose rinse in a group of individuals with different caries activities (after Stephan 1944[13])

1.4.2   The essential role of bacteria

In the mouth, the presence of bacterial plaque is essential to the production of a lesion, for it is bacterial metabolism which produces the acid from foodstuff and the plaque consistency which helps retain the acid in contact with the tooth and protected from the diluting and buffering effect of saliva. Proof of the absolute necessity for bacteria had to wait, however, until the 1950s when Orland and then Keyes and their collaborators showed that susceptible rodents on a highly cariogenic diet did not develop caries under germ-free conditions, but that caries developed in the same animals when fed the same diet after the introduction of bacteria[18, 19]. In 1960, Keyes[20] proved for the first time the infectious and transmissible nature of dental caries. He mono-infected germ-free animals with known strains of streptococci and showed that the organisms, and susceptibility to caries, became transferred to uninfected litter mates. Subsequently, the use of gnotobiotic rodents (that is, animals carrying a known flora) has done much to sort out which species of bacteria, and which combinations of species, are cariogenic to these animals and which might, therefore, be cariogenic to man[21,22]. These organisms, mostly streptococci of the viridans type, particularly the species known as *Streptococcus mutans*, and some strains of lactobacilli and actinomycetes are cariogenic in animals and man (chapter 3). Such organisms isolated from human lesions have been used to induce caries in previously caries-free monkeys maintained on diets rich in sucrose and other carbohydrates[23]; the organisms, and hence susceptibility to caries, can be transferred readily from mother to offspring, although adult cage mates, in whom the oral flora is already established, are more resistant[24].

Organisms of this type are more numerous in the mouths of caries-active than of caries-inactive persons, and their distribution within the mouth to some extent mirrors the distribution of carious lesions. It thus seems possible to regard dental caries in man as an infectious and transmissible disease, although there may be several different organisms involved. The familial pattern of caries prevalence may be partly explained by cross-infection between parents and children, although diet and other environmental factors are also important. The essential cariogenicity of these organisms lies in their ability to produce acid rapidly from carbohydrate, that is they are *acidogenic*, in their ability to survive under acid conditions, that is they are *aciduric*, and in their propensity to adhere to and proliferate upon hard tooth surfaces. Most cariogenic organisms also have the ability, through possession of the necessary enzyme systems, to synthesise large amounts of extracellular polysaccharide from dietary sugars. These polysaccharides, mostly polymers of glucose (that is, glucans of variable complexity), make up much of the interbacterial matrix of dental plaque. Plaque polysaccharides are sticky, gelatinous substances which may help bacteria adhere to the tooth and to one another, and which affect the permeability characteristics of the plaque, thus influencing the rate at which saliva can neutralise or dilute acid formed in the depths of the plaque, and slowing the diffusion away from the tooth of the products of mineral dissolution.

It is clear that dental plaque is a very heterogeneous structure which varies in composition from site to site on any given tooth surface, from tooth to tooth, and from mouth to mouth. Not all portions of enamel covered by plaque become carious, indicating important regional variations in the pathogenicity of dental plaque. Much remains to be learned of the nature and significance of these variations, which are discussed further in chapter 4.

1.4.3 The role of dietary carbohydrates: sucrose as the 'arch-criminal'

Dietary carbohydrates as substrates for acid production and for the synthesis of extracellular polysaccharides in plaque have already been mentioned. The relative cariogenicity of different carbohydrates depends on frequency of intake, on their physical form—sticky, retentive substances such as toffee being worst—and on their chemical type. Complex carbohydrates such as starch are not digested to any significant degree in the mouth. Low-molecular-weight substances, particularly sugars, are more dangerous because they can more readily diffuse into the plaque and are more rapidly metabolised by the bacteria.

Sucrose has been described as the 'arch-criminal' of dental caries[25]. It is much more cariogenic than glucose, for example, which diffuses just as readily into plaque and produces acid just as quickly. Sucrose is the most abundantly consumed sugar in modern diets and some explanation of the mechanism by which it produces damage is now available. Cariogenic microorganisms synthesise extracellular polysaccharides faster from this disaccharide than from any other sugar—faster even than from equivalent mixtures of its constituents glucose and fructose. The energy liberated from rupture of the disaccharide bond is used, with the aid of bacterial glucosyl transferases, to synthesise complex glucans from the glucose. Fructose is incorporated into fructans of the levan type which are not so chemically stable and may be metabolised to acid quite quickly.

Plaque bacteria also make, and store, intracellular polysaccharides of the glycogen type from dietary sugars. Both intracellular and extracellular polysaccharides may be used as substrates for acid production in periods when no food is being taken into the mouth. It is as important, therefore, to remove the bacteria as to restrict carbohydrate intake, and teeth might well be cleaned before meals with as much effect as after meals; indeed, all our knowledge of the pathogenesis of caries points to before-meal cleaning as the most rational oral hygiene approach to caries prevention.

1.4.4 Other theories of caries aetiology

Several theories, other than the acidogenic theory just described, have been advanced over the years to explain the cause of caries. The more important of them will be outlined here, although none has convincing experimental support[26]. Nevertheless it is important to realise that these mechanisms are by no means mutually exclusive, so that some may well operate, albeit to a minor degree, in the process of tooth destruction.

The proteolytic theory

This theory is attributed to Gottlieb who, in 1944, suggested that proteolytic enzymes liberated by oral bacteria destroyed the organic matrix of enamel so that the crystals became detached and the structure collapsed—rather like the mortar softening and weakening an old brick wall[27]. In the same year, a similar interpretation was published by Frisbie[28], and in 1949 Pincus[29] extended the concept by proposing that sulphatases of Gram-negative bacilli hydrolysed the sulphated mucosubstances of the matrix, liberating sulphuric acid, which then dissolved mineral.

While there is no doubt that a wide variety of proteolytic enzymes are produced by dental plaque, and these may be of importance in damaging soft tissue in the initiation and progression of periodontal disease[30], proteolysis is unlikely to be of prime importance in the initiation of enamel caries. Lesions cannot be reproduced in vitro with proteolytic agents although, as we have seen, organic acids can do so under appropriate conditions of diffusion limitation or buffering. Furthermore, those portions of enamel with a relatively high organic content, such as tufts and lamellae, do not show greater susceptibility to decay. Nevertheless it would be foolish to ignore the proteolytic activity which is undoubtedly present for, along with the more obvious destruction of mineral, alterations in the organic matrix of enamel undoubtedly occur[31] and must influence the progress of the lesion. These, however, are less easily detected because of the small amount of organic material present (less than 1 per cent protein by weight in sound tissue[32]). Organic changes certainly include breakdown of intrinsic enamel matrix, and we now know that some of this is acid soluble[41, 42]. In addition, there is ingress of additional organic matter derived from oral fluids and bacteria, which fills the gaps between partially dissolved apatite crystals (chapter 6). In carious destruction of cementum and of dentine (chapter 7), proteolysis is undoubtedly a much more significant event, although it may be necessary for the tissue to be first demineralised by acid, thus allowing the enzymes access for collagen and ground substance[43].

The proteolysis—chelation theory

The proteolysis—chelation theory was proposed by Schatz, Martin and co-workers in the 1950s[33], and in a large number of subsequent publications by these workers. This theory proposes that products of the proteolysis of tooth substance, and possibly also of the acquired pellicle and foods, by bacterial enzymes act as chelating agents which remove Ca ions from the tooth. The significance of this proposal is that chelation, a process whereby metallic ions are complexed to another molecule by coordinate covalent bonds, is most efficient at neutral or even slightly alkaline pH. Thus, enamel destruction could occur at times when plaque pH was close to neutrality.

The peptides and amino acids produced in this way do have chelating activity, as do a number of other molecules likely to be present in dental plaque. These latter include citrate, lactate, hydroxy and keto esters of the Embden–Meyerhoff glycolytic pathway, and intermediates of the tricarboxylic acid cycle such as citrate, and of the hexose monophosphate shunt; but all are weak chelating agents and are not present in sufficient concentration to account for the amount of demineralisation which occurs[34]. It is probable that chelators in plaque are exhausted by binding with the more readily available and more soluble calcium and other cations derived from saliva.

Nevertheless this theory is attractive in that it reconciles the conflict between whether it is destruction of matrix or mineral which is the key event, by proposing that both occur simultaneously and interdependently. Some features of the histopathology of enamel caries can be simulated in vitro with chelating agents[35], and mixtures of oral bacteria and carbohydrates permitted to undergo glycolysis and then neutralised are capable of dissolving enamel[36]. Thus, while chelation cannot be regarded as a major part of the destructive process in enamel caries, it may play a minor role for a period after plaque pH returns to neutrality following an acid pulse, such as is visualised in the Stephan curve.

The sucrose–chelation theory

Eggers-Lura (1948–68) has proposed in a series of papers that the very high sucrose concentrations often encountered in the mouths of caries-active individuals form Ca-saccharates and Ca-complexing intermediaries which require inorganic phosphate removed from the enamel by phosphorylating enzymes[37a, 37b]. This, however, is unlikely to be a significant process because of the rapidity with which sucrose is metabolised to acid and polysaccharide, and because calcium saccharates can only form at high pH, above the range usually found in the mouth[44].

Auto-immunity

Jackson and Burch, in recent years[38a, 38b], have revived the old 'intrinsic' concept of caries aetiology, by suggesting the primary event to be placed within the tooth itself, rather than on the tooth surface. They suggest that clones or regions of odontoblasts in specific sites within the pulp of specific teeth are damaged by an auto-immune process, so that the defence capacity of the overlying dentine and enamel is compromised, and conclude that caries should be regarded as a degenerative disease. The hypothesis is based on complex statistical analysis of the frequency and distribution of lesions within the mouths of a large number of individuals, and comparison with statistical analyses of known auto-immune diseases.

These authors argue that if, for example, caries develops on the mesial surface of a maxillary central incisor, it is reasonable to assume the disease will eventually involve the adjacent surface of the adjoining tooth because of a common plaque environment. However, they have shown that from the age of 22 to 60 years, the ratio of the number of attacks on single central incisors to those on both incisors remains approximately constant at 1:0.7. They conclude that the initiating events correspond to a form of somatic gene mutation in central growth control stem cells; descendant mutant cells synthesise auto-antibodies which damage specific groups of odontoblasts and thus determine the sites of caries susceptibility.

Difficulties in accepting these arguments arise from the fact that most of the data used are derived from routine clinical studies, not from rigorously conducted epidemiological trials, and it is even doubtful whether data from trials are accurate enough for mathematical analysis of this kind. Furthermore, the data are cross-sectional, not longitudinal, and Edgar states that the findings are a statistical artefact arising from selection of subjects with similar caries experience at different ages[45].

It may also be possible to reconcile the findings with events at the tooth surface, because we now know that there are marked local variations in plaque flora and thus in metabolic activity. Furthermore, an incisor which is caries-free clinically may be carious at a histological level. Finally, no histological evidence of primary damage to odontoblasts has been produced.

1.5   Pattern of Progress of the Carious Lesion

Once bacterial plaque has grown and acids, and possibly from time to time proteolytic and chelating agents, are formed within it, destruction of the tooth occurs in a highly characteristic manner. The initial enamel lesion is characterised by the important feature of sub-surface demineralisation, a narrow zone of surface enamel remaining relatively unaffected[39]. This occurs not only because the surface has a greater chemical resistance to acid, due in part to its greater fluoride content, but also because of the resistance to diffusion away from the site of liberated calcium and phosphate ions. Demineralisation of the sub-surface tissue continues, the pattern of spread being determined by structural features such as crystal and prism orientation and striae of Retzius, until it is so weakened that a cavity results. Bacteria then, and only then, gain access to tooth structure.

While these early changes are taking place in sub-surface enamel, with the causative bacteria still confined to plaque on the tooth surface, the dentine and pulp together mount a series of defence reactions (figure 1.3). The most important of these defence reactions are the laying down of reactionary dentine at the pulpal surface beneath the enamel lesion and the sealing-off of many tubules in a central zone of dentine beneath the lesion by a process of accelerated production of peritubular dentine. This latter process is known as tubular sclerosis and results, histologically, in the production of translucent dentine. At the same time, demineralisation of the dentine near the enamel–dentine junction occurs. However, because the dentine is not at this stage infected, the pulp itself is not in imminent danger

and such lesions are capable of being arrested. Treatment priorities for such lesions should, therefore, be to minimise the cariogenic challenge by control of diet and oral hygiene and the encouragement of remineralisation by topical fluoride applications.

Once a cavity has formed in the enamel, bacteria reach the enamel–dentine junction and pass along the dentinal tubules, although their progress will be delayed for a time by the presence of the translucent zone defence reaction. Initially, the organisms in dentine are mainly aciduric types like lactobacilli and streptococci, but a more mixed acidogenic and proteolytic flora soon follow. At this stage there is direct soft tissue continuity between the mouth and the neurovascular connective tissue of the pulp. The pulp therefore becomes inflamed, causing pain, and unless proper treatment is instituted the bacteria themselves will progress through the remaining dentine to infect the pulp. An infected pulp often becomes necrotic and there is then the possibility of spread of infection beyond the tooth.

Nevertheless, the pattern of progress of the disease through tooth substance is a dynamic one, and if the intensity of the attack diminishes, previously demineralised tissue may become partly remineralised. With the possible exception of rampant (nursing-bottle) caries in infants, most lesions show evidence of phasic demineralisation and remineralisation.

A detailed description of the structural changes which take place in tooth substance during the initiation and progression of a carious lesion is given in chapters 6 and 7.

1.6   Theoretical Approaches to Caries Prevention

Dental caries is a completely preventable disease, by relatively simple means, in well-motivated individuals or families. The families of motivated dentists, for example, have a strikingly lower caries incidence than the population at large[40]. To achieve effective prevention on a community level is, however, much more difficult and requires both the deployment of all the currently available methods as well as continued research for new methods.

Theoretically (table 1.1), attempts can be made to prevent caries by modifying any of the interacting aetiological factors in the top part of figure 1.5, shown earlier, or by improving some of the resistance factors in the lower part of the diagram. Thus, attempts can be made to control caries by modifying an individual's diet—first so that the diet is nutritionally adequate and teeth are well formed in utero and in childhood, secondly by restricting the amount and frequency of intake of cariogenic foodstuffs, particularly sucrose, and thirdly by the addition of inhibitory agents such as phosphates and fluorides to the diet. These approaches are described in detail in chapter 9.

Dental plaque itself can also be a prime target—either by continually removing established plaque by mechanical cleaning or chemical disinfectants, or by retarding its formation by direct attack on the growth and aggregation of constituent bacteria, particularly specific pathogens, by immunological methods. Substances which inhibit the biochemical processes in plaque of importance in caries production can also be sought. Prevention of caries by plaque control is described in detail in chapter 11.

Chapter 12 describes current methods by which the resistance of the tooth surface to demineralisation may be enhanced. These include a variety of topical fluoride applications, the sealing of pits and fissures with plastic resins, and preparations which remineralise slightly damaged tissue.

The most effective way of preventing caries on a community scale is by fluoridation of public water supplies. The mode of action of fluoride and its systemic balance is therefore considered in chapter 10.

Chapters 9–12 thus emphasise the scientific basis of caries prevention and constitute part II of the text. For several decades, methods of caries prevention have tended to be rather empirical. However, as part I of the book will show, in the past 20 years our knowledge of oral physiology and of the caries process has increased considerably, partly because dental research has benefited from the input of so many scientific disciplines. It is now possible to base methods of caries prevention on a firm scientific foundation and continued progress towards more effective and more readily applicable methods is to be expected.

References

1. Registrar General's Statistical Reviews of England & Wales, *Mortality Statistics by Cause*, Office of Population Censuses and Surveys, HMSO, London
2. Nolte, W. A. (1977). *Oral Microbiology*, 3rd edn, C. V. Mosby, St. Louis, ch. 22
3. Dental Estimates Board Annual Reports, Department of Health and Social Security, HMSO, London
4. Office of Health Economics Information Sheets, 162 Regent Street, London W1
5. *Health and Personal Social Services Statistics for England 1977*, HMSO, London, p. 20
6. Miles, A. E. W. (1969). The dentition of the Anglo-Saxons. *Proceedings of the Royal Society of Medicine*, **62**, 1311–15

Table 1.1   Approaches to caries prevention

Plaque Control:	Mechanical
	Chemical
	Immunological
Dietary Control:	Reduced frequency of carbohydrate intake
	Sucrose substitutes
	Additives

Increasing the Resistance of the Tooth:

Pre-eruptive methods —	Adequate nutrition
	— Systemic fluoride
Post-eruptive methods —	Topical fluorides
	— Fissure sealants Remineralising solutions

7. Leigh, R. W. (1935). Notes on the stoma-tology and pathology of ancient Egypt. *Journal of the American Dental Association*, **22**, 199–222

8. Jordan, H. V. and Sumney, D. L. (1973). Root surface caries: review of the literature and significance of the problem. *Journal of Periodontology*, **44**, 158–62

9. Krikos, A. (1935). The progress of decay in Greece from the most ancient times down to the present. *Transactions of the American Dental Society of Europe*. Quoted by Dunning, J. N. (1978). *Principles of Dental Public Health*, Harvard University Press, Cambridge, Mass., p. 129

10. Gray, P. G., Todd, J. E., Slack, G. L. and Bulman, J. S. (1970). *Adult Dental Health in England and Wales 1968*, HMSO, London

11. Miller, W. D. (1890). *The Microorganisms of the Human Mouth*, S. S. White Dental Manufacturing Co., Philadelphia. Repub-lished, K. Konig, (Ed.), by S. Karger, Basel, 1973

12. Williams, J. L. (1897). A contribution to the study of pathology of enamel. *Dental Cosmos*, **39**, 169, 269, 353

13. Stephan, R. M. (1944). Intraoral hydrogen ion concentrations associated with dental caries activity. *Journal of Dental Research*, **23**, 257–66

14a. Andlaw, R. J. (1968). Qualitative paper and thin layer chromatography of some non-volatile acids produced by whole human saliva. *Archives of Oral Biology*, **13**, 445–56

14b. Andlaw, R. J. (1968). Qualitative gas–liquid chromatography of some non-volatile acids produced by human whole saliva. *Archives of Oral Biology*, **13**, 457–66

15. Geddes, D. A. M. (1975). Acids produced by human dental plaque metabolism *in situ*. *Caries Research*, **9**, 98–109

16. Silverstone, L. M. (1968). The surface zone in caries like lesions produced *in vitro*. *British Dental Journal*, **125**, 145–57

17. General Dental Council, 37 Wimpole Street, London W1

18. Orland, F. J., Blayney, J. R., Harrison, R. W., Reyniers, J. A., Trexler, P. C., Gordon, H. A., Wagner, M. and Lockey, T. D. (1954). Use of germ-free animal technique in the study of experimental dental caries. *Journal of Dental Research*, **33**, 147–74

19. Fitzgerald, R. J. and Keyes, P. H. (1960). Demonstration of the aetiologic role of streptococci in experimental caries in the hamster. *Journal of the American Dental Association*, **61**, 9–19

20. Keyes, P. H. (1960). The infectious and transmissible nature of experimental dental caries — findings and implications. *Archives of Oral Biology*, **1**, 304–20

21. Harris, R. S. (Ed.) (1968). *Art and Science of Dental Caries Research*, Academic Press, New York and London

22. Stiles, H. M., Loesche, W. J. and O'Brien, T. C. (Eds) (1976). *Microbiol Aspects of Dental Caries*, special supplement to *Microbiology Abstracts*, 3 vols, Infor-mation Retrieval Inc., Washington DC and London

23. Bowen, W. H., Cohen, B. and Colman, G. (1975). Immunisation against dental caries. *British Dental Journal*, **139**, 45–58

24. Bowen, W. H. (1968). Dental caries in monkeys, in *Advances in Oral Biology*, vol. 3 (Ed. P. Staple), Academic Press, London and New York

25. Newbrun, E. (1967). Sucrose, the arch criminal of dental caries. *Odontologist Revy*, **18**, 373–86

26. Bibby, B., Gustafson, G. and Davies, G. N. (1968). A critique of three theories of caries attack. *International Dental Journal*, **8**, 685–95

27. Gottleib, B. (1944). New concept of the caries problem and its clinical application. *Journal of the American Dental Association*, **31**, 1482, 1489, 1598

28. Frisbie, H. E., Nuckolls, J. and Saunders, J. B. de C. M. (1944). Distribution of the organic matrix of the enamel in the human tooth and its relation to the histopathology

of caries. *Journal of American College of Dentists*, **11**, 243–79

29. Pincus, P. (1949). Production of dental caries: a new hypothesis. *British Medical Journal*, **2**, 358–62

30. Cowley, G. and Macphee, T. (1975). *Essentials of Periodontology and Periodontics*, 2nd edn, Blackwell Scientific Publications, Oxford and Edinburgh

31. Johansen, E. (1965). Electron microscope and chemical studies of carious lesions with reference to the organic phase of affected tissues. *Annals of the New York Academy of Sciences*, **131**, 776–85

32. Miles, A. E. W. (Ed.) (1967). *Structural and Chemical Organization of Teeth*, Academic Press, London and New York

33. Schatz, A., Karlson, K. E., Martin, J. J., Schatz, V. (1957). The proteolysis chelation theory of dental caries. *Odontologist Revy*, **8**, 308–22

34. Jenkins, G. N. (1961). A critique of the proteolysis–chelation theory of caries. *British Dental Journal*, **111**, 311–30

35. Johnson, N. W., Poole, D. F. G. and Tyler, J. (1971). Factors affecting the differential dissolution of human enamel in acid and EDTA. *Archives of Oral Biology*, **16**, 385–96

36. Mörch, T., Punwani, I and Greeve, E. (1971). The possible role of complex forming substances in the decalcification phase of the caries process. *Caries Research*, **5**, 135–43

37a. Eggers-Lura, H. (1963). Recent investigations supporting the non-acid caries theory. The biochemical properties of dental plaques and sucrose. *International Dental Journal*, **13**, 456–9.

37b. Eggers-Lura, H. (1967). The non-acid complexing theory of dental caries. Published by the author, Holbaek

38a. Jackson, D., Burch, P. R. J., Fairpo, C. G. (1972). Dental caries: distribution by age groups between the normal and distal surfaces of human permanent mandibular incisors. *Archives of Oral Biology*, **17**, 1343–50

38b. Jackson, D., Burch, P. R. J., Fairpo, C. G. (1972). The distribution of clinical dental caries between the adjacent surfaces of neighbouring mandibular incisors. *Archives of Oral Biology*, **17**, 1351–5

39. Darling, A. I. (1958). Studies of the early lesion of enamel caries with transmitted light, polarized light, and microradiography. Its nature, mode of spread, points of entry and its relation to enamel structure. *British Dental Journal*, **105**, 119–35

40. Bradford, E. W. and Crabb, H. S. M. (1962). Carbohydrates and the incidence of caries in the deciduous dentition. *Proceedings ORCA*: (The European Organisation for Caries Research). See also Idem (1961) *British Dental Journal*, **111**, 273–79

41. Robinson, C. and Lowe, N. R. (1975). Amino acid composition, distribution and origin of 'tuft' protein in human and bovine dental enamel. *Archives of Oral Biology*, **20**, 29–42

42. Weatherell, J. A. (1975). Composition of dental enamel. *British Medical Bulletin*, **31**, 115–19

43. Evans, D. G. and Prophet, A. S. (1950). Disintegration of human dentine by bacterial enzymes, *Lancet*, **1**, 290–3

44. Tatevossian, A. and Jenkins, G. N. (1974). Sucrose and the role of saccharates in enamel caries. *Caries Research*, **8**, 317–31

45. Edgar, W. M. (1974). A 15 year retrospective survey of the distributions of clinical caries attacks in human permanent maxillary incisors. *Archives of Oral Biology*, **19**, 1203–9

46. Miller, J., Elwood, P. C. and Swallow, J. N. (1975). Dental pain – an incidence study. *British Dental Journal*, **139**, 327–8

Chapter 2

The Epidemiology of Dental Caries

B. A. Burt

Program in Dental Public Health, School of Public Health, The University of Michigan, Ann Arbor, Michigan 48104, USA; formerly Lecturer in Community Dentistry, The London Hospital Medical College

Up, and after putting several things in order to my removal, to Woolwich; the plague having a great increase this week, beyond all expectation, of almost 2,000, making the general Bill 7,000, odd 100; and the plague above 6,000. Thus this month ends with great sadness upon the public, through the greatness of the plague everywhere throughout the kingdom almost. Every day sadder and sadder news of its increase. In the city dies this week 7,496, and of them 6,102 of the plague. But is feared that the true number of the dead this week is near 10 000: partly from the poor that cannot be taken notice of, through the greatness of the number, and partly from the Quakers and others that will not have any bell ring for them.

(The *Diary* of Samuel Pepys, entry for 31 August 1665)

The word 'epidemiology' is of Greek origin. It can be defined as the study of health and disease in populations, and of how these states are influenced by the environment and by ways of living. As one example of how the environment affects disease, the major causes of death in Britain at the end of the nineteenth century were diphtheria, scarlet fever, typhoid fever, tuberculosis and other bronchial conditions, all of which reflected the environment of the time. Current major disease problems, such as heart disease, cancer, kidney disease, mental disorders, venereal diseases and accidents, reflect just as accurately the environment of our times. The 'epidemiological method' means the approach to examining the states of health and disease in a community as they relate to specific factors in its environment.

Epidemiology is related to ecology, that branch of biology dealing with the interrelationships of organisms with their environment. The ecological view sees man as an organism in constant interaction with other organisms in the environment, all endlessly changing and adapting to each other so that a permanent equilibrium is never reached. It also allows for an easier understanding of the 'multifactorial' concept of disease causation, so that the 'cause' of modern disease problems is just as much bound up with stress, affluence, diet, leisure, material and moral standards as it is with microorganisms. Both dental caries and peridontal disease are examples of diseases with multifactorial causes.

2.1   The Measurement of Disease

2.1.1   Development of the epidemiological method

An *epidemic* is an outbreak of a disease condition affecting many people in a region at the same time, although 'an epidemic disease' is frequently understood to be a disease of high morbidity which is only occasionally present in a community. The word has lost much of its dramatic impact in Western* society of the 1970s; the periodic epidemics of upper respiratory infections now experienced account for few deaths and do not disrupt the pattern of life very much. It should not be forgotten, however, that up to the mid-1950s epidemics of poliomyelitis produced serious consequences in Western countries, and the great influenza epidemic of 1918/19, more properly called a *pandemic*, was responsible for some 20 million deaths around the world. In some countries, epidemics of cholera and typhoid fever still occur, although they are becoming less frequent. A cholera epidemic in Egypt in 1947 killed 10 000 people, and about that number die each year of cholera in the Indian subcontinent. In those countries, cholera is an *endemic* disease, meaning that it is constantly

---

*   Throughout this volume the terms 'Western society' or 'Western diet' are used to describe the predominant culture and diet of those countries of Western Europe or countries of principally European origin, such as the USA, Canada, Australia and New Zealand. It refers to those nations where industrialisation has produced high material living standards, and where modern diets consist chiefly of processed and manufactured foods which are mass-distributed far from their point of preparation. These diets are notable for their frequency of high-carbohydrate 'convenience' foods, and they include high quantities of sugar. In the so-called 'developing' countries, industrialisation has not developed to the point where mass-distribution of processed foods allows such high consumption of sugar as is found in the Western societies, although it is a matter of concern that this situation is rapidly changing in some of them. This distinction between Western and non-Western societies, even from this oversimplified description, needs to be recognised for the influence it has on the epidemiology of caries.

present but occurring in a relatively small number of cases.

Advances in medical treatment in Western countries have been so great in recent years that it is difficult for us to envisage the terror created by the great epidemics of other years. The Black Death of the fourteenth century, and the periodic outbursts of plague from the Middle Ages until fairly recent times, all ravaged Europe. These diseases struck so suddenly and so universally that it was no wonder that the helpless populations of the time ascribed religious significance to them. Even in the more enlightened nineteenth century, the issuing of an official prayer in November 1831 was seen as an appropriate response to the arrival of a long-feared cholera epidemic in Britain. It was probably at least as effective as the ice, hot compresses, bleeding, electric shocks, incisions in the head and other traumas and potions which were used to treat the unfortunate cholera victims.

It was in the rational study of these epidemics that epidemiology took on its present form. Pepys, as we have already seen, used the Bills of Mortality, the forerunner of death certificates, to measure the progress of the plague. He also observed that certain quarters of the City of London were affected worse than others and that the poor suffered more than the rich.

Later workers employed what could be called the scientific method, at least in embryonic form. Dr Percival Pott wrote his 'Treatise of the Chimney-Sweep's Cancer' in 1775, and Charles Thrackrah his 'The Effects of Arts, Trades, and Professions and of Civic States and Habits of Living on Health and Longevity' in 1831, the same year as the first cholera epidemic in Britain. These were times of profound social upheaval in Britain, and it was the squalor produced by industrialisation that led to Edwin Chadwick's 'Report of the Sanitary Conditions of the Labouring Population of Great Britain in 1842'. This landmark work provided the inspiration for the 'sanitary movement' in the middle of the nineteenth century and, with the second cholera epidemic providing the spur, it led to public health legislation as we know it today.

In 1854, John Snow went beyond describing the distribution of disease and actually controlled an outbreak of cholera in London by application of his epidemiological conclusions. Snow, a medical practitioner in the Soho area of London, mapped out the residences of those persons who died from cholera in the district. He noticed that they were clustered around the public water pump in Broad Street (now Broadwick Street), and after some further investigations he concluded that the cholera came from some agent in the pump's water. Snow's method of preventing people from using the contaminated water was to persuade the authorities to remove the handle of the pump, and the epidemic subsided. Snow was perhaps lucky in that the epidemic may have almost have run its course anyway, but his principles were correct.

Epidemiology has since become the science we know today, but the lessons of those pioneers must not be forgotten. They were all working before the bacterial origin of infectious diseases was recognised (Pasteur's first work was published in 1857), but time has since shown that their conclusions were substantially correct. Today, the epidemiological method is being applied to studies of chronic diseases, alcoholism, drug addiction and even motor vehicle accidents. Computers, sensitive indices and statistics have replaced the crude measurements of the pioneers, but epidemiology still requires the same enquiring minds, meticulous observations and logical deductions which they displayed.

2.1.2 Ecology and epidemiology

If we return to the broad ecological view, we can see man as a host organism set in an environment which can both harbour the agents of disease and affect man's resistance to these agents. The balance between host, agent and environment is rarely static. The interplay between them determines whether disease will be clinically present or absent, and whether it appears in an acute or chronic form.

The *host* in the biological sense is defined as the living organism which harbours a parasite or commensal. A host can be animal or plant, but the one in which we are most interested is naturally man. Man can present a wide range of susceptibility or resistance to disease, conditions which can alter through biological or social adaptation, or which can be deliberately influenced by processes such as vaccination. The *agent* of disease is often a microorganism or a group of microorganisms. A successful parasitic invasion of a host usually results in chronic disease, for this implies a state of balance where both host and agent can co-exist. If the agent overwhelms the host, as when death results from an acute bout of illness, the invasion of the parasite has not been successful. Of course, the terms 'success' or 'failure' here are used from the biological viewpoint; the view of man as a human being would see 'success' from a different perspective, that is, when the host's resistance overwhelms the invader.

The *environment* can be a more difficult area to examine. It can be defined in terms of the immediate environment of the body such as the blood stream, the mouth or a particular organ. There is also the wider social perspective— factors such as housing, education, occupation, sanitation, water supply, diet and culture, all of which can affect the disease processes in the community or the individual.

2.1.3 The uses of epidemiology

The long-term aim of epidemiology is the control and prevention of disease. So it is with other branches of the health sciences, such as clinical medicine and pathology, so what is the value of the epidemiological approach? In essence it is the recognition that biological variation can be enormous from one individual to another in any given situation. A drug that produces an effect in one individual may not produce it in another; two members of the same family can have quite different patterns of dental caries. In a study situation, biological variation can only be allowed for by examining a group of subjects in which a range of variability can be expected to be seen. Then, as a range of measurements will be obtained from the group, the science of biostatistics must be employed in order to interpret the measurements. Biostatistics has been called a rigorous way of thinking about variable phenomena, and the application of biostatistics to epidemiological measurements is a fundamental step towards the reaching of correct conclusions from the measurements made. Relationships between a disease pattern and some cultural or environmental factor, or variations between different groups in response to the same factor, can then be identified.

Epidemiology is employed to study the normal as well as the abnormal; for example, human growth rates as measured by increases in height and weight, the distribution of blood groups and eruption dates for teeth. The last-mentioned factor is a good example of where the epidemiological approach is a necessity; it is a matter of clinical observation that there is a wide variation in the times of eruption of human teeth, so the collection of data from a large number of individuals is required for the facts to be apparent.

Epidemiology as it is understood today can be said to fulfil six purposes:

(1) Provision of data which allow the determination of normal biological processes.

(2) The classification of disease and the determination of its natural history.

(3) The development of hypotheses that can explain the patterns of disease distribution in relation to specific human characteristics.

(4) The testing of hypotheses, through special studies, which relate to disease aetiology and occurrence.

(5) The evaluation of concepts and methods employed in disease control and prevention.

(6) The provision of data on disease distribution for use in planning and evaluating health care services.

An epidemiological study can assess the *prevalence* of a condition in a population, prevalence being the occurrence of a condition at a particular point in time. If the occurrence of the condition in a population is assessed at two separate points in time, the *incidence* can be determined, incidence being the increase or decrease in the occurrence of a condition over a given period. For example, if a survey determines that 40 per cent of the population of a country has dental caries, that figure describes the prevalence of the condition. If a similar study 10 years later finds that 75 per cent are affected, the difference between the two figures describes the incidence of caries over 10 years.

Studies of this kind are usually *cross-sectional*, meaning that a cross-section of the population is examined each time, but the subjects are not the same people. Cross-sectional studies are more common in dental epidemiology, because *longitudinal* studies, where the same group of subjects are followed over a period of time, are more difficult to administer. Cross-sectional studies are quite adequate for many purposes, but in recent years it has been recognised that the pattern of development of caries, that is, its natural history, can only be understood with longitudinal studies. Furthermore, estimates from cross-sectional data can be misleading because of environmental variables introduced over a period. For example, a survey in an inner London community revealed that 12.1 per cent of people aged 35–44, and 52.7 per cent of those aged 55–64, were edentulous. It would be tempting, but quite wrong, to conclude that 52.7 per cent of the present 35–44-year-olds will be edentulous in another 20 years, because the factors influencing total tooth loss are not the same for the two groups. Availability of dental care, the nature of dental practice, diet, socioeconomic groupings and attitudes towards tooth loss may all be different.

Most dental epidemiology has been concerned with caries and periodontal disease in Western societies, where both conditions are highly prevalent. In these instances, measurement of the simple presence or absence of the conditions is of limited use, as there is little practical difference between, say, 95 per cent and 98 per cent prevalence. Both conditions occur in a wide range of intensities, however, so in a situation of

high prevalence the measure of the *intensity* of the condition is more useful than a simple statement of its prevalence. Like prevalence, the degree of intensity of the conditions are known to be closely linked to a number of specific factors in the social environment.

2.1.4   Methods for measuring dental caries

Disease is essentially a qualitative entity; against a background of scientific knowledge the good clinician quite rightly exercises a degree of subjective judgement during the diagnostic and treatment planning process. The epidemiological problem is to quantitate this qualitative entity.

The most common method of measurement is by means of a *rate*—the number of occurrences in a given population. For example, the infant mortality rate in Britain in 1970 was 18.4 deaths per 1000 live births[1]. Changes in this standardised measure over the years can indicate improvements in the maternity and neonatal services, and it can also be used for comparisons with other countries. Rates can be used to measure some of the less prevalent oral disease conditions, such as oral neoplasms, but where a condition is highly prevalent its measurement by a rate is of limited value.

Dental caries can vary highly in the intensity of its attack, even in a society where it is highly prevalent. It can affect one tooth in an individual or it can affect thirty-two; each lesion can be barely discernible or it can destroy the entire crown of the tooth, so a measure of caries intensity is required for most purposes. Intensity is measured by an index, defined as: ' . . . a numerical value describing the relative status of a population on a graduated scale with definite upper and lower limits, designed to permit and facilitate comparisons with other populations classified by the same criteria and methods.'[2]

An index should be clear and simple, reproducible in the sense that different examiners can apply it in a similar way, and it should be amenable to statistical analysis. It must also have *validity*, meaning that it measures what it is intended to measure so that observed differences in measurements are likely to be true differences and not those due to constant or random errors. For example, a thermometer measures temperature in the early morning and again in the heat of the day. If the thermometer is a valid instrument, the difference between the two readings registers the true change in temperature. An index must also be *reliable*, which means that it must be consistent. As an example, a colorimetric test for a chemical reaction may be valid enough, but the experimenter's colour-matching with his set of standard test-tubes can be affected by the quality of light in the room at different times. If the matching is made only by the human eye under these conditions, then the test is almost certainly not reliable.

Indices (the plural of index, sometimes called indexes) should vary in their *sensitivity* according the purpose of the measurement. A two-year clinical trial of a caries-preventive agent in small groups of subjects will demand a more sensitive index than one which is to assess the caries prevalence in a community. It is worth adding that an index should always be used for its intended purpose. To say that one group of people has a Peridontal Index of 1.8 may be of great value for comparison with another group, but as a statistical abstraction it is of no use in assessing the quality of the disease or the treatment needs of the group.

2.1.5   Indices used in measuring dental caries

H. Trendley Dean, in the 1930s, was faced with the problem of determining the relationship between caries and fluorosis in a number of American cities. He devised an index for fluorosis; for caries measurement he computed the percentage of carious teeth in sample groups. Later he scored the number of teeth affected by caries per 100 children[3, 4].

The index most universally employed today is the Decayed–Missing–Filled index, the DMF, introduced by Klein, Palmer and Knutson in 1938 when they studied dental caries distribution among the children of Hagerstown, Maryland[5]. This index is based on the fact that the dental hard tissues are not self-healing; established caries leaves a scar of some sort. The tooth either remains decayed, or if treated it is extracted or filled. The DMF is therefore an *irreversible* index, meaning that it measures total lifetime caries experience. (By contrast, the Gingival Index is an example of a *reversible* index—it records conditions which can alter with time.)

The DMF is a simple and versatile index. The examiner records each tooth in turn as being sound, decayed, filled or missing because of caries, and the sum of the decayed, filled or missing teeth is the subject's DMF. The DMF of a group is the mean of each individual's score.

The DMF index when used without further qualification refers to the whole tooth, rather than to any particular surface or surfaces. In other words, a tooth with one decayed surface counts the same as a tooth with three decayed surfaces. This method is often called the DMFT index, but the index can also be employed as the DMFS, meaning that each individual surface of each tooth is assessed rather than the tooth as a whole. Choice of which approach to use depends on the purposes of the study; DMFS is more sensitive and is usually the index of choice in a clinical trial of a caries-preventive agent. This is because relative incidence is more likely to be detected over the limited time period of a clinical trial. On the other hand, a DMFS examination takes longer, is more likely to produce inconsistencies in diagnosis, and may require the use of radiographs to be fully accurate. For even more sensitivity in clinical trials, the 'D' component can be graded according to the extent of the carious attack. One way of doing this is to grade the caries as (a) in enamel only, (b) in enamel and dentine, and (c) with pulpal involvement.

Examination of the three DMF components can indicate the type of treatment received in the community and so provide more information than does total DMF alone. For example, look at the mean figures found in two groups of British 20–24-year-olds, shown in table 2.1. Although the total DMF scores are the same in

Table 2.1   Average values for decayed, missing and
filled (DMF) teeth in two hypothetical
groups of British persons aged
20–24 years old (from
Burt[33])

	Mean DMF	Mean D	Mean M	Mean F
Group A	11.8	1.6	3.8	6.4
Group B	11.8	0.2	0.7	10.9

each group, group B appears to have received a
higher quality of dental care than has group A.
The epidemiologist would then want to know
why; it could be through a better availability of
care, more regular dental attendance, or a different pattern of carious attack.

The DMF index, either whole tooth or surfaces, can be used to record basic prevalence,
caries incidence and the natural history of the
disease. It is used in clinical field trials of
preventive agents; if we say that water fluoridation reduces new caries by 50 per cent or
fluoride mouth-rinsing can reduce it by 30 per
cent, these statements are based on field trial
measurements which have used DMF. It can also
be used to evaluate the effect of dental care on
community dental health.

Like any index however, the DMF has its
limitations. These are:

(1)   It has been developed for use in Western
populations, and can require modification in
some non-Western groups.

(2)   It can be misleading in adults, where
teeth are often lost for reasons other than caries,
in particular because of periodontal disease.

(3)   It can be misleading in some child populations where there have been extractions for
orthodontic reasons, or where a lot of 'preventive' fillings have been placed.

(4)   The decayed component does not distinguish between early and advanced caries, nor
in an incidence study can it record the rate of
increase of caries unless it is modified to score
different grades of the carious attack.

(5)   DMF data are not related to the number
of teeth erupted, so the 'increase' in caries with

age does not always mean that the intensity of the
disease has increased—it may mean that there
are just more teeth at risk.

Several 'shorthand' methods of DMF examination have been devised; they are intended for
use in surveys where basic prevalence is being
assessed. They are based on examination of
selected teeth only, and the object is to reduce the
time taken for each examination and still provide
valid data.

One such method is described by the World
Health Organisation[6], and recommends the use
of half-mouth DMF in its basic survey technique. Here, the object is to obtain assessments
of caries prevalence in a population which has
not been previously surveyed. This technique
means that half the upper arch only is scored,
then the contralateral lower half-arch, and the
results doubled. It is quicker and easier than full-
mouth DMF, and the apparent symmetry of the
carious attack means that the data obtained are
still sufficiently valid for the purpose. Another
modification is to examine first molars and upper
central incisors only; this method was devised to
estimate total DMF in groups where caries
prevalence was moderate to high, and where the
children had been exposed to little treatment[7]. A
similar method is to examine the lower left first
molar and upper central incisors only[8]. This
latter method has been tested in Brazil and was
found to allow better inter-examiner compara-
bility than did the use of full-mouth DMF[9]. Yet
another approach gets away from DMF altogether and classifies individuals in a hierarchical
pattern according to which sites in the mouth
have been attacked. If caries is found first in the
approximal surfaces of mandibular incisors, the
individual is graded in zone 5, the most severe
zone. If caries is first found on the labial surfaces
of lower incisors, zone 4, and so on. This method
was suggested by Grainger in 1967, and is
described with some proposed modifications
after field-testing by Poulsen and Horowitz[10].

Caries in the primary dentition can be measured by the dmf index, which is the exact parallel
of DMF (the index for the permanent dentition is

always written in upper-case letters, that for the primary dentition in lower-case letters). Exfoliation is a complication, so dmf can only be used up to the age of 5 years, or else applied only to canine and molar teeth in slightly older children. There is some lack of uniformity in indices for measuring caries in primary teeth. In 1944, Gruebbel proposed the def index[103], where the 'e' meant 'indicated for extraction' and missing teeth were ignored, but def has been used where the 'e' has meant 'extracted'. Another method of getting around the exfoliation problem is to use df, where missing teeth are ignored; this is the method of choice of the World Health Organisation in its basic survey techniques[6]. Any of these methods is satisfactory so long as it is made clear just what is being recorded, and if the objectives of the study are being met.

In summary, DMF remains as the index of choice for recording the degree and intensity of carious attack. It has been modified in several different ways, and the choice of which system to use in any one study is dependent upon the objectives and design of the study.

2.2 The Ecology of Dental Caries

Caries is known to have occurred in Britain during Neolithic and Bronze Age times, although prevalence was low compared to the present day. Examination of ancient skulls has indicated that prevalence seemed to rise during the era of Roman occupation, then to fall again during Anglo-Saxon times. The diet for most people at the time was coarse, with little in the way of food preparation. Dental attrition was marked and occurred early, so that the caries that has been found most commonly was cervical and root-surface caries. The disease seems to have been rare in the deciduous dentition, although some lesions in younger persons seemed to have begun in the occlusal fissures and then declined, probably because the rate of attrition was faster than the rate of progression. The pattern of caries in Western society today, where the disease is usually first found in pit and fissure surfaces and soon afterwards on approximal surfaces, does not appear to have become common until Tudor times. Caries prevalence in Britain rapidly increased during the second half of the nineteenth century, during which time it approximated present-day levels[11, 12].

Since ancient times therefore, three distinct changes in caries occurrence in Britain can be identified. They are:

(1)   The prevalence of caries, and the intensity of its attack, has increased greatly.

(2)   Marked attrition, universal in ancient times, has practically disappeared.

(3)   The pattern of the carious attack has changed from one where it began in root and cervical areas to the present-day pattern of beginning in fissures and contact areas. The rate of development of lesions has almost certainly speeded up over the ages.

Dental caries, as a chronic disease, develops in an individual from a particular host–agent interaction which occurs in a certain set of local environmental conditions. These local conditions in turn are influenced by wider environmental conditions, the whole social–cultural environment of the community in which the individual lives. The changes in caries occurrence in Britain down the ages, just outlined, have taken place because of changes in the host–agent–environment balance. One does not have to wait for centuries to pass, however, before seeing similar changes in parts of the world today.

There are a number of instances, which we will consider in detail later, where abrupt changes in caries experience, similar to the British ones over the ages, have occurred over the space of a generation or so. These rapid increases in caries experience are found in previously isolated societies, such as Eskimos, which have now come into contact with Western culture. The evidence is that these changes have been initiated by alterations in the external environment, for they have all occurred when a society, unchanged for centuries, has been catapulted into the modern world. These external changes, in turn, appear to have led to changes in the local, intra-oral environment; previously uninfected groups are likely now to have become infected with caries-inducing bacteria. Infection, together with the abrupt departure from traditional dietary patterns, has led to drastic increases in caries among many populations which used to be considered immune from the disease.

Most of this book deals with agent factors in dental caries, and some host and local environmental factors in terms of the tooth surface, the dental plaque and the conditions which can initiate the carious process. This section of the present chapter concentrates on some of the broader environmental factors which influence the occurrence of caries in man, and it will also consider some host factors which influence the patterns of caries in a community. These can be listed as follows:

Host factors	Environmental factors
Age	Geography and soil types
Sex	Diet
Race	Effects of dental treatment
Familial and genetic patterns	

Let us now examine the relationship between dental caries and each of these factors in turn.

2.2.1   Age and dental caries

Dental caries has been described as a 'disease of children', and certainly in Western society the disease is seen early in life. In Britain, Sweden, Denmark, USA and French Polynesia, studies of children aged between 2 and 5 years show that 57–80 per cent of them already suffer from caries[13–19, 104]. Caries in the permanent dentition is found soon after the eruption of the first permanent molars, where it usually begins in the pit and fissure surfaces, and DMF scores mount steadily as more permanent teeth erupt. Among British children, half of the first permanent molars have become carious by 9 years of age[104]. Carious second molars begin to be seen at age 10, and by age 14 caries has attacked 14 per cent of upper central incisors, 19 per cent of upper lateral incisors, and 20 per cent of upper first premolars. An average DMF of 3.9 in 11-year-old British children has jumped to 8.4 by 15 years of age[104].

Berman and Slack[20] have shown that there is a sharp increase in caries activity between the ages of 11 and 15; at ages 11–12 the occlusal surfaces of the posterior teeth are the most susceptible to attack, but soon afterwards the total DMFS for occlusal and approximal surfaces is the same. The first permanent molar is the most caries-susceptible tooth in the British mouth, and 94 per cent of these have been attacked at age 14–15[20]. DMF scores continue to rise in Western societies until around age 24, where they appear to level out, and soon after this age the DMF begins to lose its validity as an index of dental caries. By adulthood, nearly all susceptible surfaces are likely to have been attacked. Factors contributing to the decline in caries incidence are likely to be the build-up of fluoride in the outer layers of enamel and perhaps the change in dietary habits assumed to come with adulthood. This latter point is not universal, however, for sudden bursts of caries activity have been observed in adults who have given up smoking and have taken to sucking sweets instead.

One caries problem found in older age-groups is that of root caries, frequently found where gingival recession has led to radicular exposure and where bacterial plaque has accumulated around the exposed roots. This form of caries is found in both Western and non-Western societies. Schamschula, Keyes and Hornabrook[21] described its occurrence in a remote adult group in New Guinea where there was very little coronal caries, and they commented on its similarity to the forms of caries in ancient peoples described earlier. They postulated that there may be certain compositions of dental plaque which are not conducive to coronal lesions but which can be associated with periodontal disease and root caries (chapter 3). They also suggest that the global prevalence of root caries may exceed that of coronal caries.

2.2.2 Sex and dental caries

It has been stated that women have a higher caries attack rate than men. Bibby has said this[22], and Dunning has inferred it in his textbook *Principles of Dental Public Health*[105], but it is a difficult claim to substantiate.

There are a number of studies on children aged between 5 and 19, in a number of different countries, which show that in any one age and race group the girls have higher DMF scores than the boys[23-28]. Most of these differences were small, however, and some were based on small numbers of subjects. Against this, other studies in different countries among people aged between 1 and 25 have failed to show any difference between the sexes in any one age and race group[13, 14, 16-18, 29-32].

Most caries epidemiological studies have concentrated on younger people because of the 'disease of childhood' attitude, because reparative and preventive programmes are aimed at children, and because schools and colleges provide the researcher with convenient groups for study. Reliable data on the progression of caries in older people are hard to come by. Dunning bases much of his argument on records from a treatment programme for employees of an insurance company and on a questionaire survey of dentists, but there is some self-selection in the choice of these samples.

It has been stated that teeth erupt earlier in girls than in boys. For example, the national survey of children in England and Wales in 1973 showed that at any one age a higher proportion of girls had particular teeth erupted. Early eruption has been suggested as one reason why girls apparently get more caries than boys. Studies in Indiana, USA, and in South Australia have shown that at ages 18 to 39 months, and again at $14\frac{1}{2}$ years, girls had more teeth erupted than boys[18, 23]. But studies of children aged 3-5 have failed to show any difference in caries prevalence or intensity between girls and boys[13, 14, 16-18, 31], so if there is any difference at this stage it is unlikely to be of any clinical importance.

A cross-sectional study in a London community showed that in all five-year age-groups from 10-14 to 35-39, females had higher DMF scores than did males[33]. They tended especially to have higher scores for filled and missing teeth, but males tended to have more untreated decayed teeth. It must be remembered here that the DMF index records treatment patterns as well as basic carious attack; as the same study showed that women had a better record of dental attendance, it is likely that the observed difference in DMF scores were at least partly attributable to the different diagnostic criteria applied by the epidemiologist and the dentists who had provided the treatment to the community. This point will be discussed in more detail later in the chapter.

This same London study found other differences between men and women, such as in oral cleanliness, choice of dentist, attitudes towards dental health, and patterns of tooth loss. Their different patterns of dental attendance could have reflected further attitudinal differences, or they could have come about because dental care was more accessible to women than to men—many of the women being housewives, whereas the men would lose income if they took time off work to go to the dentist. On the other hand, the DMF figures could indicated some real difference in caries prevalence, perhaps brought about by different dietary patterns between housewives and working men, as one study in Greenland suggested[34].

If there are real differences between men and women in their lifetime experience of dental caries, it will require more precise studies than have so far been carried out to demonstrate them. Such differences as have been demonstrated are attributable to cultural differences rather than to inherent ones, and even if there are inherent differences they are likely to be of less clinical importance than the social and cultural factors in the environment.

2.2.3 Race and dental caries

The belief that some races were more caries-resistant than others came partly from early observations of some non-European races and perhaps in part from the remains of the 'noble savage' concept of the late eighteenth century. This belief has been fading in recent years as evidence grows that racial immunity, if it exists at all, is of less importance than environmental factors.

There is considerable evidence to show that caries prevalence is much less among African, Asian and aboriginal peoples than it is among those of European origin; this evidence will be examined in detail later in the chapter. Direct comparisons of the data are of little help in the racial context, however, because they ignore the environmental variables, including social and cultural factors. Studies carried out where different racial groups share an apparently common environment, and where data are collected under the same research conditions, are more useful although they still do not answer all the questions.

Australian studies have shown that caries prevalence among Aboriginal adolescents is about half that found in Caucasoid children of the same age, and the severity is three to six times less[35, 36]. There were, however, marked environmental differences between the groups studied. In Hawaii, caries was found to be more prevalent among children of Japanese, Korean or Hawaiian parentage than among those of Chinese, European, Puerto Rican or Filipino descent[25], and in Uganda there is more caries in Asians than in the African populations studied[37]. In the latter study the Asians were urban dwellers whereas the Africans were rural. In Birmingham, England, 5-year-old Negroid children had less caries than either Asian or Caucasoid children of the same age, although different treatment patterns were noted[31].

The National Health Survey of the US Public Health Service showed a marked difference in DMF scores between white and black adults of the same age-group[45]. These differences remained even when the groups were standardised for income and education. The report did not offer any explanation for the findings. The biggest difference in comparing the D, M and F components separately was found in the F

component, indicating that white people received a different standard of care from that received by the blacks. Other studies in USA have examined black and white children living in the same geographic area. One looked at 13–14-year-old boys living in a fluoridated area; the white boys had a mean DMF of 3.5, the black boys 1.7[38] (more caries-inducing streptococci were cultured from the dental plaque of the whites than from that of the blacks). Another study compared the caries experience of the black and white students aged 14–17 in Detroit, Michigan, and Columbia, South Carolina[29]. The DMF scores among the blacks in Detroit were only slightly lower than the DMF scores of the whites in the same city, and in Columbia there was no difference. A further study in Portland, Oregon, found that black primary-school children had a higher caries experience than did the white children[24]. The latter two studies both concluded that there were dietary and cultural reasons for the absence of difference between the racial groups.

All studies on racial comparisons have difficulties, even when the different races appear to share the same locality and life style, as in the American studies. There is the problem of categorising persons of mixed race, as well as trying to determine just how common are the environmental variables such as diet. It is possible that real differences in caries experience may exist between races, but even if they do they are masked by, and are of secondary importance to, the social and cultural factors in the environment.

2.2.4   Familial and genetic patterns of caries

It is widely held by both the profession and the public that 'good teeth or bad teeth run in families'. However, it is difficult to ascertain whether any familial tendency is due to true genetic inheritance or whether it is the adoption from an early age of habits and attitudes known to affect dental health.

Mansbridge[39] compared identical and non-identical pairs of twins with unrelated pairs of children of similar age and demographic status, and concluded that whereas genetic factors could affect caries experience to some extent, the influence of environment was stronger. In the absence of further evidence, this conclusion is still accepted today. Other evidence[62] has shown that a distinct familial pattern can exist even over three generations, but it cannot be certain whether this is due to genetic inheritance, bacterial transmission from mother to child, or the perpetuation of dietary and behavioural patterns. Further research, not easy in this field, will be necessary to separate these variables.

2.2.5 Geographic variations in the prevalence of dental caries

Geography is a difficult variable to relate to caries prevalence, as many other variables are bound up with it. There is no doubt that caries prevalence does show tremendous variations from country to country, and from region to region within a country. But it can be immediately appreciated that geographic variation includes racial, climatic, dietary, cultural and economic variables as well.

Table 2.2 lists 36 different DMF scores in young age-groups, taken from 23 recent studies in 12 different countries. This represents only a fraction of the studies on caries prevalence which have been carried out; those cited are from published work in the period 1967–73. The data are arranged from the younger age-groups to the older, and the table is intended to provide a general comparison of caries prevalence in different countries. Because the studies are conducted by different examiners under differing conditions and using variable criteria for caries, it would be wrong to interpret observed differences too literally. Despite these qualifications, there is a clear pattern of higher DMF scores appearing in those countries where Western European civilisation is established, with lower scores being seen in the non-European countries.

Russell[53] has provided a great deal of data on the prevalence of caries in various parts of the

Table 2.2 Mean DMF scores for population groups in various parts of the world; studies published since 1967

Geographic locality	Age-group	Sex	Mean DMF	Ref.
USA (national sample)	11	M	2.4	46
USA (national sample)	11	F	3.2	46
Morocco (from 12 areas	12	M	1.2–3.8	28
Morocco (from 12 areas)	12	F	1.2–4.2	28
New Zealand (Palmerston North)	12	M&F	9.39*	32
USA (Rochester, NY)	12	M&F	9.48*	32
Hawaii	12	M	5.27	25
Australia (aboriginal mission)	6–14	M&F	1.05–3.04	41
Nigeria (northern villages)	10–14	M&F	1.14	49
Nigeria (European residents)	10–14	M&F	4.95	49
Scotland (Paisley)	14	M&F	13.04	48
Hawaii	14	M	7.14	25
USA (New England)	14	M&F	8.93	43
USA (South Atlantic)	14	M&F	6.38	43
Western Samoa	14	M&F	0.84	47
New Zealand (Palmerston North)	15	M&F	15.46*	32
USA (Rochester, NY)	15	M&F	15.78*	32
England (Essex)	15	F	11.71*	20
Hawaii	15	M	9.19	25
Australia (South Australia)	15	F	14.3*	23
Australia (Brisbane, Qld.)	15	F	12.7–14.4	42
England and Wales (national sample)	15	M&F	8.4	104
USA (Detroit, Mich. white students)	14–17	M	10.85	29
USA (Columbia, SC, black students)	14–17	M	11.07	29
New Zealand (national sample)	15–19	M&F	18.6*	50
Uganda (rural)	15–19	M&F	0.4	37
England (London)	15–19	M&F	9.8	33
French Polynesia	15–19	F	11.7	15
Greenland (west)	15–19	M&F	13.0†	34
Greenland (east)	15–19	M&F	7.7†	34
Canada (Ontario)	17–25	M&F	11.93	30
England and Wales (national sample)	16–34	M&F	17.1	51
England (Birmingham)	18–19	M&F	11.3	52
USA (national sample)	18–24	M	13.4	45
USA (national sample)	18–24	F	14.1	45
England (London)	40–44	M&F	18.2	33
New Guinea	40–45	M&F	2.3	44

* These studies included radiographs.
† Some estimation involved.

world. These data, collected as part of the research work of the Inter-departmental Committee on Nutrition for National Defence (ICNND) around the early 1960s, have considerable value as they were gathered by calibrated examiners under standardised conditions. The results are similar to the trends shown in table 2.1 in that the lowest caries prevalence and intensity was found in Ethiopia, Vietnamese hill tribes, Burma, Thailand and Jordan, with highest DMF scores in Chile, Colombia, urban Eskimos, white residents of Baltimore, USA, and among Aleuts in the Alaska National Guard.

A true geographic difference in caries prevalence must mean that factors such as latitude, longitude, altitude, sunshine, rainfall and mean temperature will affect caries prevalence of and by themselves. Dunning has examined this question seriously[105]. He points out that relationships can be demonstrated between regional dental caries prevalence and hours of sunshine, mean temperature, relative humidity and distance from the seacoast, although he emphasises that such relationships must be interpreted cautiously because of other unknown variables that are likely to be present. Certainly it is hard to find a theoretical basis for purely climatic variations in caries prevalence.

McPhail and Grainger[40] mapped out the world-wide prevalence of caries from several hundred sets of data for which they felt the criteria and methods of data collection were similar enough to allow reasonable comparison. They concluded that the world attack rate varies inversely with the level of social and economic development, rather than with purely geographic variables.

Broad regional variations in caries prevalence in USA have been known for some time, variations which can still be seen when obvious environmental factors such as fluoridated water are excluded from analysis. These variations can be associated with climatic differences, but it is more likely that they are related to the different cultures and life styles which result from climatic differences. The major factor is likely to be diet; in Western societies, for example, inhabitants of

colder climates may eat more processed carbohydrate than do those of warmer climates, as carbohydrates are a convenient source of warmth and energy.

One geographic variable which has attracted attention is that of soil type, the theoretical basis for this interest being because of the known association of certain trace elements with the prevalence of caries. Ludwig and Bibby[43], for example, were able to show that caries prevalence among 12–14-year-old white American children was higher in New England than in the Central Atlantic region, which in turn was higher than that in the South Atlantic states. This decrease with descending latitude they related to climate, but they were also able to relate it to soil type, in particular to the trace element selenium.

Selenium has been known for some time to be a caries-enhancing element, although the reasons for this are not clear. Hadjimarkos[54] found that the caries prevalence in 14–16-year-old children in north-west USA was directly related to their intake of selenium. He found the selenium present in varying quantities in milk and eggs, and demonstrated its presence in the human subjects from urine samples. Hadjimarkos went on to say that it was difficult to relate caries prevalence to the degree of selenium in the soil, because it is not the absolute amount of selenium which is critical but rather the factors governing its availability in the diet. He concludes, therefore, that there is little point in trying to correlate caries simply with soil type and with the level of trace elements in the soil, but exactly this procedure is being pursued by other researchers. There is some evidence to show that caries prevalence is inversely proportional to molybdenum in soil[55, 56], although a mechanism for any caries-inhibitory action of molybdenum is difficult to offer.

There are other long-term studies which suggest that soil types, perhaps because of their trace element contents, influence caries prevalence. For example in Medellin, Colombia, caries prevalence is about the same as in white urban populations in the USA. But in a nearby village there is a much lower mean DMF among the children which cannot be explained by differences in diet, fluoride or genetics. There was no clustering of caries-free individuals within the village. Some possible suggestions have been put forward as to what soil factors might be responsible for this phenomenon, but no conclusions have yet been reached[57, 58].

An even more intriguing situation has been found in Papua, New Guinea[44], where a series of studies are attempting to find reasons why in some villages there should be a total absence of caries in a region of low caries prevalence. The proportion of children and adults completely caries-free varies from zero to 100 per cent among the different villages of the region studied, and the proportion of teeth per person that are decayed varies from zero to 29.5 per cent. There is no apparent reason for these variations, meaning that no gross differences in diet, fluoride intake, or effects of dental treatment could be found. Communities with low caries prevalence in the study tended to have alkaline soils, they were associated with higher soil levels of Sr, Ba, K, Mg and Ca. Analyses of food are also being made, but the research team stresses that conclusions to date must be cautious as analyses of this kind are complex, and the interrelationships of trace elements which are probably relevant are very difficult to define. This research, however, is of extreme interest, for if the reason for the caries-immunity of a whole community could be found there may be potential worldwide implications.

It was mentioned earlier that some previously isolated societies used to be considered immune from caries, but that this apparent immunity unfortunately disappeared when they came into contact with Western culture. In fact, a major health problem in the world today is the rapid increase in caries prevalence in economically underdeveloped countries, where resources for prevention or control of the condition are virtually non-existent. This trend might demonstrate the infectious nature of dental caries. Caries is a bacterial disease, so presumably it can spread just as the plague used to and the common cold still does. Societies where caries does not

seem to be increasing, such as some of those just discussed in New Guinea, are among the most isolated populations left in the world. At the other end of the scale, caries does not seem to be increasing in high-prevalence groups such as Scandinavians, which could be due to a 'saturation' level of infection having been reached.

The epidemiological evidence to support these suggestions is scanty. The necessary longitudinal studies, and especially the joint studies in epidemiology and microbiology, remain to be done. Other sections of this book deal with the microbiology of the oral cavity, but it can be said here that its complexity, added to the chronic nature of the disease process in caries, presents special problems in epidemiological studies. But such studies must be done in due course, and they will play an important role in our understanding of the aetiology of the disease.

To summarise this section, geographic variations do exist in the prevalence and intensity of caries. There is no reason, however, why purely geographic factors such as latitude, altitude or mean annual temperature should in themselves affect the distribution of caries; almost certainly if they do have an influence it is an indirect one in that they affect culture and diet. Most geographic interest at the present centres on relating soil types to caries prevalence, because of factors in the soil thought to influence caries patterns through diet. There are 13 trace elements so far identified which are thought to influence caries one way or another[59], but nothing as yet has been proved conclusively. The potential exists, however, for important future discoveries to be made concerning the role of trace elements in the development of dental caries.

The next great frontier, following the demonstration of geographic variations in caries prevalence, is to relate the microbiology of these populations to their prevalence and incidence.

2.2.6 Diet and dental caries

Diet has been associated, either positively or negatively, with the prevalence of dental caries for centuries, and in the total field of research into caries aetiology diet has probably received more attention than any other subject.

'Diet' is defined by *Webster's New Collegiate Dictionary* as the habitual nourishment of a person, group or population; 'nutrition', on the other hand, is the act or process of being nourished, human nourishment in normal circumstances coming from the constituents of the diet. The distinction between diet and nutrition needs to be kept clear.

The diet of any society is woven into the fabric of its culture. The food that people normally eat is influenced by geography, climate, tradition, religion, costs and marketing practices, among other factors. In almost all societies, the process of eating is more than merely a way of taking in nourishment, it is a social act; mealtimes are an important part of the family's day—sharing a meal with friends is one of the oldest ways of offering hospitality. All this is stated by way of indicating that dietary practices, whether they are seen as good or bad, are deeply ingrained and are not easily changed while living conditions remain stable. Lasting dietary changes are usually accompanied by fundamental changes in a way of life.

Early theories

It was mentioned earlier in the chapter that the ideal of the 'noble savage' grew during the Age of Reason—the latter half of the eighteenth century. It was perhaps an understandable development from this ideal that the apparent freedom from caries which the so-called primitive races enjoyed would be attributed to the 'natural' diet on which they existed. Eating hard, fibrous and unprocessed food, so the theory grew, led to better development of the jaws and teeth and helped to clear food debris from the surfaces of the teeth. Western man, by contrast, ate soft, processed food, high in fermentable carbohydrate, which did not properly exercise the masticatory apparatus and which remained stuck to the teeth and so caused dental decay. With such theories prevalent, Miller's chemicoparasitic explanation for the initiation of dental caries,

which began with his work on microorganisms in 1883[79], won early acceptance.

Theories on the preventive value of hard and fibrous foods became even more widespread in the early years of the twentieth century with the writings of Wallace[73] and Pickerill[74]. Wallace was a firm proponent of 'cleansing foods'. He followed Miller in stating that accumulations of fermentable carbohydrates were the cause of caries; he further believed that such deposits could be removed by eating hard and fibrous foods, the so-called 'cleansing' or 'detersive' foods. Pickerill[74] also believed that if a meal was finished with a salivary stimulant, such as an apple, the mouth would be kept free of fermentation both by the cleansing effect of the fibrous apple, and also because of the salivary flow that the apple induced.

The chemicoparasitic theory remains the basis for present beliefs on caries aetiology, although the process is far more complex than was imagined in Miller's time. We can now see that Wallace, Pickerill and their followers were hampered by the absence of indices and statistical methods, and frequently by poor research design. Many of their conclusions, in fact, were totally subjective. The chief logical error to which the proponents of cleansing foods succumbed was that it was not the *presence* of hard and fibrous foods which led to low caries prevalence, but the *absence* of fermentable carbohydrates in the diet. At the time, however, the theories were widely accepted, and more than traces of them remain today in dental health education materials. Research over the past 20 years has identified the role of bacterial plaque in caries and shown that carrots, apples and celery have little effect on established plaque. The only remaining value of the 'detersive' foods is the indirect one, meaning that a child wanting a between-meals snack is likely to be better off with an apple than with a bag of toffees.

General nutrition or local dietary factors

The 1920s and 1930s were a period during which the vitamins and their health functions were being identified, and dietary imbalances were being associated with many disease processes. It was also a period when deficiency diseases were common in the economically depressed Western world. In Britain, rickets, the bone-malformation disease seen in children who have not received sufficient vitamin D, was probably the most common deficiency disease. Once again, the prevailing scientific climate was probably a strong influence behind the development of the nutrition theory of caries, a theory usually associated with Lady May Mellanby. Mellanby hypothesised[75] that the more perfect the structure of a tooth then the less susceptible it was to decay, and that resistance to caries could therefore be influenced by some of the factors which also controlled calcification. She related malformed and hypoplastic teeth to a deficiency of vitamin D, and then assumed that such teeth were more susceptible to caries. Mellanby's research, however, had design flaws and her conclusions were not always supported by her research results.

The nutrition theory faded in importance after some epidemiological research findings from studies conducted during World War II, and after later research emphasised the role of local bacterial plaque. Some of the nutrition theory, however, was still supported in 1952[76], although it was not completely accepted even during the 1930s. Bunting[77], for example, found that Michigan children on adequate high-sugar diets had more caries than children on inadequate low-sugar diets, and in England, Breese[78] used his own observations to dismiss the nutrition theory in a well-argued paper.

Classic epidemiological studies on diet and dental caries

Dentists have long believed that eating sweets predisposes to caries, and much of this book describes in detail the role of fermentable carbohydrates, especially sucrose, in the carious process. The traditional belief in this case has been shown to be correct, although the complex mechanism has only recently been described, and

some of it is still not fully understood. Much of the impetus for the basic research on the constituents of dental plaque and their role in the carious process came from several conclusive epidemiological studies. One of these was the longterm study by Toverud[80 – 82] on the dental health of Norwegian children before, during and after World War II. Norway was occupied for much of war, and strict food rationing was enforced for this period of some five or six years. Protein intake for all age-groups remained adequate, but carbohydrate and fat intakes were reduced. General mortality rates increased during this period; in particular there was increased mortality from infectious diseases and from gastric and duodenal ulcers in men. However, mortality from diabetes and circulatory disorders fell from pre-war levels. Among children aged 8–14, average height and weight were reduced.

Dental effects included delayed eruption of teeth, which began to be seen a year or so after rationing began and reached a peak after the war, only declining in the 1950s. Caries in the permanent dentition was dramatically reduced, the number of caries-free children aged 7–8 increasing by a factor between three and four times between 1941 and 1946 (with allowance made for the delayed eruption effect). Caries prevalence was back to 1941 levels by 1949, after rationing had been removed. Toverud clearly related the lower caries prevalence of the Norwegian children to the reduced intake of carbohydrates, and his work strongly indicated that the reduced level of general nutrition did not have an adverse effect on caries prevalence rates.

Another site for long-term study has been the island of Tristan da Cunha in the South Atlantic. This is a remote and unique community of mainly European descent, which for years lived undisturbed by the world. The people lived simply, subsisting principally on a diet of fish. The community's limited contacts with the outside world gradually increased as modern communications improved, and items of processed food inevitably began to appear in the islanders' diet. A volcanic eruption in the early 1960s necessitated the temporary emigration of the entire community to England. The islanders returned when their island was habitable again, and in recent years the establishment of some industry has created an economy and a demand for consumer foods. Much of the diet now consists of processed food, in particular processed carbohydrates.

The initial remoteness of the community followed by its increasing contacts with modern civilisation and its subsequent social changes, have presented a unique situation for studying the effects of dietary change over a period of time. The islanders were dentally examined in 1932, 1937, 1953, in England in 1962, and again on the island in 1966. Efforts were made, by the different examiners involved, to keep to standardised measurements which would allow the data to be comparable over time. The results tell a sad tale; the prevalence of caries in the first permanent molars of 6–19-year-olds, which was zero in 1932 and 1937, increased to 50 per cent in 1962 and to 80 per cent in 1966[83].

Hopewood House, an institution in the Australian state of New South Wales, was the site for a long-term study of children living in a protected environment on a basically vegetarian diet almost totally free of fermentable carbohydrate. The study began with 81 children aged 4–9 years, and continued for some 15 years. Originally, 63 of the 81 children (77.8 per cent) were completely caries-free[84] and at age 13 there were still 53 per cent caries-free compared to 0.4 per cent of the local non-institutionalised population of the same age[85]. Over the years of the study, some of the rigid dietary conditions in the institution were relaxed, but there were still 34.7 per cent of 13-year-olds caries-free when it was concluded[86]. This study could be criticised on the grounds of small numbers and some lack of rigidity in research design, but it was a study which took advantage of a real-life situation and therefore had to be conducted within these limitations. Even so, the differences between the Hopewood House children and the general population are so profound that the dental value of dietary control was adequately demonstrated.

Perhaps the best-known research project into diet and caries is the Vipeholm study[87]. This Swedish study, reported in 1954, was carried out over a period of several years in a mental institution. It raised so many ethical questions that it is unlikely to be repeated, but its results were so conclusive that repetition is hardly necessary. The inmates of the institution were divided into groups which had different amounts of refined sugar intake, varying from none to *ad lib.* intake of sticky toffees 24 hours per day. The variations in incidence of caries between the groups were enormous, and the conclusions of the study are still acceptable at the present time. They are:

(1)   Sugar consumption increases caries activity.

(2)   The risk of the sugar increasing caries activity is greater if the sugar is in sticky form.

(3)   The risk is greatest if the sugar is taken between meals and in a sticky form.

(4)   The increase in caries under uniform conditions shows great individual variation.

(5)   The increase in caries disappears on the withdrawal of sticky foodstuffs from the diet.

(6)   Caries can still occur in the absence of refined sugar, natural sugars and total dietary carbohydrates.

Further epidemiological studies on diet and dental caries

A number of other studies have examined the impact on oral health of a hitherto isolated community being exposed to a Western diet over a fairly short period of time. One of the more tragic of such groups are Eskimos, who were virtually caries-free when subsisting on their original high-protein, high-fat diet, but who rapidly developed a high prevalence of caries when they began to get confectionery through the trading posts. One study[88], showing the rapid increase in caries among Eskimos between 1933 and 1961, also showed that caries prevalence varied inversely with the degree of remoteness from the trading post.

Baume[15] found that caries prevalence in Polynesia is also related to sugar consumption. This is now over 76 kg per head per year on Tahiti, whereas in the outer islands it is only 16 kg per head per year and is associated with substantially less caries.

A recent study in Greenland[34] shows that caries prevalence there is rising, but it is much higher now in the main trading stations than in the rural areas. The authors report that caries prevalence in West Greenland increased from 58 per cent to 95 per cent between 1913 and 1945. The proportion of imported food in the diet of Greenlanders has been rising rapidly, and average sugar consumption is now around 50 kg per head per year, being higher in the west than in the east of the island.

Hargreaves[27] compared a 1937 study on the Scottish island of Lewis with his own 1967/68 survey, re-calculating the earlier data where necessary. Mean DMF scores for children aged 12–15 had approximately doubled in that period, and although total sugar consumption had fallen, confectionery consumption had sharply increased.

One of the conclusions of the Vipeholm study was that the form of the fermentable carbohydrate, chiefly sucrose, was as important as its chemical composition. Newbrun[89] also makes that point when he presents two cases of hereditary fructose intolerance, both caries-free. Glass and Fleisch[90] were unable to correlate caries incidence with consumption of breakfast cereals and suggested that factors such as time of eating, food consistency and the conditions under which it was eaten are likely to be important. Further studies have related high incidence of caries with between-meal snacks[91] and availability of sweets in school canteens[92]. Much higher sucrose-consumption scores have been found in caries-active dental students compared to caries-free students[93], and caries-activity in a group of Swedish students was more directly related to between-meal sucrose consumption than it was to socio-economic status[94].

While there is now no doubt that consumption of sweet, sticky snacks is directly related to caries

incidence, the effect of sweetened drinks is less certain. Winter *et al.*[16] found rampant caries among pre-school children to be most common when the children were given reservoir (or 'dinky') feeders of syrups, while an American study found little increase in caries with the consumption of 12 oz of carbonated soft drink daily[95]. There could be a difference in time-exposure to the sucrose here, as children can hold a reservoir feeder in their mouths for some hours. Furthermore, children in the American group were older than those in the London study.

Jackson[64] reviewed the literature on caries epidemiology in Britain between 1947 and 1962, and concluded that the decrease in caries in English children which could be attributed to sugar rationing during World War II was not as great as had been supposed. He thought that much of the apparent increase in DMF in the post-war era was due to the placing of more 'preventive' fillings, especially after the introduction of the air turbine engine in the mid-1950s. If his argument is correct, some intriguing speculations arise. Is there, for example, a level beyond which sugar consumption has no additional effect—a 'saturation' level, perhaps related to the qualitative and quantitative nature of the microbiota in the population? Are the sites in which caries most commonly begins in England, the pit and fissure surfaces of molars[20], sufficiently resistant to preventive measures that reduction in caries prevalence among the age-groups studied would always be minor? Had there been sufficient data for Jackson to make good comparisons in, say, 15–16-year-olds in whom smooth-surface caries is more prevalent[20], would he have found a greater reduction?

Additional speculations relate to the concept of 'herd immunity', meaning the gradual build-up of resistance to disease in a population through constant exposure to that disease. As an illustration, colds in Western societies are a minor inconvenience, but a lack of resistance led to American Indians and Australian Aborigines dying from colds when they first came into contact with the cold virus. Does 'herd immunity' play any part in the prevalence of caries in a population? Could societies such as Britain, where caries in its modern form has been prevalent for centuries, have developed some 'herd immunity' over that time? (The subject of herd immunity is discussed in R. Dubos' book, *The Mirage of Health*, in the list of Further Reading to this chapter.)

Other dietary vehicles have been studied in the search for an agent to prevent, or at least retard, the development of caries. The role of trace elements in caries epidemiology has already been discussed; they appear to play some part in the carious process, although exactly what and why is not yet known. The addition of inorganic phosphates to topical solutions of fluoride have been shown to increase the uptake of fluoride by the enamel surface[98] and to reduce the incidence of caries [101]. Acidulated-phosphate-fluoride solutions and gels (APF) are now in routine clinical use. Incorporation of inorganic phosphates into human diet for cariostatic purposes, however, has not produced such favourable results[97, 100], although animal studies indicate that some cariostatic benefits are possible[96]. It remains to be seen whether the preventive effects which dietary inorganic phosphates produce in laboratory animals, and which theoretically should be obtained in humans, can ever be reproduced in a practical community-wide application. Fluoride, which is a trace element, is a story unto itself and has been examined fully elsewhere[71], as well as receiving consideration in other parts of this book.

It can be seen then that many questions remain to be answered about the full relationship between diet and caries. At this time, however, it seems that diet is a dominant variable in determining the caries prevalence rates in a community, so much so that it can mask other possible genetic influences such as sex or race, or the effects of a community's geographic location. When we consider that diet is an integral part of a society's culture and is affected by other factors, which in their turn are influenced by diet and dietary habits, it can be seen that the ecology of caries is complex indeed.

Sucrose has been clearly identified as the most important dietary factor in the initiation and progress of the carious lesion[99]. Our sweet-toothed society, however, is not prepared to give up its sugar, or is unable to do so without making unacceptable changes in its life style[104]. As a result, a lot of epidemiological and laboratory research remains to be done to find how society can have its cake, eat it, and still minimize the ravages of caries.

2.2.7   The effect of dental treatment

One problem facing the epidemiologist who surveys the prevalence of caries in a community is that every filled tooth or surface counts as one 'F' unit in the DMFT or DMFS index, even though there is no way of knowing what was the condition of the tooth or surface prior to the restoration being placed. The assumption must be made that caries was present, although this may not always have been the case. A mesio-occlusal restoration in a molar, for example, counts as two filled surfaces, even though only the mesial surface may have been carious.

It was stated earlier that there can be differences in diagnostic criteria between the epidemiologist and the dentists who provide the care in a community, as indeed there can be between different clinicians, or even the same clinician at different times. These differences are likely to be most pronounced in the diagnosis of the small early carious lesion and rigid criteria must therefore be defined in epidemiological studies. Here is an example of criteria for diagnosing dental caries in pits and fissures, as used in one London study:

Decay diagnosed if:

(i)   Frank and obvious caries was visible.

(ii)   A lesion was of sufficient size to admit a probe with moderate pressure, and showed evidence of softening at the base of the lesion and/or resisted the removal of the probe.

(iii)   If an enamel opacity was sufficient to indicate undermining of the enamel, even though the enamel lesion itself was minimal.

Criteria such as these attempt to eliminate the questionable lesion as far as possible, and a short study of them will show that a lesion requires to be fairly well established before it is diagnosed as carious. On the other hand, a clinician may feel justified in filling a tooth in which the fissures just catch the point of the probe, or in one where the fissures are only lightly stained. Some clinicians place what are sometimes called 'preventive fillings' in teeth which are not carious at the time, but which they believe are likely to become so.

When a school-age population under study has received a lot of reparative dental treatment, for example in Norway or New Zealand where there are highly organised school dental programmes[60], it is likely that this type of clinical practice is more common than when the dentist : population ratio is less favourable. In the former situations, missing permanent teeth and untreated decayed teeth are uncommon, and the 'F' component comprises the bulk of the overall DMF score. In addition, frequent radiographic examination among populations receiving a lot of treatment will detect more initial caries of approximal tooth surfaces than would be found by clinical examination alone. When these initial lesions are restored they add to the DMF score, whereas the same teeth would probably have not been recorded as carious under survey conditions when radiographs were not employed.

A study in Louisville, Kentucky[61], demonstrated the differences between diagnosis reached by epidemiologists and by clinicians preparing a treatment plan. A group of children who were attending for treatment at a dental clinic were first examined by an epidemiologist. He found that children aged 6–10 averaged 0.7 decayed permanent teeth each, but their clinic records showed that the dentists providing the treatment diagnosed an average of 1.7 permanent teeth each which required treatment. Among the 11–18-year-olds, the epidemiologist diagnosed 1.74 untreated decayed teeth per subject, whereas the clinicians recorded 4.90 decayed teeth per subject requiring treatment.

The question of which set of diagnoses is nearer the absolute truth is irrelevant. The epidemiologist records the status of teeth as they are at that time, according to specific criteria; where inter-group comparisons are required, consistency in diagnosis is more important than the absolute recording of all possible lesions. On the other hand, the clinician exercises the art of dentistry as well as the science. He must look ahead and decide if it is in the interests of the patient to restore teeth now, even if overt caries is not present. The philosophy behind the two types of examination is quite different, so it is hardly surprising that the diagnosed conditions are also different.

Socio-economic status has been described as an important vehicle in community dental health and so it is, to the extent that attitudes and behaviour vary in different social classes. But the question we must ask is do people of the same age, sex, nationality, and with the same access to dental care, vary in their basic attack rate of caries?

Jackson, Murray and Fairpo[68] examined the effect that regular or irregular dental attendance had on dental health in two communities. In all age-groups where DMF is a valid measure, they found that the regular dental attenders had higher DMF values than did the irregular attenders. The regular attenders had a lower number of untreated decayed teeth, about the same number of missing teeth, and a considerably higher number of filled teeth than did the irregular attenders. They also noted that regular attendance had little effect on primary prevention of disease. In a London survey conducted around the same time[33], the higher socio-economic groups, who visited the dentist more frequently than lower socio-economic groups, had the higher DMF values. The same phenomenon has been reported in the USA[45].

So the apparent anomaly exists that people who act on the advice to 'see your dentist regularly' have higher DMF values. It is possible that such people could be a self-selected group with higher disease prevalence. However, it has been demonstrated that regular dental attendance is predominantly a function of higher

socio-economic groups[69, 70]. The answer is far
more likely to be related to the factor described
earlier, that of differing criteria between the
epidemiologists and the clinicians. When a national survey finds that irregular attenders have
more sound, unfilled teeth than regular attenders[51] it might be pertinent to ask whether some
teeth are being unnecessarily filled.

This brief discussion has centred on the effects
of dental treatment on young populations. The
question is more complex in older groups where
tooth extraction can reflect treatment for pe-
riodental disease, and/or patients' prosthetic
demands, which in turn are influenced by attitudes prevailing in the community. The important factor to accept is that the dental health
status of a community, however measured, is
influenced by the treatment it receives as well as
by the disease patterns it experiences.

2.3   Dental Caries in Great Britain

Dental caries is a major public health problem in
Britain, as it is in many other nations; the Adult
Dental Health Survey of 1968[51] found that only
three adults in 1000 had not suffered from caries
at some time in their lives. Unlike many other
countries, however, dental treatment is reasonably available to most people in Britain through
the National Health Service. As most people in
Britain use dental services, at least to some
extent[51], it is impossible to examine the epidemiology of caries without considering the effects
of the treatment services at the same time. The
existence of comprehensive data from several
recent national surveys, and the ready availability of treatment statistics from National
Health Service records from 1948 onwards,
make Britain a valuable source for the study of
caries epidemiology.

2.3.1   Prevalence of caries

It is never easy to judge whether 'teeth are worse'
in Britain than they are anywhere else. Cross-
national comparisons must be carried out with

caution, as was stated earlier, and only general
conclusions can be reached.

The studies by Hardwick[11] and Moore and
Corbett[12] have shown that caries as we know it
today was almost unknown in ancient times.
Present-day patterns of dental caries appeared
during the latter half of the last century, the same
period when cheap sugar became widely available. Figures from the time are not reliable, but
caries was obviously prevalent enough by 1885 to
provoke W. M. Fisher, of Dundee, to suggest at
the annual meeting of the British Dental
Association that legislation to secure compul-
sory attention to the teeth of school children was
required. Eventual action led to the School
Dental Service.

Some data on caries prevalence in Britain have
already been given. Caries commences early in
life; a London survey of pre-school children
found that 58 per cent of 4-year-olds had experienced caries, and a quarter of them had rampant
caries[16]. In another study, 5-year-old children
from non-flouridated areas near Birmingham
were found to average one lost tooth each
through caries[31]. The first permanent molar is
highly vulnerable to caries[51], and only 12 out of
666 girls aged 11 in clinical trials in southern
England were found to be free of caries[20]. Some
90 per cent of these girls had first permanent
molars attacked by caries at age 11.

The national survey of children in England
and Wales in 1973 produced some sobering
findings[104]. There were 63 per cent of 5-year-olds
who had active caries, and 40 per cent of 8-year-
olds who had some active caries in their permanent teeth. A perusal of figure 2.1 shows that
at all ages from 5 to 15, untreated decayed teeth
make up a considerable portion of the average
DMF score. Longitudinal studies[20, 102] show
that there is a sharp increase in caries incidence
between the ages of 11 and 14, which appears to
level out a little after that, at least up to age 17.
British studies on the young adult population are
few, and none of them is longitudinal. Treatment
statistics from the Dental Estimates Board suggest that caries incidence could still be high in the
17–24 age-group.

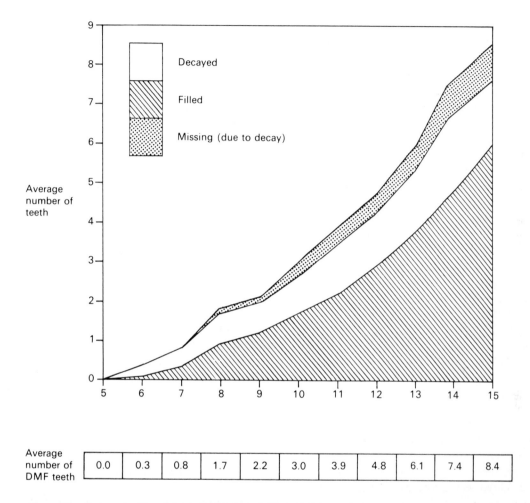

Average number of DMF teeth	0.0	0.3	0.8	1.7	2.2	3.0	3.9	4.8	6.1	7.4	8.4

Figure 2.1   Average number of decayed, missing and filled (DMF) permanent teeth in children aged 5–15, in England and Wales, 1973 (from Todd[104])

Data on whether caries prevalence and incidence are increasing or remaining static are equivocal. James, Parfitt and Roydhouse[63] concluded that caries prevalence increased between 1950 and 1961; they related this finding to the ending of sugar rationing in Britain in 1953. They argued that the restriction of sugar postponed the time of onset of caries, but once initiated the rate of increase in DMF values was the same as that seen when sugar was no longer rationed. The study by Jackson[64], previously mentioned, challenged the assumption that caries prevalence and incidence had increased sharply since the ending of sugar restriction. Jackson suggested that

much of the increase in DMF values since the end of World War II has been due to the placing of so-called 'preventive fillings'. If this is so, it is a further indication of how apparent caries prevalence can be influenced by treatment patterns.

There appears to be little regional variation in the basic caries attack rate in Britain, but there is a sharp difference in the availability of dental services[51]. As a result, the balance of D, M and F components of the DMF index varies considerably from region to region. The correlation is not simple, however, for availability of care, public attitudes, socio-economic status of the community and dental health as measured by the

DMF index are all linked in a little ecology of their own. Table 2.3 shows how the components of the DMF index, in 15–19-year-old British teenagers, varies from region to region. It is noticeable how total DMF in Hartlepool, the only fluoridated community in the group, is lower than the others, but untreated decayed teeth still account for nearly half of the DMF total. This reflects the low socio-economic status of the area and the low availability of care, factors discussed earlier in the chapter.

Table 2.3 Decayed, missing and filled teeth in groups of 15–19-year-old persons in various areas of Britain

Study location	Mean D	Mean M	Mean F	Mean DMF	Ref.
Warrington	1.8	3.0	6.1	10.8	66
London*	0.7	0.8	9.9	11.4	66
London†	1.1	1.5	7.2	9.8	33
York	1.3	2.3	8.0	11.6	67
Hartlepool‡	2.3	1.2	2.5	6.0	67

* Sample was 86 per cent persons in social classes I, II and III.
† sample was 34 per cent persons in social classes I, II and III.
‡ naturally fluoridated.

2.3.2 Treatment patterns

Despite the absence of reliable comparative data, there is little question that the dental health of the British people has greatly improved since the introduction of the National Health Service in 1948[65]. Perhaps the most profound change in dental health behaviour since 1948 has been the increased demand for dental services. Reports from the Dental Estimates Board show that the number of courses of treatment in the general dental services rose from 7 million in the first full year of the service to 23 million by the early 1970s. This increase in demand was proportionately far greater than the increase in either population or dental manpower during the same period. There is evidence now to show that during this period the rate of total tooth loss in

younger persons has sharply decreased[51], although it still occurs to an undesirable extent.

Data from the National Adult Dental Survey of 1968[51] show that the dentist : population ratio varies from 1 : 3290 in south-east England to 1 : 6070 in Wales and the south-west and to 1 : 5750 in the north; these regional variations in dentist : population ratios can be roughly linked to the different patterns of care received, as shown in table 2.3. However, why is the dentist : population ratio more favourable in one area than another? What attracts dentists to a locality or region? To what extent does availability of care stimulate demand, or are dentists attracted to an area because demand already exists?

In summary, it can be said that basic rates of attack of dental caries do not vary much, if at all, in different regions of Britain. What do vary considerably are the treatment services. Separating the different influences of care availability, community attitudes and socio-economic status on the dental health of the community is very difficult, but at the same time very important. The first step is to realise that these factors are interrelated.

2.3.3 Future trends in the prevalence of dental caries in Britain

This chapter began by introducing the ecological concept of dental caries. It follows that if the prevalence of dental caries is to be substantially reduced in the future it must be by increasing host resistance, nullifying the action of the agent, or altering the environment where the disease process takes place. If prevalence does not decrease, there remains the possibility of increasing resources to repair the diseased tissues.

Dental plaque is the environment where the bacterial agent thrives and, as described earlier, sucrose is a major factor in the development of dental plaque[89, 99]. Figures from the Board of Trade indicate that annual sugar consumption in Britain has remained at around 45 kg per head in the 1960s and 1970s, a rate of consumption which must be a major contribution towards the high caries prevalence in the country. So long as sugar remains a significant part of British culture, meaning its image as a treat, a reward and a symbol of all good things for children, then caries prevalence is likely to remain high.

Dental health education programmes for years now have been exhorting the public to eat less sugar, but despite evidence that sugar might be implicated in other disease processes, these efforts have met with little wide-scale success. Sugar consumption seems so much a part of the British way of life, and commercial sugar interests work so effectively to keep it that way, that nothing short of a major economic or social upheaval is likely to change this situation in the foreseeable future.

Host resistance may be radically increased some time in the future with the development of a vaccine against dental caries; the immunological processes involved are described elsewhere in this book. It is apparent however, that a vaccine will not be available for some time yet, if at all; more practical at the present time are methods for increasing the resistance of the tooth surface against acid-induced decalcification.

Incorporation of fluoride into the enamel has been shown to be the most effective approach to increasing resistance to caries, and a number of workable methods for this process are currently available. Fluoridation of water supplies is widely accepted as the most feasible and economic method of bringing fluoride to whole communities—the effectiveness of fluoridation in reducing the incidence of carious lesions is now beyond question[71]. Fluoridation's greatest strength is paradoxically its greatest weakness as well—the fact that it reaches a whole community without conscious action on the part of the individual. This makes fluoridation a social issue as well as a preventive health measure and, as a consequence its progress in Britain has been slow.

Other methods of incorporating fluoride into enamel, such as by topical application, mouth-rinsing, dentifrices, or by systemic alternatives such as fluoridised salt or milk, have all shown varying degrees of success. All of these methods, however, are unlikely to be effective in reducing community-wide prevalence of decay to any extent, because they require conscious action on the part of the individual and are therefore used only by motivated persons. They are also considerably less cost-effective than water fluoridation[72]. Newer preventive measures, such as the use of fissure sealants in reducing occlusal caries, are promising, but they require further evaluation before they can be confidently used in community programmes.

At present then, water fluoridation remains the only effective community-wide measure for substantially reducing the incidence of caries, and hence in time its prevalence. The social climate in Britain, however, does not favour fluoridation, and even after the 1974 reorganisation of the National Health Service its permanent acceptance has remained slow.

From what has been said to date, it is unlikely that caries prevalence will drop substantially in Britain in the foreseeable future. Some progress in fluoridation, more use of other fluorides and fissure sealants and some response to dental health education may lead to slight decreases over the next generation, but for all practical purposes current levels are only likely to be changed by deep social and economic changes.

This leaves as a final consideration the question of manpower available to treat the results of the disease. Dentist: population ratios in Britain vary by region, as previously described, and there are indications that this imbalance is getting worse rather than better. The overall dentist: population ratio is now approximately 1:3500, a figure derived from some 16000 active dentists in a population of 55 million. If, over the next 10 years or so, the population increases to, say, 57 million and the number of active dentists reaches 20000, the dentist: population ratio will be 1:2850. Even if this more favourable figure is reached, it does not automatically mean that care will be more available to all. If the proliferation of dentists in the south-east corner of England continues at its present rate, then other regions will remain short of manpower. If the apparent trend, seen in recent years, of dentists leaving the

National Health Service to practise privately continues, then large sections of the population will not have access to care.

It is quite possible that future efforts to improve the dental manpower situation will be directed towards ancillary personnel of various kinds. Building up such a corps takes time; at present there is still only one auxiliary to every 20 dentists. Questions too are being asked about the proper role and duties of auxiliary personnel, and research is being conducted to examine the most effective ways in which dentists and their ancillary staff can provide care to a community.

To summarise, it is probable that national levels of dental caries prevalence will not be reduced much in the next generation. It seems more likely that methods of providing dental care will attract more attention than will methods for preventing dental caries. Certainly, effective preventive methods are already at hand. What perhaps is required is more will on the part of the profession to see that they are applied to the whole community, and more will on the part of the community to demand and to accept them.

Further reading

Barker, D. J. P. (1973). *Practical Epidemiology*, Churchill Livingstone, Edinburgh and London, 168 pp.

Chadwick, E. (1842). *Report on the Sanitary Condition of the Labouring Population of Great Britain* (Ed. and introduced by M. W. Flinn), Edinburgh University Press, 1965, 443 pp.

Dubos, R. (1959). *Mirage of Health*, Doubleday, New York, 230 pp.

Dunning, J. M. (1970). *Principles of Dental Public Health*, 2nd edn, Harvard Univ. Press, Cambridge, Mass., 598 pp.

McMahon, B. and Pugh, T. F. (1970). *Epidemiology; Principles and Methods*, Little, Brown and Co., Boston, 376 pp.

Morris, J. N. (1967). *Uses of Epidemiology*, 2nd edn, Churchill Livingstone, London and Edinburgh, 338 pp.

Slack, G. L. and Burt, B. A. (Eds) (1974). *Dental Public Health; An Introduction to Community Dentistry*, Wright, Bristol, 338 pp.

Young, W. O. and Striffler, D. F. (Eds) (1969). *The Dentist, His Practice, and His Community*, 2nd edn, Saunders, London, XIII + 346 pp.

Yudkin, J. (1972). *Pure White and Deadly; the Problem of Sugar*, Davis-Poynter, London, 164 pp.

References

1. Department of Health and Social Security (1971). *Digest of Health Statistics 1970*, HMSO, London

2. Russell, A. L. (1964). Epidemiology and the rational basis of dental public health and dental practice, in *The Dentist, His Practice, and His Community*, 1st edn (Eds Young, W. O. and Striffler, D. F.), Saunders, Philadelphia, pp. 58–59

3. Dean, H. T. (1938). Endemic fluorosis and its relation to dental caries. *Public Health Reports*, **53**, 1443–52

4. Dean, H. T., Jay, P., Arnold, F. A., Jr., McClure, F. J. and Elvove, E. (1939). Domestic water and dental caries, including certain epidemiological aspects of oral *L. acidophilus*. *Public Health Reports*, **54**, 862–88

5. Klein, H., Palmer, C. E. and Knutson, J. W. (1938). Studies on dental caries. I. Dental status and dental needs of elementary schoolchildren. *Public Health Reports*, **53**, 751–65

6. World Health Organisation (1971). Oral Health Surveys; Basic Methods, World Health Organisation, Geneva, 51 pp.

7. McClendon, B. G., Abrams, A. M. and Horowitz, H. S. (1972). Test of a method for estimating prevalence of DMFT. *Journal of Public Health Dentistry*, **32**, 165–8

8. Viegas, A. R. (1969). Simplified indices for estimating the prevalence of dental caries-experience in children seven to twelve

years of age. *Journal of Public Health Dentistry*, **29**, 76–91

9. Lopes, E. S., Filho, H. N., Chiodi, J. and Tavano, O. (1973). Inter-examiner variability when using Viegas' simplified caries index. *Journal of Public Health Dentistry*, **33**, 7–12

10. Poulsen, A. and Horowitz, H. A. (1974). An evaluation of a hierarchical method of describing the pattern of dental caries attack. *Community Dentistry and Oral Epidemiology*, **2**, 7–11

11. Hardwick, J. L. (1960). The incidence and distribution of caries throughout the ages in relation to the Englishman's diet. *British Dental Journal*, **108**, 9–17

12. Moore, W. J. and Corbett, M. E. (1971). The distribution of dental caries in ancient British populations. I. Anglo-Saxon period. *Caries Research*, **5**, 151–68

13. Poulsen, S. and Møller, I. J. (1972). The prevalence of dental caries, plaque and gingivitis in 3-year-old Danish children. *Scandinavian Journal of Dental Research*, **80**, 94–103

14. Köhler, L. and Holst, K. (1973). Dental health of four-year-old children. *Acta Paediatrica Scandinavica*, **62**, 269–78

15. Baume, L. J. (1969). Caries prevalence and caries intensity among 12,344 schoolchildren of French Polynesia. *Archives of Oral Biology*, **14**, 181–205

16. Winter, G. B., Rule, D. C., Mailer, G. P., James, P. M. C. and Gordon, P. H. (1971). The prevalence of dental caries in pre-school children aged 1–4 years. I. Aetiological factors. *British Dental Journal*, **130**, 271–7

17. Dodd, D. M. (1974). Dental caries in five-year-old schoolchildren. *Public Health (London)*, **88**, 131–9

18. Hennon, D. K., Stookey, G. K. and Muhler, J. C. (1969). Prevalence and distribution of dental caries in pre-school children. *Journal of the American Dental Association*, **79**, 1405–14

19. Bronstein, E. (1969). A survey of caries experience among the pre-school children of Philadelphia. *Journal of Public Health Dentistry*, **29**, 24–6

20. Berman, D. E. and Slack, G. L. (1972). Dental caries in English school children; a longitudinal study. *British Dental Journal*, **133**, 529–38

21. Schamschula, R. G., Keyes, P. H. and Hornabrook, R. W. (1972). Root surface caries in Lufa, New Guinea. I. Clinical observations. *Journal of the American Dental Association*, **85**, 603–8

22. Bibby, B. G. (1970). Inference from natural occurring variations in caries prevalence. *Journal of Dental Research*, **49**, 1194–1200

23. Fanning, E. A., Gotjamanos, T. and Vowles, N. J. (1969). Dental health and treatment requirements of South Australian secondary schoolchildren. *Medical Journal of Australia*, **2**, 899–901

24. Creighton, W. E. (1969). Dental caries experience of Negro and Caucasian children in Portland, Oregon. *Journal of Dentistry for Children*, **36**, 139–43

25. Chung, C. S., Runck, D. W., Niswander, J. D., Bilben, S. E. and Kau, M. C. (1970). Genetic and epidemiological studies of oral characteristics in Hawaii's schoolchildren. I. Caries and periodontal disease. *Journal of Dental Research*, **49**, 1374–85

26. Ainamo, J. and Alvesalo, L. (1970). Caries prevalence in a Finnish rural population. *Acta Odontologica Scandinavica*, **28**, 271–81

27. Hargreaves, J. A. (1972). Changes in diet and dental health of children living in the Scottish Island of Lewis. *Caries Research*, **6**, 355–76

28. Poulsen, S., Møller, I. J., Naerum, J. and Pedersen, P. O. (1972). Prevalence of dental caries in 2,383 Moroccan school children aged eight and twelve. *Archives of Oral Biology*, **17**, 1165–75

29. Bagramian, R. A. and Russell, A. L. (1971). An epidemiologic study of dental

caries in race and geographic area. *Journal of Dental Research*, **50**, 1553–6

30. Stamm, J. W. (1973). Dental caries in 506 young Ontario adults. *Journal of the Canadian Dental Association*, **39**, 338–41

31. Beal, J. F. (1973). The dental health of five-year-old children of different ethnic origins resident in an inner Birmingham area and a nearby borough. *Archives of Oral Biology*, **18**, 305–12

32. Beck, D. J. (1967). Evaluation of dental care for children in New Zealand and the United States. *New Zealand Dental Journal*, **63**, 201–11

33. Burt, B. A. (1973). A study of the oral condition, utilisation of services, and attitudes towards dental health of a population in the East End of London, England. *Ph.D. Thesis*, Univ. of London

34. Møller, I. J., Poulsen, S. and Nielson, V. O. (1972). The prevalence of dental caries in Godhavn and Scoresbysund districts, Greenland. *Scandinavian Journal of Dental Research*, **80**, 169–80

35. Kailis, D. G. and Silva, D. G. (1971). Prevalence of dental caries in Australian aboriginal children resident in Carnarvon, Western Australia. *Australian Dental Journal*, **16**, 109–15

36. Barrett, M. J. and Williamson, J. H. (1972). Oral health of Australian aborigines: survey methods and prevalence of dental caries. *Australian Dental Journal*, **17**, 37–50

37. Møller, I. J., Pindborg, J. J. and Roed-Petersen, B. (1972). The prevalence of dental caries, enamel opacities and enamel hypoplasia in Ugandans. *Archives of Oral Biology*, **17**, 9–22

38. Littleton, N. W., Kakehaski, S. and Fitzgerald, R. J. (1970). Study of differences in the occurrence of dental caries in Caucasian and Negro children. *Journal of Dental Research*, **49**, 742–51

39. Mansbridge, J. N. (1959). Heredity and dental caries. *Journal of Dental Research*, **38**, 337–47

40. McPhail, C. W. and Grainger, R. M. (1969). A mapping procedure for the geographic pathology of dental caries. *International Dental Journal*, **19**, 380–92

41. Kailis, D. G. (1971). Dental conditions observed in Australian aboriginal children resident in Warburton and Cundeelee missions, Western Australia (August, 1968). *Australian Dental Journal*, **16**, 44–52

42. Marlay, E. (1970). Dental caries and the adolescent girl in Brisbane. *Australian Dental Journal*, **15**, 204–15

43. Ludwig, T. G. and Bibby, B. G. (1969). Geographic variations in the prevalence of dental caries in the United States of America. *Caries Research*, **3**, 32–43

44. Barmes, D. E., Adkins, B. L. and Schamschula, R. G. (1970). Etiology of caries in Papua–New Guinea. Associations in soil, food and water. *Bulletin of the World Health Organization*, **43**, 769–84

45. US Department of Health, Education and Welfare; Public Health Service (1967). Decayed, Missing and Filled Teeth in Adults, Series 11, No. 23, National Center for Health Statistics, Washington DC

46. US department of Health, Education and Welfare; Public Health Service (1971). Decayed, Missing and Filled Teeth Among Children, Series 11, No. 106, National Center for Health Statistics, Washington DC

47. Camrass, R. (1974). An oral health survey of Western Samoans. *Community Dentistry and Oral Epidemiology*, **2**, 12–19

48. Stephen, K. W. and Sutherland, D. A. (1971). A dental health study of 14-year-old school children in Paisley. *British Dental Journal*, **130**, 19–24

49. Enwonwu, C. (1974). Socio-economic factors in dental caries prevalence and frequency in Nigerians. *Caries Research*, **8**, 155–71

50. Beck, D. J. (1968). Dental Health Status of the New Zealand Population in Late

Adolescence and Young Adulthood, Wellington, National Health Statistics Centre Special Report No. 29

51. Gray, P. G., Todd, J. E., Slack, G. L. and Bulman, J. S. (1970). *Adult Dental Health in England and Wales* 1968. HMSO, London

52. Anderson, R. J., James, P. M. C., James, D. M. and Borden, H. (1971). Dental caries experience and treatment patterns; social differences in 1,252 university students. *British Dental Journal*, **131**, 67–71

53. Russell, A. L. (1966). World epidemiology and oral health, in *Environmental Variables in Oral Disease*, (Eds Kreshover, S. J. and McClure, F. J.), American Association Advancement Science, Publication No. 81, Washington DC, pp. 21–39

54. Hadjimarkos, D. M. (1969). Selenium: a caries-enhancing trace element. *Caries Research*, **3**, 14–22

55. Anderson, R. J. (1969). The relationship between dental conditions and the trace element molybdenum. *Caries Research*, **3**, 75–87

56. Losee, F. L. and Adkins, B. L. (1969). A study of the mineral environment of caries-resistant Navy recruits. *Caries Research*, **3**, 23–31

57. Rothman, K. J., Glass, R. L., Espinal, F. and Velez, H.(1972). Caries-free teeth in the absence of the fluoride ion. *Journal of Public Health Dentistry*, **32**, 225–8

58. Rothman, K. J., Glass, R. L., Espinal, F. and Velez, H. (1972). Dental caries and soil content of trace metals in two Columbian villages. *Journal of Dental Research*, **51**, 1686

59. Losee, F. L. and Ludwig, T. G. (1970). Trace elements and caries. *Journal of Dental Research*, **49**, 1229–36

60. Burt, B. A. (1974). The administration of public dental treatment programmes, in *Dental Public Health: An Introduction to Community Dentistry* (Eds Slack, G. L. and Burt, B. A.), Wright, Bristol, pp. 113–33

61. Pickles, T. H. (1970). The relationship of caries prevalence data and diagnosed treatment needs in a child population. *Medical Care*, **8**, 463–73

62. Ringelberg, M. L., Matouski, G. M. and Kimball, A. W. (1974). Dental caries-experience in three generations of families. *Journal of Public Health Dentistry*, **34**, 174–80

63. James, P. M. C., Parfitt, G. J. and Roydhouse, R. H. (1970). Caries experience during a decade. *Journal of Dentistry for Children*, **37**, 289–95

64. Jackson, D. (1974). Caries experience in English children and young adults during the years 1947–1972. *British Dental Journal*, **137**, 91–8

65. Sheiham, A. (1973). An evaluation of the success of dental care in the the United Kingdom. *British Dental Journal*, **135**, 271–9

66. Sheiham, A. and Hobdell, M. H. (1969). Decayed, missing and filled teeth in British adult populations. *British Dental Journal*, **126**, 401–4

67. Murray, J. J. (1971). Adult dental health in fluoride and non-fluoride areas: I. Mean DMF values by age. *British Dental Journal*, **131**, 391–5

68. Jackson, D., Murray, J. J. and Fairpo, C. G. (1973). Regular dental care in dentate persons; an assessment. *British Dental Journal*, **135**, 59–63

69. Burt, B. A. (1974). The use of dental services in an East London borough. *British Dental Journal*, **136**, 141–4

70. US Department of Health, Education and Welfare; Public Health Service (1972). Dental Visits: Volume and Interval Since Last Visit, DHEW Publication No. (HSM) 72–1066, National Center for Health Statistics, Washington DC

71. Burt, B. A. (1974). Fluoridation of public water supplies, in *Dental Public Health; An Introduction to Community Dentistry*,

(Eds Slack, G. L. and Burt, B. A.), Bristol, Wright, pp. 45–68

72. Davies, G. N. (1973). Fluoride in the prevention of dental caries; a tentative cost–benefit analysis. *British Dental Journal*, **135**, 131–4; **135**, 173–4; **135**, 233–5; **135**, 293–7; **135**, 333–6

73. Wallace, J. S. (1912). *The Prevention of Dental Caries*, 2nd edn, Dental Record, London

74. Pickerill, H. P. (1923). *The Prevention of Dental Caries and Oral Sepsis*, 3rd edn, Baillière, Tindall and Cox, London

75. Mellanby, M. (1934). *Diet and the Teeth*, Part III, The Effect of Diet on Dental Structure and Disease in Man, Medical Research Council and HMSO, London

76. Shaw, J. H. (1952). Nutrition and dental caries, in *Survey of the Literature on Dental Caries* (Ed. Toverud, G.), National Academy of Sciences and National Research Council, Washington DC, pp. 415–567

77. Bunting, R. W. (1935). Diet and dental caries. *Journal of the American Dental Association*, **22**, 114–22

78. Breese, F. (1934). Diet and teeth. *British Dental Journal*, **56**, 120–4

79. Miller, W. D. (1883). Agency of micro-organisms in decay of human teeth. *Dental Cosmos*, **25**, 1–12

80. Toverud, G. (1956). The influence of war and post-war conditions on the teeth of Norwegian school children. I. Eruption of permanent teeth and status of deciduous dentition. *Milbank Memorial Fund Quarterly Bulletin*, **34**, 354–430

81. Toverud, G. (1957). The influence of war and post-war conditions on the teeth of Norwegian school children. II. Caries in the permanent teeth of children aged 7–8 and 12–13 years. *Milbank Memorial Fund Quarterly Bulletin*, **35**, 127–96

82. Toverud, G. (1957). The influence of war and post-war conditions on the teeth of Norwegian school children. III. Discussion of food supply and dental condition in Norway and other European countries. *Milbank Memorial Fund Quarterly Bulletin*, **35**, 373–459

83. Fisher, F. J. (1968). A field survey of dental caries, periodontal disease and enamel defects in Tristan da Cunha. *British Dental Journal*, **125**, 447–53

84. Lilienthal, B., Goldsworthy, N. E., Sullivan, H. R. and Cameron, D. A. (1953). The biology of the children of Hopewood House, Bowral, N. S. W. I. Observations on dental caries extending over five years (1947–1952). *Medical Journal of Australia*, **1**, 878–81

85. Sullivan, H. R. and Harris, R. (1958). The biology of the children of Hopewood House, Bowral, N. S. W. II. Observations extending over five years (1952–1956). 2. Observations on oral conditions. *Australian Dental Journal*, **3**, 311–17

86. Harris, R. (1963). Biology of the children of Hopewood House, Bowral, Australia. 4. Observations on dental caries experience extending over five years (1957–1961). *Journal of Dental Research*, **42**, 1387–99

87. Gustafsson, B. E., Quensel, C. E., Lanke, L. S., Lundquist, C., Grahnen, H., Bonow, B. E. and Krasse, B. (1954). The Vipeholm dental caries study. The effect of different levels of carbohydrate intake on caries activity in 436 individuals observed for five years. *Acta Odontica Scandinavica*, **11**, 232–364

88. Curzon, M. E. and Curzon, J. A. (1970). Dental caries in Eskimo children of the Keewatin District in the Northwest Territories. *Journal of the Canadian Dental Association*, **36**, 342–5

89. Newbrun, E. (1969). Sucrose, the arch criminal of dental caries. *Journal of Dentistry for Children*, **36**, 239–48

90. Glass, R. L. and Fleisch, S. (1974). Diet and dental caries: dental caries incidence and the consumption of ready-to-eat cereals. *Journal of the American Dental Association*, **88**, 807–13

91. Weiss, R. L. and Trithart, A. H. (1960). Between-meal eating habits and dental caries experience in pre-school children. *American Journal of Public Health*, **50**, 1097–1104

92. Fanning, E. A., Gotjamanos, T. and Vowles, N. J. (1969). Dental caries in children related to availability of sweets at school canteens. *Medical Journal of Australia* **1**, 1131–2

93. Duany, L. F., Zinner, D. D. and Jablon, J. M. (1972). Epidemiologic studies of caries-free and caries-active students. II. Diet, dental plaque, and oral hygiene. *Journal of Dental Research*, **51**, 727–33

94. Martinsson, T. (1972). Socio-economic investigation of school children with high and low caries frequency. 3. A dietary study based on information given by the children. *Odontologist Revy*, **23**, 93–113

95. Steinberg, A. D., Zimmerman, S. O. and Bramer, M. L. (1972). The Lincoln dental caries study. II. The effect of acidulated carbonated beverages on the incidence of dental caries. *Journal of the American Dental Association*, **85**, 81–9

96. Keyes, P. H. (1969). Present and future methods for dental caries control. *Journal of the American Dental Association*, **79**, 1395–1404

97. Rogerson, M. J. (1973). The role of a calcium sucrose phosphate – calcium orthophosphate complex in the reduction of dental caries. *Australian Dental Journal*, **18**, 160–6

98. DePaola, P. F. and Mellberg, J. R. (1973). Caries experience and fluoride uptake in children receiving semiannual prophylaxes with an acidulated phosphate fluoride paste. *Journal of the American Dental Association*, **87**, 155–9

99. Makinen, K. K. (1972). The role of sucrose and other sugars in the development of dental caries: a review. *International Dental Journal*, **22**, 363–86

100. Jenkins, G. N. (1972). Current concepts concerning the development of dental caries. *International Dental Journal*, **22**, 350–62

101. Horowitz, H. S. (1973). Fluoride: research on clinical and public health applications. *Journal of the American Dental Association*, **87**, 1013–18

102. Sutcliffe, P. (1973). The need for treatment in 11 to 17-year-old children: a longitudinal epidemiological survey. *British Dental Journal*, **135**, 153–7

103. Gruebbel, A. O. (1944). A measurement of dental caries prevalence and treatment service for deciduous teeth. *Journal of Dental Research*, **23**, 163–8

104. Todd, J. E. (1975). *Children's Dental Health in England and Wales, 1973*. HMSO, London

105. Dunning, J. M. (1970). *Principles of Dental Public Health*, 2nd edn, Harvard Univ. Press, Cambridge, Mass.

Chapter 3

The Microbiology of Dental Caries

As was mentioned in chapter 1, there have been a number of theories concerning the aetiology of dental caries, of which the acidogenic theory has been the most generally accepted. According to this theory, caries is initiated by organic acids produced by oral bacteria as a result of their fermentative activity on carbohydrates. The credit for the 'Chemicoparasitic' or acidogenic theory is usually ascribed to W. D. Miller[1], but it is fair to say that his conclusions were based on the accumulated efforts of a number of other investigators, as well as his own, during the nineteenth century. In 1897, N. B. Williams reported his observation that the enamel of human teeth was covered with adhesive 'gelatine-like' material, consisting largely of micro-organisms, and suggested that this material might be responsible for the localisation of acid attack to certain areas of the tooth surface. Writing a year later, G. V. Black coined the phrase 'gelatinous microbial plaques' for the bacteria on the tooth surface, and supported the idea that acid-producing bacteria were the main aetiological agents in caries.

A considerable amount of work was carried out by pioneer research workers during the past century and the early part of the twentieth century[2], but these early studies will not be considered in any detail here. In this chapter, the evidence for regarding caries as an infectious disease will be discussed and some of the properties of those bacteria thought to be of importance in the disease will be described. In addition, some of the oral defence mechanisms which may operate to protect the teeth against such organisms will be considered briefly.

3.1 Evidence for the Role of Microorganisms in Caries

3.1.1 *In vitro* experiments

Early in the nineteenth century it was shown that teeth could be corroded by inorganic acids such as sulphuric and nitric acid. Experimental carious lesions were produced by the 'window

technique', in which extracted teeth were covered in wax leaving a small opening of unprotected enamel. When these prepared teeth were exposed either to dilute acids or fermenting mixtures of microorganisms, decalcification of the window areas was observed. However, this was usually complete etching of a layer of outer enamel and not the deeper partial loss of sub-surface mineral which is characteristic of the natural carious lesion.

In his famous studies, Miller incubated teeth with saliva and mixtures of different foods such as bread and sugar. This resulted in decalcification of the teeth, although once again it was of the surface-etching type. Miller also demonstrated that many different types of oral bacteria could produce enough acid to decalcify enamel, and identified lactic acid as one of the products of his incubation mixtures.

In recent years it has been shown that artificial lesions which are histologically indistinguishable from natural caries can be produced *in vitro*[3]. This has been achieved using a window technique similar to that described a 100 years earlier by Magitot, but incorporating the acid into a gel such as gelatin or cellulose. It has also been found that experimentally produced deposits of oral bacteria on the enamel surface alter the effect of acid on the tooth *in vitro*, and can produce an appearance similar to that of early natural lesions[4]. However, although it has been possible to mimic natural caries, little is known of the physical chemistry which leads to the peculiar structure of the carious lesion.

More recently, other workers have used modified artificial mouth systems[8] and continuous culture apparatus (known as a chemostat) to study the growth and physiological properties of cariogenic microorganisms such as *Streptococcus mutans*[9]. One of the advantages of such systems is that experiments can be conducted at slow rates of bacterial growth which may be more directly comparable to the normal intra-oral situation than the conventional batch culture methods traditionally used in most laboratories. However, complete and realistic *in vitro* simulation of the tooth surface microflora in all its complexity remains to be achieved.

Some research workers have gone to great lengths to simulate oral conditions in the laboratory, and several 'artificial mouths' have been designed for caries studies. A historical review of the early *in vitro* studies leading up to the development of the artificial mouth has been provided by Pigman[5, 6]. Although these more elaborate experiments allow better control of the *in vitro* environment in which the tooth is placed, it is arguable that they have not really contributed greatly to our understanding of the caries process. Several types of bacteria, particularly streptococci, have been shown to produce enamel demineralisation in the artificial mouth, while others, such as *Candida albicans*, *Leptotrichia dentium* (now called *Bacterionema matruchotii*) and *Actinomyces odontolyticus* apparently did not[7].

It appears, therefore, from *in vitro* experiments that several types of bacteria can produce enough acid from carbohydrate substrates to decalcify tooth enamel. Furthermore, in the presence of added acid, bacterial deposits modify the rate of decalcification to produce a subsurface lesion closely resembling natural caries.

3.1.2 Reduction of caries by antibiotics

Several studies have shown that antibiotics can reduce the incidence of dental caries, both in experimental animals and in man. In animal experiments, a reduction in caries has been achieved by administration of penicillin in the diet or drinking water[10], and in man by brushing the teeth with a penicillin-containing dentifrice.

In one clinical trial of a penicillin dentifrice, in which the subjects' toothbrushing was unsupervised, no reduction in caries incidence was observed[11]. However, subjects using the same concentration of 1000 units of penicillin per gramme of toothpaste in a supervised brushing regimen showed a slight reduction in caries (16 per cent) compared to control subjects using an ordinary paste. In another study, with supervised toothbrushing, a significant caries reduction of 55 per

cent was achieved after one year, the figure increasing to 58 per cent reduction in the second year of the trial[12].

Epidemiological studies on children receiving long-term administration of penicillin for medical reasons indicate a significantly reduced caries incidence in this group when compared to untreated children in the same populations. In one retrospective study, a reduction of 55 per cent in DMFS of penicillin-treated subjects compared to controls was recorded after $2\frac{1}{2}$ years[13], and in another investigation, where subjects were compared to siblings, the caries reduction was 56–69 per cent[14].

The clearly demonstrated fact that penicillin can reduce the incidence of caries strongly indicates that the disease is of microbial origin, since it is difficult to explain the cariostatic effect of an antimicrobial agent on any other basis. These observations also indicate that the causative bacteria are likely to be Grampositive, since penicillin is most active against these organisms.

At first sight it might appear that antibiotics offer an attractive method of preventing dental caries. However, as will be discussed in a later chapter, there are several contra-indications to the widespread use of antibiotics for this purpose, particularly the danger of side effects, development of hypersensitivity reactions to the drugs, and the overgrowth of antibiotic-resistant microorganisms.

Further, more detailed consideration of the effect of antibiotics on dental caries can be found in two recent reviews[15, 16].

3.1.3 Caries in experimental animals

Until 1954 there was no conclusive evidence that bacteria were essential for the initiation of caries. In that year, Orland and co-workers[17] demonstrated that completely germ-free rats of a caries-susceptible line failed to develop caries even when fed a cariogenic, high-sucrose diet. By implanting bacteria into the mouths of these germ-free animals, caries was produced.

Unfortunately, the precise identity of the

strains of bacteria used in these pioneer experiments is not known, except in general descriptive terms such as 'an enterococcus' and 'a proteolytic rod', and the original strains are no longer available for further study. However, these experiments established a basic method by which dental caries can be studied in an animal model system. Such experimental systems have subsequently been widely adopted in dental caries research for studying the microbial aetiology of the disease. They can also be used to good effect for estimating the caries-enhancing properties of various dietary substrates and for testing potential cariostatic or preventive measures.

The term 'gnotobiotic' means, literally, 'known life'. It is applied to the situation where the composition of the microbial flora of an experimental animal is completely controlled by the investigator. Thus, animals can be raised and maintained in a completely sterile or germ-free environment. Subsequently, these mouths may be inoculated with one or more known varieties of bacteria. Many of the studies on experimental caries have been carried out using mono-infected animals which have only one known species of bacteria inhabiting the mouth. Mixed flora studies, where combinations of two or more species are introduced into the oral cavity, are more difficult to monitor and control, but have occasionally been undertaken.

Another condition which is sometimes utilised in animal studies is referred to as 'relative gnotobiosis'. In this case a conventionally raised animal, which carries a normal oral flora, is treated with antibiotics (such as erythromycin or streptomycin) in order to suppress the indigenous microorganisms. Then a test strain of bacteria, known to be resistant to the particular antibiotic employed, is introduced into the mouth of the animal. Thus the oral flora of such animals may be dominated by an erythromycin-resistant strain of streptococcus, although the exact composition of the remainder of the (suppressed) flora is not known. 'Conventional' animals are those which carry the 'normal flora' of the particular animal species, although this is often not known in any detail. 'Specific pathogen free' animals are those which are guaranteed not to be harbouring particular pathogenic microorganisms, but here again the supposedly non-pathogenic indigenous microflora is not generally specified.

Since the original studies on germ-free and mono-infected rats, many other reports have appeared in the literature to confirm and extend Orland's findings. In addition to rats of several varieties, caries can be produced experimentally in hamsters, gerbils, white-tailed rats and monkeys. Keyes and Fitzgerald and their colleagues, working at the National Institute for Dental Research in the USA, demonstrated that particular dextran-producing streptococci, subsequently shown to belong to the species *Streptococcus mutans*, were highly cariogenic in mono-infected animals[18, 19]. They also showed, in hamsters, that caries-producing microorganisms could be transmitted from one animal to another, either by caging them together or via infected faeces[20]. The streptococcal strains used originally were isolated from animals, but subsequently similar strains of human origin were found by several workers to produce caries in gnotobiotic animals[21-25].

Many strains of bacteria representing several species have now been tested for their cariogenic potential in animals and the literature on the subject is extensive[26, 27]. It is clear, in some cases, that a given bacterial strain may be cariogenic in one animal species but not in others. Thus it may be misleading to extrapolate the results obtained in one animal and assume that the same situation would apply in other animals, or in man[28].

Although much useful information has been gained from studies on caries in rodents, there are obviously fundamental differences between the situation in the rodent mouth and that of man. Primates are in many ways preferable to rodents for experimental caries studies, since their dentition and the pattern of caries attack is similar to that of man. In addition, it is possible to maintain primates on a diet which closely resembles that consumed by humans, and the microbial flora of the mouth of monkeys is also quite similar to that of man.

Caries research on monkeys has been limited to a small number of centres, largely due to the high cost of maintaining a suitable colony of animals and also because of the considerable technical problems involved in such an enterprise. Pioneers in this field have been the staff at the Royal College of Surgeons Research Establishment, in Kent, where a series of experiments have been carried out since the 1960s. It has been demonstrated that caries can be induced in monkeys (*Macaca fascicularis*) which are infected with cariogenic streptococci[29] and many of the observations made originally on rodents have been confirmed in primates. Since the monkey appears to provide such an excellent model for human caries, this experimental system is being used increasingly for studies on prevention of caries by various means, including immunisation (chapter 11). In addition to *M. fascicularis*, the rhesus monkey (*M. mulatta*) is also of value for caries research[30].

The majority of gnotobiotic animal experiments have been designed to test the caries-inducing effects of mono-infections with specific bacteria, usually streptococci. A very interesting recent development at the University of Nijmegen has been the introduction of combinations of different bacterial species in the mouths of animals[31]. In these studies it has been observed that the normal cariogenic effect of implanting strains of *Streptococcus mutans* into the rodent can be reduced by simultaneously introducing a strain of *Veillonella*, which is capable of utilising lactate produced by the streptococcus. It is to be hoped that many more investigators will turn their attention to the interrelationships of bacteria in the oral cavity and their relevance to dental disease.

The appearance of caries in rodents and in monkeys is shown in figures 3.1 and 3.2.

3.2 Microorganisms Shown to be Cariogenic in Animals

Most of the published studies on gnotobiotic

animals have been concentrated on the cariogenic potential of streptococci, especially the species *Streptococcus mutans*. However, a few investigators have reported the production of caries by other genera. It is important to remember that the situation in which a germ-free or relatively gnotobiotic animal is mono-infected with a pure culture of bacteria is a highly artificial one. Under natural conditions, caries occurs in a very complicated microbiological environment in which the caries-producing organisms are associated with large numbers of other bacteria of a variety of species. In addition, the animals used in caries experiments are usually fed a diet containing over 50 per cent sucrose, and this is quite unlike their natural diet.

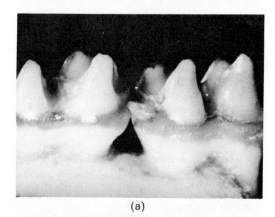

(a)

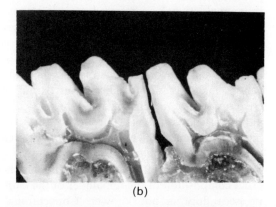

(b)

Figure 3.1 Appearance of dental caries in rodents.
(a) Gross appearance of caries in molars of a hamster
(b) Section of carious posterior teeth of a rat

negative rods which are characteristically both acidogenic (acid producers) and aciduric (acid tolerant). Their unique ability to survive and grow at low pH levels is utilised in selective culture media such as Tomato Juice agar and Rogosa (MRS) medium, where the pH of about 5.0 inhibits the growth of most other bacteria and allows the recognition of lactobacillus colonies.

For many years lactobacilli were widely considered to be the causative agent of human caries. Lactobacilli can be isolated from human saliva and from dentinal caries, but their numbers are usually extremely low in dental plaque. At least three reports have been published in which strains of *Lactobacillus* were shown to be capable of inducing caries in gnotobiotic rats. One of these strains was *L. acidophilus*, the second was *L. casei*, and the other report was of an unnamed *Lactobacillus* species[26, 32]. A number of other *Lactobacillus* strains tested have failed to produce caries under the experimental conditions employed.

The evidence available to date indicates that at least some lactobacilli are capable of producing caries when inoculated into the mouths of germ-free animals. It is not possible to make realistic comparisons between the cariogenic potentials of lactobacilli and streptococci, since few workers have systematically studied them in this way. However, from his observations on dental caries in monkeys, Bowen[29] has suggested that 'the importance of these microorganisms (lactobacilli) in the aetiology of dental caries cannot be discounted'.

3.2.2 Streptococci

Streptococci are Gram-positive, catalase-negative cocci, sometimes appearing as short rods, which may form chains under certain conditions of growth.

The original streptococcus used in the first gnotobiotic animal studies by Orland and co-workers was described as an enterococcus, but the precise identity of this strain is not known. Several other known enterococci (i.e. Lancefield Group D streptococci, normally found in the

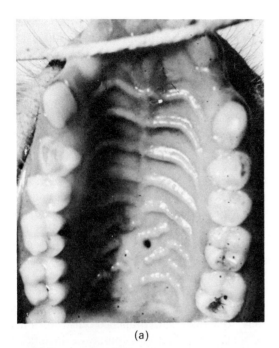

(a)

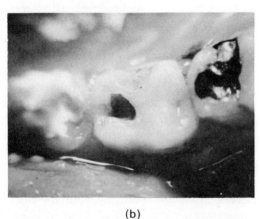

(b)

Figure 3.2 Appearance of dental caries in monkeys. (a) Upper jaw of monkey (*Macaca fascicularis*) showing caries in molar teeth. (b) Appearance of carious molar in monkey. (Photographs by courtesy of Dr. G. Colman, Royal College of Surgeons, Research Establishment, Downe.)

In the following sections, some of the bacterial types which have been found to produce caries in animals will be considered.

3.2.1 Lactobacilli

Lactobacilli are Gram-positive, catalase-

gut) have subsequently been shown to be caries inactive in gnotobiotic rats.

Those species which are known to produce caries in experimental animals are *S. mutans, S. sanguis*, and *S. salivarius**. Of these *S. mutans* has been the most extensively investigated and appears to be more effective than the other species in producing caries in mono-infected animals.

The name *S. mutans* was given to streptococci isolated from human carious teeth by Clarke in 1924. Although Clarke's findings were confirmed by one or two other workers in the 1920s, the species was almost completely forgotten until the experimental animal caries studies got under way more than 30 years later. During the past decade a great deal of research has been carried out on the properties of *S. mutans* and the recent literature on the subject is very extensive.

Dozens of strains of *S. mutans*, originally isolated from both man and animals, have now been tested for cariogenicity in rats, hamsters and monkeys. In many laboratories all over the world it has been conclusively demonstrated that strains of *S. mutans* are cariogenic in suitable mono-infected animals. It also appears from some experiments that the chances of successful implantation of test strains are enhanced by feeding the animals with a high sucrose diet.

A few strains of *S. sanguis* and *S. salivarius* have been shown to produce caries in experimental animals, although other strains of these species apparently are not cariogenic. The amount of caries produced is generally less than that caused by *S. mutans* infections. *S. sanguis* induces caries in rats but not in hamsters, probably due to the fact this species is less easily established in the hamster mouth.

The relative caries-inducing ability of a number of streptococci has been tested in albino hamsters by Krasse and Carlsson[28].

Their results showed that all 10 strains of *S. mutans* tested produced highly significant amounts of caries in the animal model system used, and that 6–7 of the *S. salivarius* strains produced a lesser, but still significant, degree of caries. None of the other species tested, which included examples of *S. sanguis, S. mitior* and *S. bovis*,

produced caries, but neither were they successfully implanted in the mouth of the hamsters. The authors concluded their interesting report with the following statement: 'These facts show the obvious limitation of animal caries-models in elucidating the specific role of various micro-organisms in human caries. This also means that the designation "cariogenic" and "non-cariogenic" streptococci should only be used when referring to specific animal experiments. Comparison of characteristics between "cariogenic" and "non-cariogenic" strains collected from various experiments leads to more confusions than useful information'. We have been warned!

3.2.3 Actinomyces

Actinomyces are pleomorphic, Gram-positive rods, sometimes with branched cells, which may be anaerobic, micro-aerophilic or facultative. Catalase-negative and catalase-positive species are found within the genus.

In recent years, several studies have been made on the ability of strains of *Actinomyces* to produce periodontal destruction in hamsters and other animals. During these experiments it was also noted that the infecting organisms caused root surface caries, although enamel surfaces were generally not involved. Two of the species which have this pathogenic potential are *A. viscosus* (originally named *Odontomyces viscosus*) and *A. naeslundii*. *A. viscosus* was first isolated from the mouth of hamsters, but the species can also be isolated from humans although there are serological differences between strains of animal and human origin. *A. naeslundii* resembles *A. viscosus* in many respects and the two species are often difficult to distinguish in the laboratory by conventional biochemical and physiological tests. Serological cross-reactions between these named species also occur[33].

Recently, filamentous organisms isolated from human root surface cavities have been characterised and several of these isolates were shown to be *Actinomyces* species. One strain of *A. viscosus* and one of *A. naeslundii* from this source were

* Recently strains of *S. milleri* have also been shown to be cariogenic in gnotobiotic rats[84, 85].

used to mono-infect gnotobiotic rats, and all the animals developed severe periodontal infections and root surface caries.

Whether or not there is a specific microbial aetiology for root surface caries which differs from that responsible for enamel lesions is far from certain at present. However, since *Actinomyces* species are extremely common in human supragingival plaque, and also from gingival plaque in some situations, their possible role in the aetiology of both caries and periodontal disease should not be discounted.

3.3 Microorganisms Associated with Caries in Man

3.3.1 Lactobacilli

During the 1920s, several investigators reported an apparent correlation between the numbers of lactobacilli in the mouth and dental caries. It was observed that these organisms could usually be isolated from carious cavities and people with active caries had higher counts of lactobacilli in their saliva than caries-free subjects. Restoration of open lesions led to a reduction of the salivary lactobacillus count. The method of assessing the number of aciduric bacteria in saliva, or 'Lactobacillus Count' as it is usually called, was adopted as a 'caries-activity test'. Such tests are considered in greater detail in a later section of this chapter.

Although the correlation between the salivary Lactobacillus Count and caries was reasonably consistent on a statistical basis when large groups of subjects were considered, it did not always hold good in the individual case. Unfortunately, the presence of high numbers of any particular organism in the mouth after caries has been detected does not necessarily constitute proof that the organism in question caused the disease. It is possible that established carious lesions provide a particularly suitable environment for the growth and multiplication of lactobacilli and that, therefore, their high numbers might occur as a *result* of caries.

The observed fact that lactobacilli occur in relatively small numbers in dental plaque indicates that they may not be a major aetiological agent in the *initiation* of enamel caries. However, where micro-colonies of lactobacilli do occur in plaque they may well contribute to the carious process.

The real importance of lactobacilli in the initiation of caries in man cannot be stated with any certainty at present. Almost certainly they play an important part in the destruction of dentine in established lesions.

3.3.2 Streptococci (particularly S. mutans)

Following the observations made upon the ability of *S. mutans* to produce dental caries in experimental animals, several investigators have looked for an association between this species and caries in humans. Thus, in the past few years a number of reports have appeared of epidemiological surveys in which dental caries scores have been correlated with the presence of *S. mutans* in the mouth. The majority of these studies have been *cross-sectional* in design, which means that subjects have been examined and samples taken at one particular time. Such studies may show an association between a disease, such as dental caries, and a particular microorganism, but they are not capable of demonstrating a cause and effect relationship. In *longitudinal* studies, a given population of individuals is examined sequentially over a period of time, so that the *incidence* rather than the *prevalence* of the disease can be measured and correlated with other findings, such as the presence of numbers of *S. mutans* (or any other bacterial species). Such studies may give a better indication of the significance of particular microorganisms in dental caries. However, very few of the published investigations have, to date, been of the preferable longitudinal type.

In one of the earlier studies, carried out in Sweden[34] presumptive *S. mutans* occurred in plaque material from about 80 per cent of 235 people examined, sometimes constituting as much as 80–90 per cent of the total cultivable streptococci in the samples. No significant correlation was established between the incidence of these 'caries-inducing' streptococci and previous caries experience, either in school children or dental students. However, there was a significant correlation between active caries cavities and the number of *S. mutans* detected. Forty of the subjects were re-examined a year later, and those who had developed four or more smooth surface lesions tended to have significantly higher levels of *S. mutans* in their plaque.

Studies on several populations in the USA, South America and the Netherlands have shown a correlation between the numbers or isolation frequency of *S. mutans* and the DMF caries index, whereas no such relationship has been reported with other streptococcal species[35–38]. Commonly in these studies, the numbers of *S. mutans* colonies observed on a selective medium such as Mitis-Salivarius agar (MSA) are expressed as a percentage of the (presumptive) total streptococcal count on that medium. Such methods tend to bias the results in favour of the particular streptococci which can readily be recognised on these high-sucrose culture media, and often the remainder of the flora, which may in fact greatly outnumber the streptococci, is completely ignored.

A simplified summary of the results reported from one study on the isolation frequency and prevalence of *S. mutans* from carious and caries-free surfaces in the same mouth is given in table 3.1.

Table 3.1   Isolation frequency of *Streptococcus mutans* at different sites from two groups of naval recruits (from Shklair, Keene and Cullen[39])

Tooth sites	Caries-active group (%)	Caries-free group (%)
Approximal	71.7	33.6
Occlusal	69.6	37.1
Buccolingual	30.4	12.9

This study also showed that *S. mutans* appears to be isolated more frequently from approximal and occlusal sites than from the buccal or lingual smooth surfaces.

In a further investigation by the same workers, it was demonstrated that subjects carrying *S. mutans* in their mouths were more likely to have developed caries a year later than non-carriers of this species[40]. Ten out of 17 initially caries-free naval recruits who were found to be *S. mutans* carriers had developed at least one carious cavity a year after the initial examination. None of the four subjects not carrying detectable *S. mutans* showed evidence of caries development during the same period of observation.

One of the few published longitudinal studies was carried out on 12 Negro children in the USA[41]. Plaque samples were collected from pits, fissures and approximal surfaces at intervals of 3, 6 and 12 months following an initial baseline examination and caries increments were assessed periodically for 18 months; levels of *S. mutans* and lactobacilli in the plaque samples were assessed. *S. mutans* was isolated from all sites which developed caries during the period of observation, whereas not all carious sites yielded positive lactobacillus cultures. Mean levels of both *S. mutans* and lactobacilli were found to increase before the detection of carious lesions in pits and fissures and at approximal areas, but the numbers of lactobacilli only became significant after the development of carious cavities.

A recently reported longitudinal study on 54 pre-school children in Denmark[42] failed to show an unequivocal correlation between the presence or numbers of *S. mutans* and the development of caries at the approximal surfaces of primary molar teeth. However, in a few of the small number of subjects who developed approximal caries, relatively high levels of this organism were found 6–12 months before caries detection. Significant changes in the ratio of aerobic to anaerobic organisms in relationship to the development of caries were reported in this study.

Another recent cross-sectional study from the USA has shown further evidence of an association between *S. mutans* and dental decay in three groups of children[43]. Statistically significant correlations were demonstrated between the concentrations of *S. mutans* in material collected from single occlusal fissures and the presence of clinically detectable decay at those sites. Less clear, but still significant, correlations were obtained between levels of this organism in pooled occlusal and pooled approximal plaque samples and caries prevalence. No clear association was shown between salivary concentrations of *S. mutans* and caries, although such a relationship has been reported in some other investigations. When discussing the significance of their results, the authors of this report acknowledge the shortcomings of cross-sectional investigations, and state: 'This dilemma (i.e. the presumptive cause and effect relationship) may be resolved by more precise longitudinal studies which show that "*S. mutans*" colonisation precedes caries and by elimination studies which show that surfaces rid of "*S. mutans*" have lower caries experiences than surfaces which retain "*S. mutans*"'.

Interim results from a longitudinal study on 11–15-year-old schoolchildren in the London area have so far failed to show a clear relationship between the presence of *S. mutans* and the initiation of caries at specific approximal sites[82, 83]. After a two-year period of observation, it appeared that the isolation frequency and prevalence of *S. mutans* increased after the radiographic detection of carious lesions, rather than before. No isolations of *S. mutans* were made at any time from two of the fifteen reported sites which developed caries[83].

More recent findings from the same study suggest that large increases in the relative numbers of *S. mutans* at particular sites may be associated with the progression of enamel lesions, as opposed to their initiation. From the data now available it would appear that more attention should be given to the cariogenic potential of various combinations of plaque bacteria. This may prove to be more relevant than the mere presence or absence of one particular species.

The results of further longitudinal studies on human caries are awaited with great interest. If it can be shown that human caries is caused specifically by infection with *S. mutans*, this provides the basis for specific prophylaxis and treatment of the disease directed against that organism. As discussed in a later chapter, two theoretically possible approaches are specific chemotherapy and immunisation. If, on the other hand, dental caries is found to be a clinical syndrome which can be produced by colonisation with several different combinations of bacteria, the problems of finding suitable antibacterial prophylactic measures will be considerably greater. Since longitudinal studies on dental caries, by design, take several years to complete, it will be some time before the essential data required become available.

3.3.3 Other microorganisms

The evidence from human studies concerning the role of organisms other than streptococci or lactobacilli in dental caries is limited. In theory, any acid-producing organism present in plaque may contribute towards the carious process. This is especially likely if the bacteria are concentrated in a micro-colony immediately adjacent to the enamel surface. The ability to induce caries in mono-infected animals, although indicative of a high cariogenic potential, is probably not an essential prerequisite for bacteria to contribute towards caries in the normally complex microbial environment of the tooth surface.

As mentioned in the section on caries in animals, certain *Actinomyces* species appear to be able to produce a particular type of caries experimentally, and there is some evidence that these organisms may be involved in root surface caries in man[44, 45]. This type of caries occurs in older subjects than the more common enamel caries of childhood and adolescence, and attacks exposed cementum. Further studies are required in order to establish the relationship between *A. viscosus*, and possibly other Gram-positive rods, and root surface caries.

In addition to positive relationships between particular bacterial species and human caries, it is possible that some organisms may exert a modifying or protective effect. Thus, for example, high levels of *Veillonella* in plaque may reduce the harmful effects of other organisms which produce lactic acid. As already mentioned, such phenomena have been demonstrated in animal experiments but remain to be shown in humans.

3.3.4   Summary of studies on microbial aetiology of dental caries

A major problem in dental caries research is the highly complicated nature of the oral microbial flora. This complexity makes it difficult to decide which particular microorganisms to look for, and which ones to ignore, when attempting to relate bacterial species to the development of caries. However, from the large number of published studies on the relationship of bacteria to dental caries, certain conclusions can be drawn:

(1)   Studies on gnotobiotic animals have shown that many strains of *Streptococcus mutans*, of both animal and human origin, are highly cariogenic under suitable experimental conditions.

(2)   Some other bacteria, to a lesser extent, are also capable of inducing caries in some animal model systems. Among those species shown to have this ability are strains of *S. sanguis*, *S. salivarius*, *S. milleri*, *Lactobacillus acidophilus*, *L. casei*, and *Actinomyces naeslundii* and *A. viscosus*.

(3)   The cariogenic potential of streptococci in animals may be modified by the presence of other microorganisms such as *Veillonella* species in the mouth.

(4)   Cross-sectional surveys on human populations have indicated an association between the presence of *S. mutans* and the degree of caries experience.

(5)   Few longitudinal studies on humans have been undertaken, but there is some evidence of a relationship between colonisation of teeth by *S. mutans* and the incidence of caries. Further, more

extensive, longitudinal studies are required. Such studies should include examination of other microorganisms in addition to *S. mutans*.

(6)   In some situations, such as root surface caries, other bacteria (for example, *Actinomyces* species) may play a significant role in the initiation of caries.

3.4   Some Properties of Caries-inducing Organisms

All the bacteria which have been implicated in dental caries are capable of producing acid from carbohydrates. Streptococci and lactobacilli, in particular, will reduce the pH of glucose broth to below 5.0 in conventional culture-systems. *Streptococcus mutans* strains generally produce a terminal pH in batch cultures in the range 4.2–4.6. Lactic acid is the expected end-product of fermentation of these bacteria, although other products are found when strains are grown under conditions of carbon-limitation[46]. Similar variations in the types of acid produced in dental plaque in vivo, under different conditions of carbohydrate availability, have also been demonstrated[47].

In addition to their ability to produce acid, *S. mutans* and *S. sanguis* possess two further properties which may be relevant to their cariogenic potential:

(1)   Both species produce extracellular glucose polymers (glucans) from sucrose.

(2)   Both species display an ability to adhere to and grow upon hard surfaces such as glass, wire or teeth.

The latter property can easily be demonstrated in the laboratory, and artificially produced deposits of such bacteria have been used experimentally in an attempt to simulate dental plaque. The formation of adherent surface deposits is not confined to streptococci, and several filamentous bacteria, including some actinomyces, also share this property. The relative ability of different bacterial species to adhere to and colonise hard and soft tissue surfaces may be an important factor in the formation of dental plaque and is considered further in chapters 4 and 5.

A great deal of research has been carried out on the extracellular polysaccharides produced by oral streptococci, especially *S. mutans*, and also on the enzymes involved in their synthesis. Strains of *S. mutans* appear to produce both water-soluble and water-insoluble glucans, with varying structures (chapter 5). It has been demonstrated that mutant strains of *S. mutans* which have lost the ability to produce insoluble extracellular glucans are less cariogenic in gnotobiotic animals than the parent strain from which the mutants were derived[48]. Such evidence indicates that the production of these polymers may play an important role in the cariogenicity of some bacterial strains. Although the extracellular glucans produced by *S. sanguis* strains differ in some respects from those of *S. mutans* it is not known if this is the only reason why *S. sanguis* appears to be less cariogenic.

In order to study the relationship between bacteria and any disease, it is necessary to have suitable taxonomic criteria so that the organisms can be identified with certainty. In studies on the relationship of oral bacteria to dental caries, much reliance has often been placed on colonial morphology under particular cultural conditions. This has been especially common with investigations on the streptococcal flora, since extracellular polysaccharide-producing species such as *S. mutans*, *S. sanguis* and *S. salivarius* often produce characteristic colonies on culture plates containing sucrose. However, these species can exhibit a variety of colonial forms which may lead to mistaken identification in some cases. It is always desirable to confirm the *presumptive* identity of bacteria, based on colonial morphology, by other, more reliable tests.

In chapter 4 some of the properties of the numerous types of bacterium found in the mouth are discussed, including a description of a relatively simple scheme which can be used to identify most oral streptococci. Physiological characteristics which allow recognition of *S. mutans* include the following:

mannitol fermentation—almost invariably positive
sorbitol fermentation—usually positive
production of extracellular glucans—positive
hydrolysis of aesculin—usually positive
production of ammonia from arginine—almost invariably negative (apart from occasional serotype *b* strains)

As outlined earlier, a considerable amount of interest has been shown in the potential role of *S. mutans* in dental caries. Many investigators have studied the properties of this streptococcus, including some who have concentrated on the antigenic structure and serological divisions that can be made within the species. A Swedish worker (Bratthall) described five serological types[49], designated *a*, *b*, *c*, *d* and *e*, and the number of types has now been extended to seven[50]. A good measure of agreement has been found between those serotypes, the chemical composition of the cell walls, and genetic types based on DNA base ratios and hybridisation studies[49-53].

More detailed studies on the immunochemistry of the type-specific polysaccharide antigens of representative strains of most of the known serotypes have now been reported[54]. Such information is of value in the development of precise serological typing schemes for epidemiological investigations, since it may be that certain serotypes are more pathogenic than others in particular populations. In addition, an understanding of these antigens is essential for studies on immune responses to *S. mutans* in animals or humans.

Characteristics of other microorganisms present in the mouth, and which may be involved in dental caries, are given in the next chapter.

3.5 Caries-activity Tests

For many years, research workers and clinicians have searched for a suitable laboratory test to use as an indicator of caries activity, either in individual patients or groups of subjects. Some of the potential uses of such a test are listed below (after Socransky[55]):

(1)   Determination of the need for caries control measures.

(2)   An indicator of patient cooperation.

(3)   Aid in timing of recall appointments.

(4)   Guide to the desirability of placing extensive restorations.

(5)   Help in the determination of prognosis.

(6)   Guide to the orthodontist when undertaking appliance therapy.

In addition to these clinical applications, a reliable caries-activity test would be extremely useful in the selection of patients for studies on caries and the screening of potential cariostatic agents. A suitable test should ideally be simple, rapid and relatively cheap to perform, should correlate closely with the caries experience of the individual subject, and should be reproducible.

Numerous test systems have been described in the literature, most of which are intended to be carried out on samples of saliva. Some of the types of test are listed below:

(A)   Biochemical properties of saliva:
    pH
    buffer capacity
    uptake of oxygen
    oxidation–reduction potential
    alpha amylase activity
    urea concentration
    hyaluronidase activity

(B)   Acidogenic potential of salivary constituents:
    enamel dissolution (Fosdicke)
    pH (Dewar)
    pH and titratable acidity (Wach)
    double colour indicator (Rickles)
    colour indicator (Snyder)

(C)   Viable counts of bacteria in saliva:
    acidogenic bacteria (Davies, Slack and Tilden)
    lactobacillus count (Hadley: Rogosa)
    Streptococcus mutans

Some of these tests have shown a reasonably good correlation with dental caries, while others have shown little or none. It is arguable that since caries is initiated at the plaque enamel interface, and since it is known that the salivary microflora does not necessarily reflect the microbial population of plaque, it is unreasonable to expect such tests on saliva to bear much relationship to caries. It should also be remembered that caries is a multifactorial disease and that the composition of saliva is only one of the variables concerned.

The two tests which have been most widely used are the Snyder colorimetric test and the lactobacillus count, and these will be described briefly here. In the Snyder test, a measured volume of paraffin-stimulated saliva is inoculated into a semi-solid culture medium of low pH (approximately 5.0), which contains glucose and bromocresol green as a pH indicator. The inoculated medium is incubated for 3 days at 37°C and examined daily to see if the colour changes from green-blue to yellow-brown, indicating that acid has been produced. This gives a simple indication of the number of aciduric and acidogenic bacteria present in the saliva, and the rapidity with which colour change occurs is taken as an indication of caries activity. This test appears to correlate better with caries activity than many of the others, at least on a group basis, and fulfils the desirable criteria of speed and simplicity. However, it is not considered to give sufficiently accurate predictive results on an individual basis to be adopted as a universally applied test.

The salivary lactobacillus count, first described in 1933 by Hadley, has been widely employed by many investigators. This test is more elaborate to perform than the simple colorimetric tests, and depends upon counting the number of viable lactobacilli in 1 ml of saliva. Serial dilutions of saliva are made, and aliquots of each dilution are spread on the surface of selective media such as Tomato Juice agar or Rogosa's lactobacillus medium. Each of these media has a low pH of about 5.0 which inhibits the growth of most non-aciduric bacteria and allows colonies of lactobacilli to be recognised easily. After incubation, the numbers of presumptive lactobacillus colonies are counted and the concentration of these organisms in the original saliva sample can be calculated.

Different studies have shown reasonable correlations between lactobacillus count and past caries experience, but poor correlations have been found when the test is used to predict future caries increments. This is unfortunate, since it is the predictive ability of such tests which would be most useful. Both the Snyder test and the lactobacillus count are measuring essentially the same thing (i.e. numbers of aciduric organisms in saliva) and a good case can be made for using these tests for monitoring the progress of diet therapy, particularly when good oral hygiene procedures have been adopted[56]. Several investigators have shown that the lactobacillus counts in saliva are significantly reduced once open carious cavities have been restored and dietary carbohydrate intake is restricted.

In view of the evidence implicating *S. mutans* in the aetiology of caries, discussed earlier in this chapter, it would seem reasonable to use this organism as the basis of some caries-activity tests. A few workers have attempted to correlate salivary levels of *S. mutans* with caries activity. In two such studies, a positive correlation was found, but this was not confirmed in a more recent report[43].

However, the latter study did show significant correlations between the presence of *S. mutans* in plaque and caries experience. It would appear, at the moment, that further experimental work is required before a caries-activity test based on the presence or numbers of *S. mutans* in saliva and/or plaque can be recommended as a routine procedure.[57]

3.6 Protective Mechanisms Against Cariogenic Microorganisms

In many population groups there is a wide range of caries experience, which may be due to different levels of resistance among individuals or to difference in the cariogenic challenge. Some individuals remain free from caries throughout their lives, even though they may live in a community where the disease is prevalent. As explained in chapters 1 and 2, the reason for this apparent immunity is usually not known, although various factors such as diet, fluoride intake, enamel structure, race and poorly defined genetic factors may be important. Racial differences in caries susceptibility often appear to be related to dietary customs, since so-called 'primitive communities' living on simple, unrefined diets and enjoying a low caries rate, tend to succumb to extensive carious attacks once they have been exposed to modern 'civilised' diets. (chapter 9).

Within the oral cavity, a number of protective mechanisms exist to control the invasion by and activities of potentially harmful microorganisms. Some microorganisms are able to survive quite happily in the presence of these factors, so that a normal resident microflora becomes established in the mouth during the first few months of life. Once this has occurred, invasion and colonisation by extraneous microorganisms is usually prevented by a combination of the chemical and physical actions of saliva and competitive antagonism by the indigenous flora. Thus, it is relatively uncommon for the many organisms which are inhaled or ingested every day to become permanently established in the mouth. Similarly, it is difficult to implant bacteria experimentally into the mouths of animals or humans with a normal oral flora, unless conditions are altered in some way.

The antimicrobial factors present in oral secretions include non-specific factors and specific immunological agents. Some of these may have an influence upon the incidence of caries.

3.6.1 Non-specific antimicrobial factors

Salivary flow

It is well established that events which eliminate or markedly reduce the flow of saliva, giving rise to the condition known as xerostomia (dry mouth), predispose to the rapid development of caries. In experimental animals this effect has been demonstrated by surgical removal of the salivary glands, resulting in a marked increase in the caries scores compared to normal control animals maintained on the same diet. However, such drastic surgical measures may produce a number of different alterations in the animals, both systemic and local, so that it is difficult to establish which are the most important factors influencing the development of caries.

In humans, xerostomia may occur following irradiation of the salivary glands or surrounding tissues during the treatment of malignant tumours of the head and neck. Reduction of salivary flow is also found in several other conditions, such as obstruction of the salivary ducts, Sjörgren's syndrome, as a result of surgical treatment, or following therapy with certain drugs. There have been many well-documented cases of rampant caries occurring in later life in patients who develop xerostomia, particularly after irradiation treatment. In these cases the deterioration of oral health may be extremely rapid and dramatic. This type of caries may occur in patients with little or no previous experience of the disease, and widespread cervical lesions are characteristically produced[58, 59].

It is not known exactly which functions of saliva are most important in protection against dental caries. The physical, chemical or biological characteristics may be significant in this respect, and numerous workers have attempted to correlate one or other of the known properties of saliva with caries experience. The physical washing and irrigation effects appear to be necessary for maintenance of a clean mouth and are most important in mastication and swallowing. The buffering effects of saliva (chapter 5), based mainly on bicarbonate—carbonic acid and phosphate buffer systems, are likely to be a major importance in relation to caries. Attempts have been made to establish a relationship between caries incidence and a variety of salivary components, including urea, ammonia, calcium, phosphate and amylase, but so far no clearly significant associations have been found.

All studies on the relationship of salivary factors to dental disease are frustrated by the practical problems involved in collection and analysis of specimens. Flow rates vary in different individuals, in different glands and in response to different stimuli, and the chemical composition of the saliva may be altered by such variations. Thus, some of the contradictory results on salivary components in the literature may be due to variations in flow rate and methods of collection of saliva.

Chemical factors

Several non-immunological, antibacterial factors have been described in oral secretions, and although the biological significance of these is not fully understood, they may play some part in protection of the oral tissues.

Lysozyme is a hydrolytic enzyme which cleaves the linkage between N-acetylglucosamine and N-acetylmuramic acid. Such linkages occur in the cell wall mucopeptide (peptidoglycan) of bacteria. Some species of bacteria, such as *Micrococcus lysodeikticus*, are extremely sensitive to lysis by this enzyme. Other organisms are less sensitive or even completely resistant to its action. In some situations, lysozyme may be involved in antibody-complement mediated lysis of bacteria. Lysozyme is widely distributed, being found in saliva, nasal secretions, tears, tissue and body fluids, and in egg whites. Microorganisms which colonise the mouth are generally resistant to the action of lysozyme, and so it seems unlikely that this enzyme plays a significant role in protection against dental caries. However, it may be a useful factor in preventing colonisation of the mouth by extraneous microbes.

Lactoperoxidase is a haemoprotein enzyme, found in high concentration in colostrum, which also occurs in saliva. It has an antibacterial effect against certain bacteria which do not produce catalase, including lactobacilli and streptococci. The enzyme requires thiocyanate as a cofactor and reacts with hydrogen peroxide, which accumulates in susceptible microorganisms. In some of the literature, the lactoperoxidase—thiocyanate system has been referred to as the 'anti-lactobacillus factor'[60]. The precise role, if any, of lactoperoxidase in protection against dental caries has not been conclusively established as yet, although interest in this possibility has been re-stimulated by recent studies in the Netherlands[61].

There are known to be bacterial agglutinating factors in saliva which show some specificity towards particular species (such as *Streptococcus mutans*) and serotypes. These agglutinins appear to be glycoproteins and are not apparently immunoglobulins[62, 63]. Whether these salivary components have a protective function or, conversly, actually contribute towards colonisation of the tooth and accumulation of plaque, is not fully understood at present.

In addition to the soluble fractions of saliva, cellular elements can also be demonstrated. Leucocytes are derived either from the gingival crevice via the crevicular fluid or from the mucous membrane surfaces of the mouth. There is no clear evidence to show that these cells play a significant part in the defence mechanisms of the mouth against dental caries. More detailed reviews of the protective role of saliva can be found in the list of recommended Further Reading at the end of this chapter.

3.6.2 Immunological mechanisms in the mouth

It has sometimes been argued that the enamel surface of the tooth is effectively 'outside' the tissues of the body and that, consequently, immunological or other defence mechanisms would be unlikely to play a role in protection against caries. However, recent evidence indicates that this view may not be entirely correct and several mechanisms of possible significance have been described. During the past few years a great deal of research has been carried out on immunological aspects of dental diseases, and much of this work has been reviewed recently elsewhere[64, 65].

There are two routes by which either anti-bodies or immunologically active cells might reach the plaque—tooth surface interface; one is the saliva and the other via the crevicular fluid. Theoretically, both humoral (antibody-mediated) or cell-mediated immune responses could be involved, and these can be either local or systemic. Until now, most of the reported studies on the immunology of caries have been confined to antibody responses rather than cell-mediated immunity.

Salivary antibodies

It has been known for several years that there is a special secretory-immunological system, distinct from systemic responses, which operates locally as part of the defensive mechanisms of mucous membranes[66]. Immunoglobulin A(IgA), which is found in relatively low proportions in serum, is the predominant class of antibody found in fluids such as saliva, tears, colostrum, nasal and gastrointestinal secretions. Within the salivary glands the IgA molecules are secreted by plasma cells, while another protein, referred to as 'secretory component', is produced in the epithelial cells lining the ducts. Some studies on the total concentration of IgA in saliva in subjects with varying dental caries experience have indicated that there might be an inverse relationship between IgA level and DMF score[67,68]. This contrasts with the situation in periodontal disease, where increasing amounts of inflammation and tissue destruction appear to be accompanied by higher salivary IgA levels[69,70]. However, the observations on a negative correlation between caries experience and salivary IgA levels have not been confirmed by all investigators. The differences between the results reported from different laboratories may be partly due to variations in the techniques used for collection and handling of saliva specimens. At high salivary flow rates, a lower concentration of IgA is found than at low flow rates[71,72].

In one recent investigation, both the concentration of IgA and the flow rate were estimated in a number of subjects, so that a 'parotid IgA secretion rate' could be calculated[73]. In this case a significant negative correlation was found between the DMF index and IgA secretion rate, whereas no such correlation could be established from the same data when IgA concentrations alone were taken into account. The authors of this report concluded that there is probably a true association between caries susceptibility and the output of parotid IgA. However, since the opposite trend was observed when IgA secretion rates were plotted against the Periodontal Index, it seems likely these relationships will be obscured when both diseases are present concurrently.

There is only a limited amount of information available at present concerning the presence of specific antibody activity in saliva and its role in caries. In one study, antibodies were found in whole saliva against a crude glucosyltransferase enzyme* (GTF) preparation from a strain of *Streptococcus mutans*[74]. A positive correlation was observed between the antibody-titred measure and the DMF of subjects in whom no active caries could be detected. Thus it could be postulated that the salivary antibody titre may reflect the whole-life caries experience of the individual and not have a protective function. On the other hand, significantly lower salivary antibody titres against GTF were recorded in subjects who had untreated carious lesions, suggesting that there may be a fall in titre associated with the onset of caries.

Further studies are required before the significance of salivary antibodies in the prevention of caries can be fully assessed. Some new light on this problem is likely to be shed by the studies on immunisation against caries in experimental animals which are currently being undertaken in several laboratories.

Serum antibodies

A number of investigators have demonstrated the presence of circulating antibodies in the blood against a variety of different oral microorganisms. Interpretation of such data is difficult, since antigenically related organisms may be present in the intestinal tract or elswhere in the body. Serological cross-reactions between different bacteria are common, particularly with some widely distributed antigenic determinants such as those present in cell wall or membrane teichoic acids[75,76].

Differences in serum antibody titres to cell wall preparations and crude ultrasonicates of *Streptococcus mutans* have been demonstrated between subjects with high and low caries experience[77-79]. Patients with higher DMF scores were found to have lower antibody titres than those with a lower DMF. A significant negative correlation was also found between serum haemagglutination titres of IgM and IgA antibody classes to crude GTF enzyme and the DMF caries score[74]. There appears to be no obviously consistent relationship between the levels of serum and salivary antibodies in these studies.

The investigations referred to in this section have been confined mainly to observations made on relatively small groups of human subjects. The present wave of experiments on prevention of dental caries by immunisation, described later in chapter 11, should help to establish the mechanisms by which immunological protection may be afforded and provide additional information on the relative importance of systemic and local salivary responses. The possible place of cell-mediated immune responses in dental caries remains to be examined.

Possible mechanisms by which antibodies may operate to inhibit caries include:

(1) Prevention of adherence of bacteria to the tooth surface and/or plaque.

(2) Inhibition of specific enzymes (such as the glucosyltransferases which are responsible for the synthesis of extracellular polysaccharides from sucrose).

(3) Inactivation of metabolism of bacteria (such as fermentation of carbohydrates).

(4) Inhibition of growth or killing of bacteria.

(5) Opsonisation of bacteria.

---

*   This enzyme is required for synthesis of extracellular polysaccharide and is discussed in detail in chapter 5.

An immunologically mediated bacteriocidal effect is unlikely to occur, since this requires the availability of complement which is not present in saliva, although it is found in crevicular fluid. There is little evidence to indicate that the presence of antibodies to oral bacteria markedly affects their ability to produce acid[80,81].

An interesting suggestion has been made that caries of smooth surfaces may be affected predominantly by serum antibodies, which are present in crevicular fluid, while salivary antibodies may exert their influence mainly on pit and fissure caries[65]. This hypothesis remains to be tested.

Further reading

Bibby, B. G. and Shern, R. J. (Eds) (1978). *Methods of Caries Prediction*. A Special Supplement of Microbiology Abstracts, Information Retrieval Inc., Washington D.C. and London

Newbrun, E. (1978). *Cariology*. Williams and Wilkins Co., Baltimore

Kleinberg, I., Ellison, S. A. and Mandel, I. D. (Eds) (1979). *Saliva and Dental Caries*. A Special Supplement of Microbiology Abstracts, Information Retrieval Inc., New York and London

Stiles, H. M., Loesche, W. J. and O'Brien, T. C. (1976). *Microbial Aspects of Dental Caries*. A Special Supplement of Microbiology Abstracts, Information Retrieval Inc., Washington D. C. and London

References

1. Miller, W. D. (1890). *The Micro-organisms of the Human Mouth*, S. S. White Dental Manufacturing Co., Philadelphia. Republished, K. König (Ed.), by S. Karger, Basel, 1973

2. Schroeder, H. E. and De Boever, J. (1970). The structure of microbial dental plaque, in *Dental Plaque* (Ed. McHugh, W. D.), E. and S. Livingstone, Edinburgh and London, pp. 49–75

3. Silverstone, L. M. (1968). The surface zone in caries and in caries-like lesions produced *in vitro*. *British Dental Journal*, **125**, 145–157

4. Hardie, J. M., Silverstone, L. M. and Bowden, G. H. (1971). Modification of acid attack on enamel surfaces *in vitro*, by aggregations of bacteria. *Caries Research*, **5**, 290–304

5. Pigman, W, Elliot, H. C. and Laffre, R. O. (1952). An artificial mouth for caries research. *Journal of Dental Research*, **31**, 627–33

6. Pigman, W. (1968). *In vitro* simulation of dental caries using bacteria, in *Art and Science of Dental Caries Research* (Edited Harris, R. S.), Academic Press, New York and London, pp. 319–30

7. Sidaway, D. A. (1970). The bacterial composition of natural plaque and the *in vitro* production of artificial plaque, in *Dental Plaque* (Ed. McHugh, W. D.), E. and S. Livingstone, Edinburgh and London

8. Coulter, W. A. and Russell, C. (1976). pH and Eh in single and mixed culture bacterial plaque in an artificial mouth. *Journal of Applied Bacteriology*, **40**, 73–87

9. Ellwood, D. C., Hunter, J. R. and Longyear, V. M. C. (1974). Growth of *Streptococcus mutans* in a chemostat. *Archives of Oral Biology*, **19**, 659–64

10. McClure, F. J. and Hewitt, W. L. (1946). Relation of penicillin to induced rat dental caries and oral *Lactobacillus acidophilus Journal of Dental Research*, **25**, 441–3

11. Hill, T. J. Sims, J and Newman, M. (1953). The effect of penicillin dentifrice on the control of dental caries. *Journal of Dental Research*, **32**, 448–52

12. Zander, H. A. (1950). The effect of pencillin dentifrice on caries incidence in school children. *Journal of the American Dental Association*, **40**, 569–74

13. Littleton, N. W. and White, C. L. (1964). Dental findings from a preliminary study of

children receiving extended antibiotic therapy. *Journal of the American Dental Association*, **68**, 520–5

14. Handleman, S. L., Mills, J. R. and Hawes, R. R. (1966). Caries incidence in subjects receiving long term antibiotic therapy. *Journal of Oral Therapeutics and Pharmacology*, **2**, 338–45

15. Bibby, B. G. (1970). Antibiotics and dental caries, in *Dietary Chemicals vs. Dental Caries*, Advances in Chemistry Series 94 (Ed. Gould, R. F.), American Chemical Society, Washington, DC

16. Loesche, W. J. (1976). Chemotherapy of dental plaque infections. *Oral Sciences Reviews*, **9**, 65–107

17. Orland, F. J., Blayney, J. R., Harrison, R. W., Reyniers, J. A., Trexler, P. C., Gordon, H. A., Wagner, M. and Luckey, T. D. (1954). Use of germ-free animal technique in the study of experimental dental caries. 1. Basic observations on rats reared free of all microorganisms. *Journal of Dental Research*, **33**, 147–74

18. Fitzgerald, R. J. and Keyes, P. H. (1960). Demonstration of the etiologic role of streptococci in experimental caries in the hamster. *Journal of the American Dental Association*, **61**, 9–19

19. Fitzgerald, R. J., Jordan, H. V. and Stanley, H. R. (1960). Experimental caries and gingival pathologic changes in the gnotobiotics rat. *Journal of Dental Research*, **39**, 923–35

20. Keyes, P. H. (1960). The infections and transmissible nature of experimental dental caries—findings and implications. *Archives of Oral Biology*, **1**, 304–20

21. Zinner, D. D., Jablon, J. M., Aran, A. P. and Saslaw, M. S. (1966). Comparative pathogenicity of streptococci of human origin in hamster caries. *Archives of Oral Biology*, **11**, 1419–20

22. Gibbons, R. J., Berman, K. S., Knoettner, P. and Kapsimalis, B. (1966). Dental caries and alveolar bone loss in gnotobiotic rats infected with capsule-forming streptococci of human origin. *Archives of Oral Biology*, **11**, 549–60

23. Edwardsson, S. (1968). Characteristics of caries-inducing human streptococci resembling *Streptococcus mutans*. *Archives of Oral Biology*, **13**, 637–46

24. Krasse, B. (1966). Human streptococci and experimental caries in hamsters. *Archives of Oral Biology*, **11**, 429–36

25. Guggenheim, B. (1968). Streptococci of dental plaques. *Caries Research*, **2**, 147–63

26. Fitzgerald, R. J. (1968). Dental caries research in gnotobiotic animals. *Caries Research*, **2**, 139–46

27. Konig, K. G. (1968). Design of animal experiments in caries research, in *Art and Science of Dental caries Research* (Ed. Harris, R. S.), Academic Press, New York and London

28. Krasse, B. and Carlsson, J. (1970). Various types of streptococci and experimental caries in hamsters. *Archives of Oral Biology*, **15**, 25–32

29. Bowen, W. H. (1968). Dental caries in monkeys. *Advances in Oral Biology*, **3**, 185–216

30. Lehner, T., Challacombe, S. J. and Caldwell, J (1975). An experimental model for immunological studies of dental caries in the Rhesus monkey. *Archives of Oral Biology*, **20**, 299–304

31. Mikx, F. H. M., Hoeven, J. S. van der., Konig, K. G., Plasschaert, A. J. M. and Guggenheim, B. (1972). Establishment of defined microbial ecosystems in germfree rats. 1. Effect of the interaction of *Streptococcus mutans* or *Streptococcus sanguis* with *Veillonella alcalescens* on plaque formation and caries activity. *Caries Research*, **6**, 211–21

32. Fitzgerald, R. J., Jordan, H. V. and Archard, H. O. (1966). Dental caries in gnotobiotic rats infected with a variety of *Lactobacillus acidophilus*. *Archives of Oral Biology*, **11**, 473–76

33. Fillery, E. D., Bowden, G. H. and Hardie, J. M. (1978). A comparison of strains of

bacteria designated *Actinomyces viscosus* and *Actinomyces naeslundii*. *Caries Research*, **12**, 299–312

34. Krasse, B., Jordan, H. V., Edwardsson, S., Svensson, I. and Trell, L. (1968). The occurrence of certain 'caries-inducing' streptococci in human dental plaque material. *Archives of Oral Biology*, **13**, 911–18

35. Littleton, N. W., Kakehashi, S. and Fitzgerald, R. J. (1970). Recovery of specific 'caries-inducing' streptococci from carious lesions in the teeth of children. *Archives of Oral Biology*, **15**, 461–3

36. Shklair, I. L., Keene, H. J. and Simons, L. G. (1972). Distribution and frequency of *Streptococcus mutans* in caries-active individuals. *Journal of Dental Research*, **51**, 882

37. Rogers, A. H. (1973). The ecology of *Streptococcus mutans* in carious lesions and on caries-free surfaces of the same tooth. *Australian Dental Journal*, **18**, 226–8

38. Hoerman, K. C., Keene, H. J., Shklair, I. L. and Burmeister, J. A. (1972). The association of *Streptococcus mutans* with early carious lesions in human teeth. *Journal of the American Dental Association*, **85**, 1349–52

39. Shklair, I. L., Keene, H. J. and Cullen, P. (1974). The distribution of *Streptococcus mutans* on the teeth of two groups of naval recruits. *Archives of Oral Biology*, **19**, 199–202

40 Keene, H. J. and Shklair, I. L. (1974). Relationship of *Streptococcus mutans* carrier status to the development of carious lesions in initially caries free recruits. *Journal of Dental Research*, **53**, 1295

41. Ikeda, T., Sandham, H. J. and Bradley, E. L. Jr. (1973). Changes in *Streptococcus mutans* and lactobacilli in plaque in relation to the initiation of dental caries in Negro children. *Archives of Oral Biology*, **18**, 555–66

42. Mikkelsen, L. and Poulsen, S. (1976). Microbiological studies on plaque in relation to development of dental caries in

man. *Caries Research*, **10**, 178–88

43. Loesche, W. J., Rowan, J., Straffon, L. H. and Loos, P. J. (1975). Association of *Streptococcus mutans* with human dental decay. *Infection and Immunity*, **11**, 1252–60

44. Sumney, D. L. and Jordan, H. V. (1974). Characterization of bacteria isolated from human root surface carious lesion. *Journal of Dental Research*, **53**, 343–51

45. Syed, S. A., Loesche, W. J., Pape, H. L., Jr., and Grenier, E. (1975). Predominant cultivable flora isolated from human root surface caries plaque. *Infection and Immunity*, **11**, 727–31

46. Yamada, T. and Carlsson, J. (1975). Regulation of lactate dehydrogenase and change of fermentation products in streptococci. *Journal of Bacteriology*, **124**, 55–61

47. Geddes, D. A. M. (1975). Acids produced by human dental plaque metabolism *in situ*. *Caries Research*, **9**, 98–109

48. De Stoppelaar, J. D., Konig, K. G., Plasschaert, A. J. M. and van der Hoeven, J. S. (1971). Decreased cariogenicity of a mutant of *Streptococcus mutans*. *Archives of Oral Biology*, **16**, 971–5

49. Bratthall, D. (1970). Demonstration of five serological groups of streptococcal strains resembling *Streptococcus mutans*. *Odontologisk Revy.*, **21**, 143–52

50. Perch, B., Kjems, E. Ravn, T. (1974). Biochemical and serological properties of *Streptococcus mutans* from various human and animal sources. *Acta Pathologica et Microbiologica Scandinavica, Section B*, **82**, 357–70

51. Coykendall, A. L. (1970). Base composition of deoxyribonucleic acid isolated from cariogenic streptococci. *Archives of Oral Biology*, **15**, 365–68

52. Coykendall, A. L. (1974). Four types of *Streptococcus mutans* based on their genetic, antigenic and biochemical characteristics. *Journal of General Microbiology*, **83**, 327–38

53. Hardie, J. M. and Bowden, G. H. (1974).

Cell wall and serological studies on *Streptococcus mutans. Caries Research*, **8**, 301–16

54. Linzer, R. (1976). Serotype polysaccharide antigens of *Streptococcus mutans*: composition and serological cross-reactions, in *Immunologic Aspects of Dental Caries* (Eds. Bowen, W. H., Genco, R. J. and O'Brian, T. C.), Information Retrieval Inc., Washington, DC and London

55. Socransky, S. S. (1968). Caries susceptibility tests. *Annals of the New York Academy of Sciences*, **153**, 137–46

56. Sims, W. (1970). The interpretation and use of Synder tests and lactobacillus counts. *Journal of the American Dental Association*, **80**, 1315–19

57. Ellen, R. P. (1976). Microbiological assays for dental caries and periodontal disease susceptibility. *Oral Sciences Review*, **8**, 3–23

58. Llory, H., Dammron, A. and Frank, R. M. (1971). Changes in the oral flora following bucco-pharyngeal radiotherapy. *Archives of Oral Biology*, **16**, 617–30

59. Brown, L. R. Dreizen, S., Handler, S. and Johnston, D. A. (1975). Effect of radiation-induced xerostamia on human oral micro flora. *Journal of Dental Research*, **54**, 740–50

60. Dogon, I. L., Kerr, A. C. and Amdur, B. H. (1962). Characterization of an antibacterial factor in human parotid secretions, active against *Lactobacillus casei. Archives of Oral Biology*, **7**, 81–90

61. Hoogendoorn, H (1974). The effect of lactoperoxidase–thiocyanate–hydrogen peroxide on the metabolism of cariogenic microorganisms in vitro and in the oral cavity. *Doctoral Thesis*, Univ. of Delft

62. Gibbons, R. J. and Spinnell, D. M. (1970). Salivary induced aggregation of plaque bacteria, in *Dental Plaque* (Ed. McHugh, W. D.), E. S. Livingstone, Edinburgh and London, pp. 207–16

63. Magnusson, I., Ericson, Th. and Pruitt, K. (1976). Effect of salivary agglutinins on bacterial colonization of tooth surfaces. *Caries Research*, **10**, 113–22

64. Mergenhagen, S. E. and Scherp, H. W. (Eds) (1973). *Comparative Immunology of the Oral Cavity*, DHEW Publications No. (NIH) 73–438, US Department of Health, Education and Welfare, National Institutes of Health, Bethesda, Maryland

65. Lehner, T. (1975). Immunological aspects of dental caries and periodontal disease. *British Medical Bulletin*, **31**, 125–30

66. Brandtzaeg, P. (1974). Immunoglobulin systems of oral mucosa and saliva, in *The Oral Mucosa in Health and Disease* (Ed. Dolby, A. E.), Blackwell Scientific Publications, Oxford

67. Lehner, T., Cardwell, J. D. and Clarry, E. D. (1967). Immunoglobulins in saliva and serum in dental caries. *Lancet*, **1**, 1294–7

68. Zengo, A. N., Mandel, I. D., Goldman, R. and Khurana, H. S. (1971). Salivary studies in human caries resistance. *Archives of Oral Biology*, **16**, 557–60

69. Brandtzaeg, P., Fjellanger, I. and Gjeruldsen, S. T. (1970). Human secretory immunoglobulins—I. Salivary secretions from individuals with normal or low levels of serum immunoglobulins. *Scandinavian Journal of Haematology,* Supplement 12

70. Lindstrom, F. D. and Folk, L. E. A. (1973). Salivary IgA in periodontal disease. *Acta Odontologica Scandinavica*, **31**, 31–4

71. Mandel, I. D. and Khurana, H. S. (1969). The relation of human salivary γ A globulin and albumin to flow rate. *Archives of Oral Biology*, **14**, 1433–5

72. Brandtzaeg, P. (1971). Human secretory immunoglobulins VII: Concentration of parotid IgA and other secretory proteins in relation to the rate of flow and duration of secretory stimulus. *Archives of Oral Biology*, **16**, 1295–1310

73. Orstavik, D. and Brandtzaeg, P. (1975). Secretion of parotid IgA in relation to gingival inflammation and dental caries experience in man. *Archives of Oral Biology*, **20**, 701–4

74. Challacombe, S. J., Guggenheim, B. and Lehner, T. (1973). Antibodies to an extract of *Streptococcus mutans*, containing glucosyltransferase activity, related to dental caries in man. *Archives of Oral Biology*, **18**, 657–68
75. Hardie, J. M. and Bowden, G. H. (1976). Some serological cross-reactions between *Streptococcus mutans*, *Streptococcus sanguis* and other dental plaque streptococci. *Journal of Dental Research*, **55**, c50–c58
76. Knox, K. W. and Wicken, A. J. (1973). Immunological properties of teichoic acids. *Bacteriological Reviews*, **37**, 215–57
77. Kennedy, A. E., Shklair, I. L., Hayashi, J. A. and Bahu, A. N. (1968). Antibodies to cariogenic streptococci in humans. *Archives of Oral Biology*, **13**, 1275–8
78. Lehner, T., Wilton, J. M. A. and Ward, R. G. (1970). Serum antibodies in dental caries in man. *Archives of Oral Biology*, **15**, 481–90
79. Challacombe, S. J. (1974). Serum complement–fixing antibodies in human dental caries. *Caries Research*, **8**, 84–95
80. Sims, W. (1970). The concept of immunity in dental caries 1. General considerations. *Oral Surgery, Oral Medicine, Oral Pathology*, **30**, 670–7
81. Sims, W. (1972). The concept of immunity in dental caries II. Specific immune responses. *Oral Surgery, Oral Medicine, Oral Pathology*, **34**, 69–86
82. Bowden, G. H. Hardie, J. M., McKee, A. S., Marsh, P. D., Fillery, E. D. and Slack, G. L. (1976). The microflora associated with developing carious lesions of the distal surfaces of the upper first premolars in 13–14 year old children. *Microbial Aspects of Dental Caries*, Stiles, H. M., Loesche, W. J. and O'Brien, T. C. (Eds.) Special supplement of Microbiology Abstracts vol. 1, 223–41, Information Retrieval Inc., Washington, DC and London
83. Hardie, J. M., Thomson, P. L., South, R. J., Marsh, P. D., Bowden, G. H., McKee, A. S., Fillery, E. D. and Slack, G. L. (1977). A longitudinal epidemiological study on dental plaque and the development of caries – interim results after two years. *Journal of Dental Research* **56**, c90–c98.
84. Drucker, D. B. and Green, R. M. (1978). The relative cariogenicities of *Streptococcus milleri* and other viridans group streptococci in gnotobiotic hooded rats. *Archives of Oral Biology*, **23**, 183–7
85. Drucker, D. B. and Green, R. M. (1979). Potential of streptococci for inducing dental caries in gnotobiotic rats, in *Pathogenic Streptococci* (Ed. Parker, M. T.), Reed Books Ltd, Surrey, pp. 206–7

Chapter 4

The Formation, Structure and Microbial Composition of Dental Plaque

4.1 Introduction and Definition

As explained in chapter 1, dental plaque is the name given to the aggregations of bacteria and their products which accumulate on the tooth surface. The term 'gelatinous microbial plaque' was first employed by Black in 1898 to describe the felt-like masses which he and several other early investigators observed on the teeth. Reference to much of the older literature, together with detailed summaries of more recent ideas and knowledge on dental plaque, can be found in the book edited by McHugh[1]. No attempt will be made to review in detail the many original papers on this topic which have been published since the late nineteenth century, but it is the aim of this chapter to give an account of our current understanding of the development, structure and microbial composition of human dental plaque.

Plaque collects rapidly in the mouth, although the actual rate of formation varies from one individual to another. If the deposit is not removed from the tooth surface within a few hours, it builds up into a thick, adherent layer which cannot easily be removed by mouthrinsing or with a jet of water from a syringe. More loosely-adherent, creamy-white material, which may be removed with a stream of water, may also be seen to collect on the teeth, particularly in people with poor oral hygiene.

This material often referred to as 'materia alba' consists of the most superficial layers of dental plaque (i.e. mainly bacteria), together with food and cellular debris derived from leucocytes and desquamated epithelial cells. Since the distinction between 'plaque-proper' and materia alba is difficult to define precisely, it is simpler to confine clinical descriptions of accumulated deposits on the teeth to the terms supragingival and subgingival dental plaque. Such plaque deposits may be of varying thickness and extent.

Dental plaque which has been left undisturbed for a prolonged period (i.e. weeks or months) may become calcified and is then referred to as *calculus* (or tartar). Calculus varies in its distri-
bution, quantity and appearance in different individuals and different parts of the mouth, but is always preceded by plaque accumulation. Particularly heavy calculus deposition often occurs near to the openings of the major salivary glands, so that the lingual surfaces of the lower incisors and the buccal aspects of the maxillary molars may be especially affected. Bacterial plaque continues to form on the surface and around the periphery of calculus deposits, where it may be protected from attempts at oral hygiene.

4.2 Clinical Appearance and Distribution of Dental Plaque

When plaque accumulates on the crowns of the teeth, the natural, smooth, shiny appearance of the enamel is lost and a dull, matt effect is produced. As the plaque builds up, the mass of bacteria becomes more readily visible to the naked eye. The presence and distribution of plaque in the mouth can be visualised most clearly by the use of dyes or disclosing solutions (such as erythrocin) which stain the deposits. Several different disclosing preparations are commercially available in solution or tablet form for this purpose*. The technique of disclosing plaque with coloured dyes has been used for research purposes, but is also particularly valuable for demonstrating plaque deposits to patients as an aid to oral hygiene, and can be used as a check on toothbrushing efficiency, either at home or in the dental surgery.

Plaque normally collects most rapidly and extensively in inaccessible areas of the mouth, such as interproximally and in the pits and fissures. These areas have often in the past been called 'stagnation areas', but nowadays the alternative term 'uncleanable areas' is preferred by some clinicians. In the mouth of people with poor oral hygiene, dental plaque may accumulate extensively over all the surfaces of the teeth.

Dental plaque which accumulates on the tooth

* See also chapter 11

above the level of the gingival margin is referred to as supragingival plaque, while that found below this level is called subgingival plaque. The extent of subgingival deposits, which frequently become calcified, depends upon the depth of the gingival crevice or periodontal pocket. Some investigators have designated the plaque deposits immediately adjacent to the gingival margin as 'gingival plaque'. In this situation, which is a narrow, transitional zone between clearly supra- and subgingival plaque, epithelial cells and leucocytes may be particularly noticeable in microscopic preparations.

4.3   Clinical Measurements of Plaque and Oral Debris

For clinical purposes, and especially for epidemiological surveys or clinical trials, it is useful to have a method of quantifying or scoring the amount of plaque present in the mouth. Several different systems have been described for this purpose and the choice of the most suitable scheme depends upon the particular requirements of the user. For epidemiological studies it is important that the debris scoring system should be reproducible, both by the same examiner on different occasions and between examiners. A full description of some of the more commonly used indices can be found in the references given at the end of this chapter[2-7].

The simplest estimates are those in which an arbitrary classification of oral cleanliness is used, the condition being described subjectively as good, fair or poor. The whole mouth may be assessed in this way to give an overall impression, or different segments of the dentition may be scored separately. Several plaque or oral cleanliness indices rely on partial recording methods, in which only a few selected teeth are examined, and the observations on those areas are extrapolated to produce a score for the whole mouth. Similar sampling techniques are also used on occasions for estimating the amount of periodontal disease present.

A commonly used scheme is the Oral Hygiene Index of Greene and Vermillion[4]. In this system the upper and lower arches are divided into 12 areas (right, left, anterior, buccal and lingual), each of which is assessed separately for the presence of debris (plaque, stain and food debris) and calculus. The areas are scored for debris as follows:

0 — No debris or stain present.
1 — Soft debris covering not more than one-third of the tooth surface, or the presence of extrinsic stains without other debris, regardless of surface area covered.
2 — Soft debris covering more than one-third, but not more than two-thirds, of the exposed tooth surface.
3 — Soft debris covering more than two-thirds of the exposed tooth surface.

A similar scale is used for scoring calculus deposits. The overall Oral Hygiene Index is calculated by adding the individual scores recorded and dividing by the number of segments examined. Debris and calculus scores are commonly pooled, although they may also be reported separately.

Another commonly used scoring system is the Plaque Index of Loe[5]. According to this index, mesial, distal, buccal and lingual aspects of each tooth are given a score from 0 to 3, depending upon the thickness of the plaque present rather than the area of tooth covered. In epidemiological surveys, this Plaque Index (PI) is often used together with the Gingival Index (GI) of Loe and Silness[6].

The choice of appropriate indices for scoring dental plaque, periodontal disease and caries depends upon several factors, including the purpose of the investigation, the number of subjects to be examined and the conditions under which examinations are to be carried out[7]. No single index is universally suitable for all epidemiological surveys and clinical trials.

4.4   Factors Which Affect Plaque Formation

The rate of formation of dental plaque varies in different individuals, as does its qualitative and quantitative microbial composition. Some of the factors which may influence the amount and type of plaque which develops are listed in table 4.1.

Table 4.1   (after Egelberg[8])

Physical Environment	Availability of nutrients
Anatomy and position of the tooth	Saliva
Anatomy of surrounding tissues	Gingival fluid
	Remnants of epithelial cells and leucocytes
Structure of the tooth surface	Diet
Friction from diet and masticatory movements	
Oral hygiene procedures	
Presence of restorations or appliances	

In addition to the normal anatomical factors, such as the differences in habitat between pits and fissures, smooth and approximal surfaces, malocclusions may predispose areas of the mouth to excessive plaque accumulation. In particular, overcrowding of teeth may give rise to areas which are especially difficult to clean adequately. Similarly, orthodontic or prosthetic appliances may interfere with oral hygiene procedures and encourage plaque formation. Patients wearing appliances should be instructed carefully in the application of suitable cleaning methods and checked regularly to ensure that plaque control is adequate.

Restorations with overhanging edges or rough surfaces, especially large approximal fillings, crowns or bridges, are potential traps which may enhance plaque formation. Adequate cleaning of the edges of such restoration is impossible for the patient until overhangs and other faults are corrected.

From these examples it can be seen that many routine dental treatment procedures, if not carried out to a high standard, may predispose to accumulation of dental plaque or render the mouth increasingly difficult to clean. Clinicians

need to be aware of this damaging potential of their treatments and take the necessary steps to avoid subsequent problems arising from inadequate plaque control.

Roughness of a enamel surface and small developmental or acquired surface defects, such as microscopic pits or cracks, are likely to encourage the accumulation of plaque bacteria. Such defects are completely inaccessible to normal toothcleaning methods and could provide a ready source of organisms to recolonise an otherwise clean surface. Unfortunately, there is little that can be done to counteract these factors, and in most cases their presence would be undetected anyway.

Theoretically, the amount of plaque which collects on the teeth may be controlled to some extent by the degree of friction produced during mastication. Although this may have been an important factor in earlier generations, and may still play some role in primitive peoples, the nature of modern civilized diets makes this of dubious significance. Inspection of early skulls shows considerably more evidence of attrition of the teeth, indicating a diet which contained large amounts of roughage. Modern diets do not normally contain much in the way of fibrous components, and most of our food is eaten cooked rather than raw. The few published studies on the so-called 'detergent effect' of raw apples, carrots or similar foods have not shown a marked reduction in plaque levels, caries or gingivitis scores[9, 10].

Oral hygiene, including toothbrushing and inter-dental cleaning aids, can reduce the level of plaque virtually to zero under ideal conditions. As will be discussed later, in chapter 11, complete elimination of plaque deposits can control the incidence of caries and periodontal disease. However, it is difficult for most people to attain such excellent oral hygiene, either for physical reasons or because they are insufficiently motivated to spend the requisite time and effort. Thus, in most individuals imperfect tooth cleaning procedures are used which may modify the formation of plaque. Commonly this will lead to large accumulations of well-established, older plaque in those areas which are difficult to clean, whereas the more accessible sites will be reforming plaque after each toothbrushing. In this way, the mouth will usually contain plaques at several different stages of development at any given time.

The contribution made to the nutrition of oral bacteria by saliva, gingival fluid and cell remnants is difficult to evaluate, and there is little information available on these aspects of oral ecology. However, the availability of gingival crevice exudate may explain, at least in part, the differences between the microbial flora of the gingival area and other sites in the mouth[11]. Subgingival plaque does seem to form more rapidly in individuals with gingivitis, and hence an increased flow of crevicular exudate.

Without doubt, a major factor influencing plaque formation is the composition of the diet, although some plaque is still formed in animals fed by a stomach tube, thus bypassing the mouth[12]. Studies on early plaque formation in humans under different dietary regimes have been reported[13]. Subjects consuming a mixed protein – fat diet, a glucose diet or a fructose diet showed the teeth to be covered with pellicle at 1 day, with a few discrete colonies of bacterial growth. After 2 days the buccal surfaces were covered with a thin, relatively amorphous, plaque layer which increased in thickness by the third day. The plaque appeared to be thicker following periods of high glucose intake compared to that formed during protein – fat diet or fructose diet periods. However, a markedly different appearance was observed during experimental periods of high sucrose intake. In this case, no pellicle was seen after 1 or 2 days. Individual bacterial colonies were seen to develop, primarily localised to cracks and furrows in the enamel surface. These colonies of plaque growth, which were larger than those observed during the other (non-sucrose) dietary periods, were considered to resemble the appearance of some polysaccharide-producing streptococci when grown on sucrose-containing culture media in the laboratory.

These studies on the differences between early plaque formed on the tooth in vivo during different dietary periods were based on visual observations using a stereomicroscope. Other studies, using cultural techniques, have shown that the relative numbers of polysaccharide-producing streptococci in plaque increase during periods of high sucrose intake. Similarly, in animals, the establishment of species such as *Streptococcus mutans* may be facilitated by high sucrose intakes. Thus, from both animal and human experiments it has been demonstrated that dietary factors may influence the formation of dental plaque and that sucrose may favour the growth of certain species.

A recently reported study on the effect of diet on the development of human dental plaque showed that a high sucrose intake had no demonstrable effect on the total amount of plaque which accumulated during the 4- and 12-day study periods employed. However, during the sucrose-rich dietary regime the total microbial density and the numbers of *Streptococcus mutans* and lactobacilli increased[14].

4.5 Formation and Development of Dental Plaque

On eruption into the oral cavity, the teeth are initially covered with developmental, primary enamel cuticle and cellular components of the reduced enamel epithelium—Nasmyth's membrane. These constitute a $1-5\,\mu$m thick layer which is soon lost and probably contributes little to the surface integuments of the tooth after the first few days following eruption. The acquired, post-eruptive surface deposits include various structureless organic layers, referred to as cuticle or pellicle, in addition to dental plaque.

4.5.1 Theoretical considerations and mechanisms of plaque formation

Several different mechanisms are thought to play a significant part in the initial colonisation of tooth surfaces by bacteria and their subsequent development into dental plaque[15]. These include:

(1) Adherence of bacteria to pellicle and/or exposed enamel surface.

(2) Adhesion between bacteria, either of the same or different species.

(3) Growth of bacteria, either from small cracks or defects in the enamel surface, or from those cells which have initially become attached to the tooth.

The various adhesive mechanisms which exist in plaque serve to maintain the integrity of the material and prevent its removal by normal physiological processess and gentle forces such as mouthrinsing. The surface properties of plaque bacteria are particularly important in this respect, and each species has its own characteristic surface polymers. These polymers vary in chemical and antigenic properties and may carry different charges. Several oral bacteria produce extracellular polysaccharides which may play an important role in initial colonisation of the teeth and also contribute towards the inter-microbial plaque matrix (see below and chapter 5).

Oral streptococci have been studied particularly, as several species form extracellular glucans or fructans in the presence of sucrose. However, other bacteria, including certain *Neisseria* species and some anaerobic Gram-positive rods, produce extracellular polymers which may also be important in plaque formation, and these are not necessarily dependent upon the availability of sucrose.

The ability of different oral bacteria to adhere to various surfaces has been studied extensively by Gibbons, Van Houte and their colleagues in Boston[16, 17]. These workers have shown that some organisms adhere preferentially to teeth surfaces, while others favour epithelial cells for attachment. Certain important plaque constituents, especially *Streptococcus mutans*, appear to have only weak adhesive properties on their own and presumably rely on initial colonisation by other species. The production of extracellular polysaccharides from sucrose may, in some cases, be responsible for retention of organisms rather than initial adherence to the plaque. The relative adhesive properties of some species are shown in table 4.2.

Table 4.2 Ability of bacteria to adhere to oral surfaces as related to their proportions found indigenously (after Gibbons[16])

	Proportions found indigeneously			*Experimentally observed adherence*		
	tooth	tongue	cheek	tooth	tongue	cheek
Streptococcus mutans	Low to high	low	low	low to high	low	low
Streptococcus sanguis	high	moderate	moderate	high	moderate	moderate
Streptococcus salivarius	low	high	moderate	low	high	moderate
Neisseria species	low	low	low	low	low	low
Veillonella species	low	high	low	low	high	low

Recently, several groups of research workers have concentrated on elucidating the mechanisms of adherence of *S. mutans* to various surfaces. Since this particular species is considered to be of great importance in the aetiology of caries (chapter 3), an understanding of its mode of attachment to the tooth may lead to the development of methods which interfere with this process and reduce the level of colonisation

of the tooth. This is one of the theoretical mechanisms by which an anti-caries vaccine might work (chapter 11). At the present time, despite some elegant published studies, the precise method of attachment of *S. mutans* and other plaque bacteria is not fully understood, but work on this interesting phenomenon continues in several laboratories. It appears, however, that the affinity of this organism for hard tooth surfaces, even in the presence of sucrose, is not as great as was once thought, and that its prevalence in dental plaque is dependent upon factors such as interaction with other microorganisms.

The formation of dental plaque on teeth is analogous to the development of microbial films in many other natural habitats. Five stages have been proposed during the deposition of such films on surfaces[82].

(1) Polymer sorption (that is, adsorption of macromolecules, as observed in pellicle formation from saliva).
(2) Chemical attraction of mobile bacteria.
(3) Reversible sorption of bacteria to the surface.
(4) Irreversible sorption.
(5) Development of a secondary microflora.

Stages one to four take place in the mouth within a few hours, while the secondary community develops over a period of several days. During the irreversible phase attached organisms may produce extracellular polymers which aid in their retention; this phenomenon is known as polymer-bridging[83]. As mentioned above, the extracellular glucose polymers produced by some oral streptococci may be of greater importance in the irreversible phase than during initial attachment to the tooth surface.

4.5.2 Pellicle formation

When a thoroughly cleaned and polished tooth is exposed to saliva it rapidly becomes coated with an amorphous organic layer, usually referred to as the *acquired pellicle*. In fact, several pellicle or cuticle structures have been described in the literature and these have been investigated from the point of view of their structure, mode of formation and chemical composition.

It is generally agreed that the acquired pellicle is derived principally from salivary components and it has been shown experimentally that the presence of bacteria is not essential since salivary glycoproteins are absorbed to hydroxyapatite in the test tube[18]. Investigations into the nature of the acquired surface integuments are technically very difficult because of their intimate contact with enamel. As has been pointed out by Saxton[19], research workers have attempted to overcome these practical problems in three basic ways:

(1) Separation of pellicle from the surface enamel by dilute hydrochloric acid (a flotation technique), followed by chemical or structural examination.
(2) Dehydration and embedding *in situ*, followed by decalcification of the tooth, either with dilute acid or ethylenediamine tetra-acetic acid (EDTA).
(3) Formation of pellicle on various artificial surfaces, in vivo, such as plastic strips, which can easily be removed from the mouth when required.

It is now apparent from the several, sometimes contradictory, published reports on the composition of pellicle that the method used may significantly influence the results of subsequent analyses.

Structure of pellicle

At the light microscopic level, pellicle appears to be a structureless, homogeneous layer $0.3 - 1.0$ μm thick, although deposits up to 5 μm have occasionally been described. McDougall[40] was one of the first to describe pellicle, which he invariably found to be present beneath approximal plaque when examining sections in the light microscope. However, using the electron microscope, other workers have occasionally observed plaque bacteria in direct contact with surface enamel, without an intervening pellicle or cuticular layer[20].

Several investigators have used transmission or scanning electron microscopy to study the structure of the acquired pellicle. Meckel[21] described the following surface layers;

(1) Primary enamel cuticle (developmental, lost soon after eruption).

(2)   Sub-surface cuticle.
(3)   Surface cuticle.
(4)   Pellicle.

The distinction between (3) and (4) was based upon the staining of these layers, and most other workers consider these together as one entity—the acquired surface pellicle. There is also a tendency in the literature to refer to very thin layers as cuticles and thicker deposits as pellicles. Other workers[22] have also observed the presence of a sub-surface, dendritic cuticle layer on approximal surfaces, but not on buccal surfaces, and it has been suggested that this phenomenon may be related to early loss of enamel material at caries-susceptible sites. The idea that etched enamel might be repaired by exposure to saliva had also been suggested earlier by other workers[23] (chapter 12.3.2).

The outer edge of the acquired pellicle, adjacent to the inner plaque layer, may show a scalloped outline when examined in sections at very high power[22, 24], the recesses, indicating areas occupied originally by bacteria.

Formation and composition of pellicle

Pellicle forms very rapidly on a clean tooth surface within minutes of exposure to the oral environment. It increases in amount for about $1\frac{1}{2}$ hours and then appears to level off to a fairly constant thickness[25], its composition apparently not varying greatly from one tooth to another. As mentioned previously, pellicle is thought to be derived mainly from glycoproteins in saliva, which several workers have shown to be selectively absorbed to both synthetic hydroxyapatite crystals and natural enamel. Reported differences in the detailed chemical composition of pellicle are probably related to the various methods used for collection of samples and the techniques used for analysis.

Chemically, pellicle appears to be composed of undegraded salivary glycoproteins which are made up of amino acids and sugars. Varying amounts of different amino acids have been detected in pellicle by different investigators. For example, samples obtained by scraping from the enamel contained more than twice as much serine[25] as that estimated in acid-insoluble pellicle obtained by the acid flotation method favoured by some workers[22, 24]. Readily detectable levels of the amino acid diaminopimelic acid and the amino sugar muramic acid were reported in one study[26], although this finding has not been confirmed by others, at least in early pellicle specimens. The significance of this observation is that these particular components are characteristic of bacterial cell walls, but are not found in saliva or other material of human origin.

It would seem that, initially, the selective adsorption of salivary components is the important mechanism in pellicle formation, but that at later stages, when bacteria have begun to accumulate, the distinction between pellicle and plaque material is difficult to define. The differences in chemical composition reported in the literature indicate how difficult it is to separate pellicle and plaque for the purposes of analysis.

Several mechanisms have been suggested for the deposition of salivary glycoproteins on to the enamel surface; these include the effects of surface charges (for example, negatively charged terminal sialic acid groups), the concentration of calcium ions (increased Ca^{2+} may precipitate glycoprotein) and pH effects (decreased pH favours the adhesion of proteins to hydroxyapatite). The results of several chemical studies indicate that acidic amino acids adhere more abundantly than basic amino acids.

Although the composition of the enamel surface is important, structurally and chemically similar pellicle layers may be deposited on artificial surfaces placed in the mouth, such as plastic films, and these have been widely used for experimental studies. However, one recent study has shown that pellicle formed more rapidly on hydroxyapatite crystals in the mouth than on the epoxy resin splints on which the crystals were held[27]. Thus, when comparing the results of different studies on pellicle composition, it is important to take into account the surface on which the material was deposited.

In addition to the suggestion that pellicle formation may act as a repair mechanism for small surface defects produced by acid damage, it may also play a role in colonisation of the tooth by plaque bacteria. Thus it has been postulated that the pellicle may act as a substrate for the growth of certain bacteria, or alternatively that it might aid the adsorption and adhesion of bacteria to the tooth surface. Whether or not these or other mechanisms operate, formation of a pellicle layer normally precedes the colonisation of the enamel by bacteria.

4.5.3   Bacterial succession during plaque formation

Once dental plaque has developed for several days or weeks it contains large numbers of a wide variety of bacterial types. Before this stage is reached, often referred to as 'mature' or 'established' plaque, it is possible to demonstrate that the microflora builds up in numbers and complexity in a reasonably ordered and reproducible fashion[28, 84, 85].

Several workers have studied the pattern of colonisation as plaque develops on previously clean surfaces in the mouth, usually over short periods of up to 7–14 days. Some of these studies have been based on microscopy, either at the light or electron-microscopic level, others have utilised counts of viable bacteria, while a few investigators have employed both methods concurrently. A variety of surfaces have been used, including natural teeth *in situ*, extracted human teeth or artificial teeth carried on a fixed bridge or removable appliance, and various other artificial devices held in the mouth, such as plastic films and agar gels. The advantage of the various artificial devices in such studies is that they can be removed from the mouth fairly easily at the appropriate times for sectioning or culture, whereas plaque that has formed on natural teeth is more difficult to sample and handle reproducibly. On the other hand, it is arguable that plaque which grows on artificial surfaces may differ from that on natural teeth. Fortunately, the results obtained using different techniques

are reasonably similar for short-term plaque development studies and so it is possible to present a simplified summary of the sequence of events.

As described above, the newly cleaned tooth surface is rapidly covered with a thin film of pellicle, largely of salivary origin, which soon becomes colonised by bacteria. This initial colonisation has been studied both culturally and by means of the scanning electron microscope.[29] The earliest organisms to be found are predominantly coccal in form. Cultural studies have shown that both Gram-positive and Gram-negative cocci are present, and these may be aerobic or facultative. Gram-positive rods have also been isolated from early plaque. Streptococci form a prominent proportion of the earliest colonisers, but other organisms, such as *Neisseria* species, also play a significant role in initial plaque development[30]. It is thought that most of these are derived from saliva, but outgrowth from enamel defects may also contribute.

More recent studies have indicated that *Streptococcus sanguis* is a prominent organism amongst the earliest colonisers of the tooth surface[86, 87]. *Actinomyces viscosus* has also been found consistently in early plaque, together with *S. mitis, Staphylococcus epidermidis, A. israelii, Peptostreptococcus* sp. and *Veillonella alcalescens*[87]. Some species have been reported as occuring regularly in mixtures of two or more intimately associated organisms or 'suspected pairs'.[87]

After the plaque has developed undisturbed for a day or two it becomes thicker and a greater variety of morphological types of bacteria are found, including filamentous forms which start to appear at about the third day. The proportion of the total flora made up of rods and filaments increases with time so that by 7–14 days the plaque may appear in sections to be composed largely of filaments. However, even at this stage high numbers of cocci and rods can be cultivated.

This sequence of plaque development from a predominantly coccal type at the beginning to a mixed, filamentous flora a few days later has been shown by numerous investigators[31, 32]. An example of the data obtained from such studies is shown in figure 4.1.

As well as the shift in morphological types of bacteria seen during early plaque development, there is also a shift towards increasing anaerobiosis as the plaque builds up in mass and complexity. Thus, anaerobes such as *Fusobacterium*, *Veillonella*, *Actinomyces*, *Bacteroides*, etc., appear in increasing numbers after the initial colonisation by aerobic and facultative species. Correspondingly, the relative numbers of aerobes, such as *Neisseria* and *Rothia* (formerly known as *Nocardia*), appear to decrease (figure 4.1). The changes in anaerobic conditions during plaque development have been demonstrated clearly by Kenney and Ash[33], who showed that the oxidation – reduction potential

drops from an initial value of $+200$ mV to about -112 mV after seven days. Such successional changes in both microbial composition and physiological conditions are associated with the development of gingivitis and may also be relevant to the initiation of other disease processes.[84]

4.5.4 Formation of the matrix of dental plaque

The microorganisms in dental plaque are embedded in an organic matrix which occupies the space between individual bacterial cells or microcolonies and accounts for approximately 30 per cent of the total plaque volume. It is thought that the matrix has a significant effect on the ecology of the plaque and may also be important in caries; by acting as a diffusion-limiting membrane, potentially harmful bacterial products such as lactic acid may be retained in high concentrations at particular sites where they can initiate caries. The same diffusion-limiting effect may also slow down the arrival of buffers from saliva, thus delaying their neutralising action.

The origin of the plaque matrix is thought to be twofold. Part of the organic material is protein and is derived principally from salivary glycoproteins, while the remainder consists of extracellular polysaccharides produced by the bacteria themselves. The discovery that plaque matrix contains bacterial polysaccharides, largely glucose polymers, has led to a great deal of research work on the production of such extracellular materials, especially with some of the oral streptococci, and this is described in some detail in chapter 5.

A simplified summary of some of the main factors in the production of the plaque matrix has been suggested by Leach[34], and this is represented in figure 4.2. According to this theory, the protein component of the matrix is deposited by enzymatic removal of the terminal sialic acid residues on the side-chains of salivary glycoprotein molecules. Several oral microorganisms produce an enzyme, neuraminidase, which effects this reaction. The altered glycop-

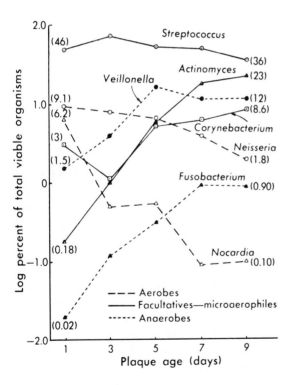

Figure 4.1 Graph showing shift in relative proportions of selected organisms in developing dental plaque. Samples taken from labial surfaces of upper and lower incisors of six adult male subjects (graph reproduced by courtesy of Dr H. L. Ritz[31] and the editor of *Archives of Oral Biology*)

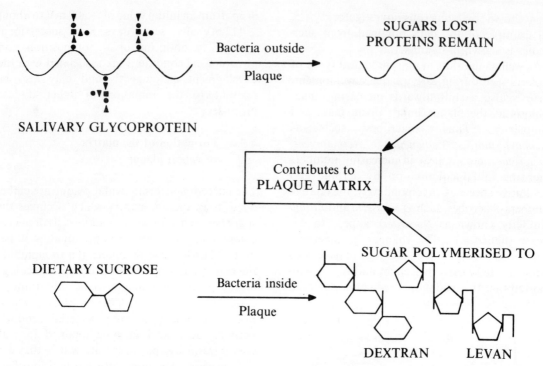

Figure 4.2 A diagrammatic representation of proposed enzymically controlled reactions that lead to the formation of the principal protein and carbohydrate components of the matrix of dental plaque (diagram reproduced by the courtesy of Dr S. A. Leach[34] and E&S Livingstone Ltd.)

roteins, minus their sialic acid moieties, are apparently in a less soluble configuration and consequently are deposited around the microorganisms.

The carbohydrate components of the matrix are derived mainly from the several different extracellular polysaccharides produced by plaque bacteria, usually from sucrose (chapter 5). Since the chemical composition of plaque matrix is complex and is derived from several sources, it is difficult to discover which components have been derived from which particular microorganisms in vivo. Because of such problems, research workers have examined the production of extracellular polysaccharides by pure cultures of bacteria in vitro, and extrapolated their findings to the situation which exists in the mouth. *Streptococcus mutans* has been studied in great detail in this respect. Strains of this species have been shown to produce several types of extracellular polysaccharides from sucrose, including

both soluble and insoluble glucans, and fructose polymers. These polysaccharides are produced by means of extracellular enzymes which cleave the disaccharide sucrose molecule and utilise either the glucose or fructose moieties for polymer formation. These enzymes, glucosyl and fructosyl transferases, are sometimes referred to as dextransucrase or levansucrase.

The water-soluble extracellular glucan is an α-1,6 linked polymer, usually referred to as dextran. Dextrans are produced by several other microorganisms (not only oral bacteria), in addition to *S. mutans*, including *S. sanguis*, *S. mitior*, *S. bovis* and *Leuconostoc mesenteroides*. This last organism is the usual source of dextrans produced commercially, for which there are a number of important applications.

S. mutans also produces insoluble extracellular glucans, which have different linkages between the glucose units, such as α-1, 3 or α-1, 4. The insoluble α-1, 3 glucan produced by a particular strain of *S. mutans* (strain number OMZ 176) has been studied in great detail[35], and this polysaccharide is called 'mutan'. Several workers have isolated the extracellular enzymes responsible for polysaccharide production from bacterial strains and have been able to synthesise the glucans from sucrose in the test-tube, using such enzyme preparations in the absence of live bacteria. Such investigations have allowed detailed structural analysis of pure preparations of microbial polysaccharides to be made.

S. sanguis and some strains of *S. mitior* also produce extracellular glucose polymers from sucrose[36, 37]. Since these species are often present in high numbers in dental plaque, it is probable that in many situations they contribute more polysaccharide material to the plaque matrix than *S. mutans*.

Fructan or levan is the polysaccharide characteristically produced by *S. salivarius*, although small amounts of fructose polymers are also produced by strains of *S. mutans* and other streptococci. It is likely that the amount of this polymer formed in dental plaque is low, since *S. salivarius* usually occurs in small numbers on the tooth surface. In any event, levan seems to be very much more labile than the glucans and is rapidly broken down and utilised as a substrate by oral microorganisms.

A detailed chemical study of the carbohydrate composition of pooled dental plaque[38], collected from 3500 school children, showed that fresh plaque contained approximately 80 per cent water. This water content was similar to that obtained in several previous reports. Approximately 30 per cent of the plaque dry weight was water-soluble and 67 per cent was insoluble. The soluble and insoluble fractions contained 6.9 per cent and 11.3 per cent carbohydrate, respectively. This investigation revealed that about 1.35 per cent of the plaque dry weight could be accounted for by water-insoluble matrix polysaccharides, containing predominantly α-1, 3 linkages (i.e. mutan-like in structure). A surprisingly high level (5.6 per cent) of low-molecular-weight, soluble carbohydrates was found, and the authors concluded from this that

the microbial activity in plaque is not limited by the supply of fermentable substances. Little evidence was found for the presence of levan material in the plaque matrix, thus confirming the results of other studies.

As indicated in the preceding discussion, most work on the origin of plaque matrix carbohydrates has been confined to the streptococci. However, for the sake of completeness, it should be mentioned that several other groups of bacteria produce extracellular materials which may contribute to the plaque matrix. These include *Neisseria*, *Actinomyces* and *Lactobacillus* species, and several anaerobic organisms. An interesting inhabitant of the tongue, *Micrococcus mucilagenosus* (formerly known as *Staphylococcus salivarius*) is sometimes isolated from plaque, and this organism produces a highly viscous, extracellular heteropolysaccharide[39].

It is clear from the available knowledge that the plaque matrix is highly complex, and may vary both chemically and structurally in different locations, depending upon the microorganisms present. Formation of the streptococcal extracellular polysaccharides is clearly influenced by the availability of dietary sucrose, but other controlling influences are little understood at present.

4.6 Structure of Established Dental Plaque

As described above, dental plaque builds up in complexity over a period of days from a predominantly coccal flora to a highly mixed microbial mass which appears to be highly filamentous when examined under the microscope. Some particularly fine illustrations of the morphological features of plaque development on epoxy resin crowns have recently been published[41].

Sections or smears of mature plaque examined under the light microscope clearly show the complexity of the structure (figure 4.3). Filamentous forms often appear to be particularly profuse in older specimens, and these are

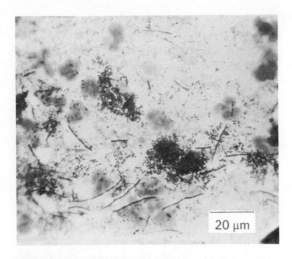

Figure 4.3 Gram-stained smear of dental plaque. This shows some of the variety of morphological types of bacteria seen in mature plaque

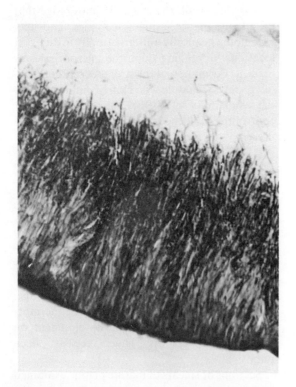

Figure 4.4 Gram-stained section of established plaque showing predominantly filamentous bacteria which are arranged perpendicular to the enamel surface. Some loosely attached micro-organisms can be seen at the outer surface of the plaque

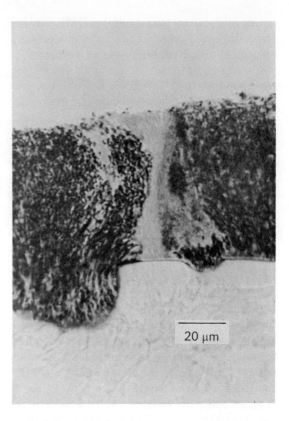

Figure 4.5 Gram-stained section of dental plaque. This field illustrates the appearance of morphologically similar bacteria which can be seen as discrete microcolonies within the plaque

commonly arranged parallel to one another, at right-angles to the tooth surface (figure 4.4). At different points along the length of a section it is possible to recognise discrete microcolonies of morphologically similar bacteria. (figure 4.5) In the studies by Listgarten[41], referred to above, vertical columns of similar microorganisms were demonstrated. When filamentous forms were observed after a few days, they appeared initially to colonise the surface of the predominantly coccal plaque and subsequently seemed to invade and replace the underlying bacteria.

The organisms at the base of the plaque, nearest to the enamel, are usually more closely packed than those towards the outer plaque–saliva interface, where the bacteria often appear

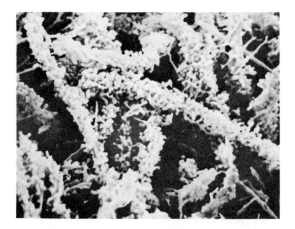

Figure 4.6 Scanning electron micrograph of mature dental plaque showing micro-organisms described as 'corn-cobs'

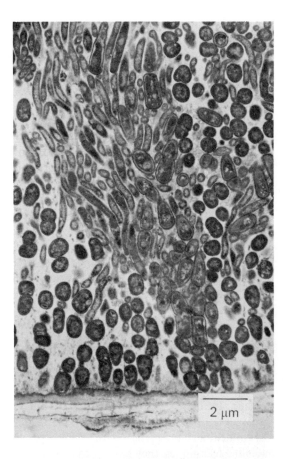

Figure 4.8 Transmission electron micrograph of dental plaque showing a mixture of bacteria of different morphological types

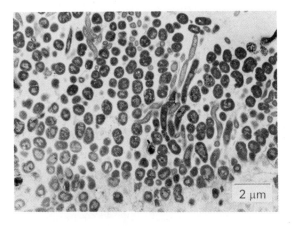

Figure 4.7 Transmission electron micrograph of dental plaque showing predominantly coccal flora

more loosely bound. In this situation, distinctive bacterial aggregations, often referred to as 'corn-cobs', have been described by several workers[42]. These consist of a central filament covered with a dense layer of coccal forms (figure 4.6). Until recently, the identity of the microorganisms showing this type of arrangement has not been known, but morphologically different forms of corn-cob have been described[40], indicating that several microbial species may be involved in the formation of such structures. One group of workers has now provided evidence which sug-

gests that these corn-cobs consist of a central filament of *Bacterionema matruchotii* surrounded by streptococci[90].

Several authors have published elegant pictures illustrating the structure of plaque at the electron microscopic level[43,44]. Both transmission and scanning methods have been employed, and special techniques such as freeze-etching and electronhistochemistry have also found a place. All such studies underline clearly the extreme complexity of the tooth surface microflora and emphasise the variations which may occur at different sites (figures 4.7 and 4.8). Although it is possible to recognise differences in the morphology of bacteria within plaque and make observations on their cell wall structure, it is not usually possible to identify microorganisms to the genus or species level by standard microscopic techniques. A possible exception to this is in the case of spirochaetes, which have a sufficiently distinctive morphology to allow them to be differentiated from other organisms.

Some special techniques are available for specific labelling of bacterial antigens and these allow direct identification under the microscope. At the light microscope level the fluorescent antibody technique may be used for this purpose. In this method, antisera containing antibodies to bacterial antigens are coupled with a fluorescent dye, such as fluoroscein isothiocyanate, and used as a specific stain. Bacteria stained with such a conjugated antiserum are examined under the microscope, using an ultraviolet light source, and if they have reacted they will fluoresce brightly. This technique has been used by a few workers for examination of plaque to demonstrate the localisation of specific bacteria, but as yet has been limited to the examination of a small number of species. At the electron microscopic level an analogous technique exists, in which specific antibodies are coupled to ferritin or peroxidase. Because of the considerable technical difficulties associated with these specific labelling techniques, they have not yet been used extensively for studies on dental plaque. However, within the past few years there has been a rapid increase in our knowledge of the antigenic structure of some oral bacteria, notably *S.mutans*, and it is likely that this information will enable further developments to be made in the identification and localisation of bacterial antigens within plaque.

In addition to observations on the microorganisms in plaque, electron microscopic studies have allowed studies to be made on the structure of the inter-microbial matrix material. In some instances, this appears to have fibrillar structure similar to that of extracellular polysaccharides produced by known bacteria in culture[77]. Histochemical techniques have been used to demonstrate variations in the amount of intra- and extra-cellular polysaccharide material synthesised by plaque bacteria under different die-

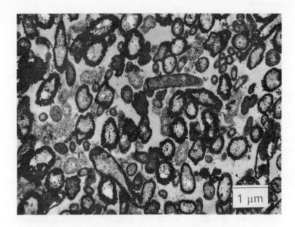

Figure 4.9   Transmission electron micrograph of section of dental plaque stained to show intracellular and extracellular polysaccharide. The polysaccharides appear as darkly-stained black material

tary conditions in vivo[45] (figure 4.9).

Structural studies on plaque associated with dental caries have not so far revealed any striking differences when compared to plaque overlying sound enamel.

4.7   Bacteriology of Established Dental Plaque

4.7.1   Quantification of dental plaque microorganisms

There are a number of intrinsic technical difficulties in examining and quantifying the microbial composition of plaque. These include:

(a) Method of collecting samples from the tooth surface.

(b) Method of dispersion of plaque specimens.

(c) Methods of counting and identifying microorganisms present: (i) microscopic counts, (ii) viable count.

Sample collection

A variety of different collection techniques have been described, and the suitability of a particular method depends upon the exact site to be examined. The easily accessible smooth surface (buccal and lingual) can be sampled with standard dental instruments such as scalers or excavators, and these present no real problems. For approximal surfaces, either dental floss or a specially made device constructed from abrasive tape may be used[46]. Plaque from pits and fissures can be obtained by means of sharp probes or small pieces of tapered orthodontic wire held in a haemostat. Because of the adherent and tough nature of plaque specimens; cotton wool throat swabs are not particularly suitable for obtaining plaque specimens.

In some studies, samples of plaque are weighed so that subsequent analyses can be related to unit weight (for example, total number of bacteria per milligramme). Wet weight measurements need to be made immediately after the sample is collected in order to avoid loss of water by evaporation, and can only be carried out accurately on samples of 1 mg or more. This is quite possible with large, pooled samples from several sites but is not feasible for single-site specimens. In the latter case, subsequent counts are usually related to the original sample (for example, viable count per floss sample).

Immediately after plaque collection, the samples are usually placed in a small volume of some transport medium. The composition of this transport fluid should preserve the viability of the microorganisms to be enumerated, and normally includes a reducing agent such as cysteine or dithiothreitol to aid in the preservation of anaerobes. Ideally, samples should be processed in the laboratory within the shortest possible time after collection. Where this period extends unavoidably to more than two hours, there is a danger that growth of some bacteria in the transport media will distort the microbiological picture and for this reason some transport media contain growth inhibitors.

Dispersion of plaque specimens

Accurate quantification of the numbers of bacteria in a given plaque specimen, either by direct microscopic or viable counting technique, depends upon adequate dispersion of clumps of bacteria to give an even suspension of individual cells. This is especially important for viable counts, where each colony counted is assumed to be derived from a single bacterial cell. In practice, it is impossible to tell whether an individual colony has grown from one cell, a chain of cells or a clump, and the term 'colony-forming units' is often used. It is largely because of problems in achieving adequate dispersal of plaque that accurate and reproducible quantification is difficult.

At the present time, no method of dispersal is universally accepted by all workers and in the end the method chosen is a compromise between the best physical disruption and optimum maintenance of viability of the organisms. Methods which have been used include shaking with glass beads, grinding in a glass tissue homogeniser, a blender, and ultrasonic probes. The last method probably achieves the best disruption but may also kill a number of Gram-negative organisms. Whichever technique is adopted, best recoveries of viable organisms are obtained when care is taken to avoid undue exposure of anaerobes to oxygen in the atmosphere. For this reason, manipulations are sometimes undertaken in an oxygen-free anaerobic chamber or under a stream of oxygen-free gas.

Methods of counting

(i) Microscopic counts Direct counts of suspended plaque bacteria, either stained or unstained, can be made on special slides (for example, Helber chamber, Petroff – Hauser chamber). These chambers are similar to those used for counting blood cells, and depend upon filling the chamber accurately with a known volume of suspension and counting the number of cells in several squares of a grid. By simple arithmetic, the number of cells in the original suspended sample can then be calculated. By such methods, dental plaque has been shown to contain approximately $2-2.5 \times 10^8$ bacteria per mg wet weight.

(ii) Viable counts The principle of viable cou-

nts is extremely simple. A series of dilutions of the original suspension of organisms are made, and measured aliquots of each dilution are dispensed on to the surface of culture plates. The drop of liquid is spread all over the surface of the plate with a sterile bent glass rod and, after appropriate incubation, each colony is counted. From the colony count and dilution factor, the number of organisms or, more precisely, colony-forming units (CFUs) in the original suspension can be calculated. Variations of this technique, such as pour plates and roll tubes, in which the organisms are mixed with molten agar before pouring, are also used, but in each case the underlying principle is the same.

The success of this method depends upon providing cultural conditions suitable for the particular organisms concerned. Such conditions include suitable culture media, temperature and atmospheric conditions. Since plaque usually contains a large variety of bacterial species, some aerobic, some facultative, and others strictly anaerobic, it is necessary to provide a variety of media and gaseous conditions when attempting a complete count. No single set of cultural conditions is optimum for growth of all the bacteria present. Commonly, some non-selective medium (such as blood agar) is included in an attempt to grow the majority of species, together with a number of selective media to allow isolation and recognition of particular species.

The proportion of the total microscope count which can be recovered in viable counts is to a large extent a function of the success of the anaerobic techniques employed. In table 4.3 the results of several investigations are illustrated, using different techniques. The most fastidious technique (roll tube) employed allowed a 70 per cent recovery, while careful conventional methods, using anaerobic jars and bench-top manipulations, gave from 8 to 50 per cent recovery[47-54].

In a recent investigation, several methods were compared in an attempt to increase the recovery of viable bacteria from supragingival plaque[88]. Failure to recover microorganisms was attributed to three main causes; inadequate disper-

sion, adhesion to glassware used in dilution and spreading, and inability of culture media to support growth of all types of bacteria present. In this study, optimum recovery was achieved when samples were dispersed under anaerobic conditions by sonic oscillation in pre-reduced one-quarter strength Ringers solution (supplemented with 1 per cent sodium metaphosphate, 0.05 per cent L-cysteine and 0.0001 per cent resazurin). Incubation of specimens plated on 5 per cent sheep blood agar plates in Brewer jars containing 80 per cent N_2, and 10 per cent CO_2 allowed recovery of 60 per cent of the total microscopic count. Use of additional media and cultural conditions permitted the recovery of a further 15 per cent of the organisms present. It was estimated that 5 % of the organisms were lost due to adsorption to glassware and that approximately 10 per cent of the bacteria remained in undispersed clumps.

Table 4.3   Recovery of anaerobic bacteria from dental plaque–viable anaerobic count expressed as percentage of total microscopic count (based on several published reports[47-54])

Per cent recovery	Technique
18.4	Anaerobic jar
33	Anaerobic chamber
24	Anaerobic jar
70.4	Roll tube
50	Anaerobic jar
8–18	Anaerobic jar
32–54	Anaerobic chamber

The number of anaerobes counted in plaque samples as related to wet weight in several independent studies are shown in table 4.4, and range from 4.0 to 7.9×10^7 per mg. The ratio of anaerobic to aerobic viable counts also varies according to the methods used, and values ranging from approximately 2:1 to 12:1 have been reported by different workers. Clinical estimates of the amount of plaque in a mouth can be correlated with the actual weight of plaque present and the microscopic count[55].

Table 4.4 Anaerobic bacteria in dental plaque—relationship of anaerobic viable count to wet weight

No. of samples	Mean count per mg ($\times 10^7$)	Technique	Ref.
10	4.6	CO	47
97	5.0	CO	48
40(G)	4.0	CO	49
18(G)	5.0	CO	50
8(G)	5.4	CO	51
8(G)	17.9	RT	51
16	11.3	CO	52
33	12.3	CO	53
11	10.0	CH	54

Symbols:
  G = gingival plaque specimen used.
  CO = conventional anaerobic jar technique.
  RT = roll-tube (Hungate) technique.
  CH = anaerobic chamber technique.

4.7.2 Differential microbial composition of established dental plaque

Probably of greater interest than the total numbers of organisms present in plaque is the differential microbial composition. The variety of types of bacteria which can be found in almost any sample of dental plaque from any site in the mouth is bewilderingly large and complex[56, 57]. The genera most commonly isolated from plaque are listed in table 4.5. Most of the genera are represented by several different species.

Many investigations have reported figures which give an idea of the overall quantitative composition of dental plaque. Most commonly these are expressed as percentages of the total (usually anaerobic) viable count, but may also be related to the microscopic count or unit weight of the samples. Despite considerable differences in the sampling procedures and laboratory methods used there is a reasonable degree of agreement between reports.

It can be seen from table 4.6, that the numerically dominant groups of bacteria are the Gram-positive rods and filaments which consist largely of *Actinomyces* species, and the streptococci. Both of these large groups include several different species, which may be microaerophilic, facultative or strictly anaerobic. Anaerobic Gram-negative cocci belonging to the genus *Veillonella*, and anaerobic Gram-negative rods (mainly *Bacteroides* species), can reach quite high levels, but there is considerable variation between the relative number of these organisms reported in different studies. Aerobic Gram-negative cocci (*Neisseria* species), fusobacteria, haemophili and several other genera are commonly isolated, but these organisms generally comprise a small percentage of the total cultivable flora.

Detailed studies on plaque collected from the distal surfaces of upper first premolars have shown a similar distribution of bacteria to that given in table 4.6. The results obtained in two

Table 4.5 Microorganisms commonly present in dental plaque

Gram-positive		*Gram-negative*	
cocci	rods and filaments	cocci	rods and filaments
Streptococcus	Actinomyces	Neisseria	Bacteroides
Peptococcus	Lactobacillus	Branhamella	Fusobacterium
Peptostreptoccus	Bacterionema	Veillonella	Haemophilus
Staphyloccus	Rothia		Vibrio (Campylobacter)
Micrococcus	Arachnia		Leptotrichia
	Bifidobacterium		Capnocytophaga
	Eubacterium		Selenomonas
	Propionibacterium		Spirochaetes

Table 4.6   The microbial flora of dental plaque—overall composition based on published surveys*

Type of organisms	Per cent viable count (range)
Streptoccocci	17–38
Gram-positive rods and filaments	22–52
Neisseria	0–2
Veillonella	1–13
Gram-negative anaerobic rods	0–17
Fusobacteria	0–7

* These figures have been assembled from five independent surveys by different authors, who have used a variety of sampling methods and laboratory procedures[46, 54, 58-60].

Table 4.7   The microbial composition of approximal dental plaque—results of 59 samples from ten 14-year-old children (from Bowden Hardie and Slack[46])*

Genera	Mean per cent	Range
Streptococci	23	0.4–70.0
Gram + Rods (mainly Actinomyces)	42.1	4.0–81.0
Gram – rods (mainly Bacteroides)	7.8	0–66.0
Neisseria	1.5	0–44.0
Veillonella	13.1	0–59.0
Fusobacterium	0.4	0– 5.4
Individual species		
S. mutans	2.2	0–23.0
S. sanguis	5.9	0–64.0
S. salivarius	0.7	0–33.0
S. milleri	0.5	0– 7.0
A. israeli	16.5	0–78.0
A. viscosus/naeslundi	19.1	0–74.0

* Selected organisms expressed as percentage of total viable count; samples obtained from distal surfaces of upper first premolar teeth.

Table 4.8   Further studies on the microbial composition of approximal dental plaque—results on 291 samples from 50 subjects (from Bowden, Hardie and Slack (1976), unpublished data)

Type of organisms	Mean per cent (of viable count)	Isolation frequency %
Streptococci	14	100
Gram-positive rods and filaments	45	100
Anaerobic Gram-negative rods	18	98
Veillonella	17	94
Neisseria	3	99
Fusobacterium	1	55
Rothia	0.5	40
Lactobacilli	0.3	36
Black-pigmented Bacteroides	8	35
Bacterionema	0.6	16

wide (table 4.7), underlining the intrinsic difficulties of obtaining accurate and reproducible viable counts from mixed bacterial populations. The isolation frequencies shown in table 4.8 indicate that, in addition to streptococci and actinomyces, *Veillonella*, *Neisseria* and *Bacteroides* species are almost invariably present. Other species and genera are detected less frequently in plaque samples, but this may either be a true reflection of their occurrence or possibly due to the technical problems of isolating bacteria which are present only in very small numbers, since these may be obscured by overgrowth of the more numerous species present. Some compensation for the latter problem can be made by judicious use of selective media, but it is probable that many organisms present in low concentrations are missed.

Site variations in bacterial composition

Several investigators have shown that the quantitative composition of plaque can vary quite markedly at different sites in the mouth, or even at different points on the same tooth[28, 56, 61]. The best documented differences are probably those related to the plaque which is formed in or adjacent to the gingival crevice. In this situation

recent investigations are shown in tables 4.7 and 4.8.

Once again, the Gram-positive rods predominate, but the streptococcal counts are rather lower than those in most previously published reports. It can be seen that the range of values obtained for any individual type of bacteria is

Table 4.9 Variations of cultivable plaque flora on 3 sites of the same tooth*

Subject	Site	Streptococci	Actinomyces	Bacteroides	Fusobacterium	Veillonella
1	A	11.4	0.04	8.5	0.85	11.4
	B	65.5	5.7	9.0	11.4	0
	C	0.4	0.6	0.08	0.26	73.0
	Mean	25.7	2.1	5.9	4.2	28.1
2	A	8.6	85.3	0.65	0	1.7
	B	71.5	18.7	8.0	0.93	0
	C	14.3	56.6	0	0	16.6
	Mean	31.2	53.5	2.9	0.3	6.1
3	A	30.0	14.0	2.0	0	23.0
	B	65.0	7.0	25.0	3.0	14.0
	C	64.0	25.0	0	0.5	10.0
	Mean	53.0	15.3	9.0	1.2	15.6
Mean for all sites		36.6	23.6	5.9	1.9	16.6

* Figures expressed as percentage of total viable count. Site A = contact area; site B = gingival crevice below contact; site C = buccal surface.

the proportion of anaerobes is generally higher, and increased numbers of fusobacteria, bacteroides, vibrios and spirochaetes have been reported.

An example of the variations in quantitative composition which may occur on a single tooth is given in table 4.9. In this experiment, plaque material from three adjacent sites, approximately 2–3 mm apart, was removed from the surface of freshly extracted teeth and the microbial composition of each was compared. It can be seen that there are obvious variations in the relative numbers of the bacterial types from one site to another, but that some of these differences may be obscured when mean values are calculated. The differences in the relative proportions of cultivable bacteria counted in this and other studies reflect the observed morphological variations in plaque composition that can be demonstrated by microscopic examination.

Repeated collection of plaque samples from a particular site over a period of time shows fluctuations in the relative numbers of bacteria present, although part of this may be due to unavoidable experimental errors. However, there is also some evidence of persistence of particular species of bacteria at certain sites, and

sometimes there appears to be a remarkable degree of stability in their numbers. The localisation and persistence of *S. mutans* has been investigated, and this species does seem to remain fixed at some sites, while other comparable areas in the same mouth may not become colonised. An example of the localised distribution of this particular streptococcus is shown in table 4.10[62].

In summary, from the large number of published accounts of the microbial composition of dental plaque, the following general conclusions may be drawn:

(1) The microbial flora is highly complex. In any sample of plaque a large variety of bacterial species can be isolated.

(2) The overall quantitative composition appears to be similar if the results of many different estimations are averaged. This similarity between plaque examined by different workers is especially marked if relatively large, pooled samples have been used.

(3) More specific and detailed studies, in which plaque samples are collected from relatively small well-defined sites on the tooth surface, indicate that each microenvironment

Table 4.10　Percentage of *Streptococcus mutans* on approximal molar surfaces sampled at weekly intervals (from Gibbons et al.[62])

Subject	Site	Week				
		1	2	3	4	5
14	A					
	B	4	12		20	8
	C					
	D	25	36	48	26	32
24	A					
	B					
	C					
	D	36	8	1	2	
5	A	38	20	40	18	52
	B	12	30	1	6	78
	C	36	8		8	64
	D	76	20	2		72

* A, B, C and D represent four different sites in the same mouth.

may harbour a unique and characteristic microflora.

It is clearly of the utmost importance for these regional variations, and their relationship to disease, to be better understood.

4.8　Some Characteristics of the Predominant Groups of Plaque Bacteria

4.8.1　Streptococci

For various reasons, streptococci have probably been studied more intensively than any other genera amongst the oral microflora. As mentioned in chapter 3, one species in particular, *Streptococcus mutans*, has received a considerable amount of attention in recent years. However, despite the large number of published papers, the taxonomy and nomenclature of streptococci still cause some confusion.

Streptococci are characteristically found inhabiting mucous membranes, and several species are regularly found in the mouth. Although they comprise a significant proportion of the total plaque flora, in some situations they are commonly outnumbered by Gram-positive rods of various kinds, as will be described below. The majority of strains of streptococci found in the mouth are of the greening (alpha-haemolytic) types and have often been referred to simply as '*Streptococcus viridans*'. However, this term is highly misleading since it includes several readily distinguishable species, and its use should be discontinued. Beta-haemolytic streptococci, such as the pathogenic species *S. pyogenes* (Lancefield Group A) are not generally found in plaque, although they can be isolated from the saliva of patients suffering from streptococcal sore throats. Some characteristically oral species, including strains of *S. mutans* and *S. sanguis*, can be found occasionally which produce complete (beta)-haemolysis on blood agar plates, but these can fairly easily be distinguished from haemolytic streptococci belonging to Lancefield group A.

Our understanding of the greening or viridans-type streptococci has been increased in recent years, thanks especially to the studies of Colman and Williams[65], and Carlsson[66]. Based on the work of these and other workers, the following species may be recognised amongst the oral streptococci[67]: *S. mutans*, *S. sanguis*, *S. mitior*, *S. salivarius* and *S. milleri*. One characteristic of several of these species is that their microscopic appearance may be highly variable or pleomorphic and on occasions they may be mistaken for Gram-positive rods.

These species can be identified in the laboratory by relatively simple means (table 4.11), and other named species, such as *S. faecalis*, may also occasionally be isolated from plaque. However, there remain other streptococci whose properties do not appear to conform to the known or expected species and further work is required in order to characterise these and facilitate their identification.

Streptococcus mutans

This species was first described in 1924 by

Table 4.11   Simple scheme for identification of oral streptococci (from Hardie and Bowden[67])

	S. mutans	*S. sanguis*	*S. mitior*	*S. milleri*	*S. salivarius*
Fermentation of:					
mannitol	+	−	−	−	−
sorbitol	+[a]	−	−	−	−
Hydrolysis of:					
arginine	−[b]	+	−	+	−
aesculin	+[a]	+	−	+	+[a]
Production of:					
acetoin	+	−	v	+	v
glucan	+	+	+[a]	−	−
H_2O_2	−[c]	+	+	−	−

Symbols:

+ = most strains positive.
− = most strains negative.
v = variable results.

[a] = some negative strains known.
[b] = serotype *b* strains positive.
[c] = some positive strains known.

Clarke[68], and has been extensively studied in recent years. The name *mutans* was given because this species characteristically charges from a round, coccus shape to a rod shape under certain growth conditions, such as low pH.

Some of the properties which are useful for identification purposes are shown in table 4.11. This streptococcus ferments a wide variety of carbohydrate substrates, producing a terminal pH in the region of 4.2–4.6 in broth cultures. A particular characteristic of *S. mutans* is the production of extracellular polysaccharides of the glucan type from sucrose. Bratthall[69] demonstrated that there are at least five serologically distinct types of *S. mutans* (designated *a – e*), and more recently the number of proposed serotypes has been increased to seven[70]. Most of the type antigens demonstrated in the serological differentiation of these serotypes have now been shown to be cell wall carbohydrates[78]. Over the past two or three years, several investigators have begun the complex task of unravelling the antigenic structure of *S. mutans* and several type-specific and cross-reacting antigens have been isolated and characterised from a few representative strains. The difference in antigenic structure and cell wall composition of *S. mutans* serotypes have been shown to correlate well with genetic differences, by means of DNA base ratio and DNA homology studies[71].

Since *S. mutans* is thought to be particularly important in the aetiology of dental caries (chapter 3), this species continues to be the subject of detailed investigations in many research laboratories all over the world. In addition to its relevance to dental caries, several reports have also been made of infective endocarditis due to this species.

Streptococcus sanguis

This is another oral species which produces extracellular glucans from sucrose. Originally the species was isolated from the blood cultures of patients with endocarditis, and several years later it was shown to be one of the predominant species in dental plaque. *S. sanguis* does not colonise the mouth of infants until about the age of 6 months, when the first teeth erupt, but from then on it is universally present in plaque. The interesting studies on adherence of organisms to different surfaces, described elsewhere in this chapter (section 4.5.1) have shown that *S. sanguis* adheres strongly both to enamel and to epithelial cells. It is thought that *S. sanguis* is of particular importance in the early stages of colonisation of the clean tooth surface. Identification of *S. sanguis* by biochemical and physiological tests is relatively straightforward (table 4.11). Most strains are alpha-haemolytic, but occasional beta-haemolytic strains are also found. The serology of *S. sanguis* is complex and not completely understood at present, but most strains react with Lancefield Group H antisera and there is some published evidence which indicates that the group H antigen may be a teichoic acid. However, further work on the various antigens possessed by different strains of *S. sanguis* is required in order to clarify some of the confusion which still exists in this area.

Streptococcus mitior

Strains allocated to this species include some which were previously referred to as *S. sanguis* serotype II, and others which have been called *S. mitis*. The latter 'species' name was never very well defined and several organisms with different properties have been included in the species.

Many oral strains of *S. mitior*, like *S. sanguis*, produce an extracellular polymer of the dextran type from sucrose. Both species tend to produce hard, adherent colonies on sucrose-containing agar media and can usually be distinguished from *S. mutans* on the basis of colonial morphology on such media. However, all these species tend to produce several colonial variants on sucrose media, and they may also alter in appearance between initial isolation and subsequent subcultures. Hence, it can often be misleading to base identification on colonial morphology alone, and presumptive isolates should always be checked by other tests.

S. mitior, together with *S. sanguis*, often comprise the numerical majority of the streptococci in plaque. Their significance in human caries is not known, but like other species they occur as the causative agent in endocarditis from time to time.

One of the characteristics of *S. mitior* strains is absence of significant amounts of rhamnose in their cell wall, and although they share some common antigens with *S. sanguis* and other species, they are serologically distinct.

Streptococcus salivarius

This species is generally not found in very high numbers in plaque, but can be found as a dominant part of the streptococcal flora of the tongue and other soft tissue, and in saliva. It has been shown experimentally that strains of *S. salivarius* adhere well to epithelial cells, but poorly to hard tissues.

Colonies of *S. salivarius* are often recognised by their large, mucoid appearance on sucrose agar. This particular morphology is due to the production of another extracellular polymer, fructan or levan, from sucrose.

Identification of *S. salivarius* is facilitated by the colonial appearance just described, but other characteristics are not particularly clear-cut, as the results of many commonly used tests tend to be negative or variable. At least two serotypes are known to exist, one of which reacts with Lancefield Group K antisera. On blood agar, strains of *S. salivarius* are usually non-haemolytic, but occasional beta-haemolytic strains are also found.

Because of the low numbers of *S. salivarius* in plaque, it is not thought that this species is of great significance in caries. However, as mentioned in chapter 3, one or two strains have been shown to produce some caries in experimental animals.

Streptococcus milleri

This species had not been recognised as part of the oral flora until comparatively recently, but it is now known to be present frequently in dental plaque. It can be recognised fairly easily by biochemical tests (table 4.11), but serologically it is extremely heterogeneous. Strains reacting with antisera to Lancefield Groups F, G, C and A have been allocated to the species, together with other strains which fail to react with any of the Lancefield grouping sera.

The importance of *S. milleri* in dental caries or other oral conditions is not known at present, but in other parts of the body this organism seems to be associated with localised collections of pus, such as brain and liver abscesses.

It is interesting that *S. milleri* strains are often isolated on a selective medium containing sulphonamide which was designed for isolations of *S. mutans*, and this may have caused some confusion in earlier studies[72]. The name *S. milleri* is not currently accepted by all workers, particularly in the U.S.A., and several alternatives can be found in the literature (for example, *S. anginosus*).

More detailed reviews on oral streptococci may be found in the list of further reading at the end of this chapter.

Other gram-positive cocci

In addition to the streptococci, which are generally facultative anaerobes with varying degrees of dependence upon carbon dioxide in the atmosphere, strictly anaerobic cocci belonging to the genera *Peptococcus* and *Peptostreptococcus* have been reported in plaque. The organisms are not always isolated from plaque samples using conventional anaerobic techniques and it is not easy to comment on their significance. However, they may be isolated from infected root canals and purulent infections of the mouth and jaws.

Catalase-positive cocci such as *Staphylococcus* and *Micrococcus* species are sometimes isolated from plaque, although usually in comparatively low numbers. One organism, *M. mucilagenosus* (formerly called *S. salivarius*), which is found primarily on the tongue and in saliva may occasionally be found in plaque. This interesting species produces copious amounts of an extremely viscous extracellular heteropolymer[38].

4.8.2 Gram-positive rods and filaments

A wide variety of Gram-positive rods are found in plaque, and collectively these often constitute the numerically dominant organisms isolated. They include aerobic, facultative and anaerobic species, many of which may be pleomorphic and display variable staining characteristics. Spore-forming Gram-positive rods belonging to the genera *Bacillus* or *Clostridium* have been reported only occasionally and are not isolated with any frequency from plaque samples collected from British subjects. It is possible that there may be some geographical variations in their distribution. Clostridia have been isolated from the mouths of mentally retarded individuals living in an institution in the U.S.A.[73]

Actinomyces

Representatives of this genus are the most common and numerous Gram-positive rods found in the mouth. They are characteristically micro-aerophilic or anaerobic, although some strains grow quite well aerobically. Microscopically, *Actinomyces* cells are often pleomorphic and may display branching and filamentous forms. They do not produce spores. Most species are catalase-negative, with the exception of *A. viscosus*. The animal pathogen, *A. bovis*, which causes lumpy jaw in cattle, has never been isolated with any certainty from human sources. The species found in the human mouth are *A. israelii*, *A. naeslundii*, *A. viscosus* and *A. odontolyticus*; in addition to their presence in plaque and possible involvement in caries and periodontal disease, some of these species are the causative agents of actinomycosis[63].

A. israelii This species is common in dental plaque and is also the most common cause of human actinomycosis. Of the different *Actinomyces* species it is the most dependant upon anaerobic conditions for growth. Two serologically distinct types can be recognised within the species[64].

A. naeslundii This species is also sometimes isolated from cases of actinomycosis and has been shown to cause periodontal destruction and bone loss in experimental animals. Together with

A. viscosus, which it closely resembles, *A. naeslundii* comprises the most commonly isolated type of *Actinomyces* in dental plaque.

A. viscosus   Apart from the catalase reaction, this species is very similar to *A. naeslundii* in most of its properties. The original animal isolate was called *Odontomyces viscosus*, but similar isolates were subsequently found in humans. The animal and human strains are serologically distinct. *A. viscosus* strains have been shown to produce periodontal destruction and root surface caries in animals.

A. odontolyticus   This species was first isolated from carious dentine, and characteristically produces reddish-brown colonies on blood agar plates. It is isolated less frequently and in lower numbers from human plaque than the other *Actinomyces* species described above.

Arachnia propionica

This organism resembles very closely *Actinomyces israelii* and may be difficult to distinguish when isolated from pathological specimens. It can be differentiated on the basis of acid end-products from glucose fermentation, since *Arachnia* produces propionic acid whereas *Actinomyces* species produce acetic, lactic and succinic acids. These products are usually estimated by means of gas–liquid chromatography. *Ar.propionica* has only occasionally been described from plaque samples and is probably of minor significance.

Lactobacillus

Lactobacilli are Gram-positive, catalase-negative, facultatively anaerobic rods. In the past they were one of the favourite candidates as the causative agent of caries because their numbers in the mouth tend to increase with the amount of caries present. In many plaque samples, especially from caries-free surfaces, their numbers are extremely low. Several species of *Lactobacillus* may be isolated from the mouth,

some homofermentative and some heterofermentative. Probably the most commonly found varieties in plaque are *L. casei* and *L. acidophilus*, both of which are homofermentative, but heterofermentors (which produce gas as well as acid from glucose) also occur. These organisms produce a low terminal pH in carbohydrate media (that is, they are acidogenic), and they can also survive and grow in a low pH environment (aciduric). Their aciduric potential is utilised in several selective media for lactobacilli, such as Tomato Juice agar and Rogosa's medium, both of which have a low pH which inhibits the growth of most other bacteria.

Bifidobacterium

These organisms have only occasionally been isolated from the mouth. They are anaerobic, Gram-positive rods, typically with bifid ends. In the past they have often been referred to as anaerobic lactobacilli. When grown in glucose broth the major end-products are acetic and lactic acids in a ratio of greater than 1:1. These organisms are more commonly found in the intestines, where they occur in large numbers.

Propionibacterium

These catalase-positive, anaerobic, Gram-positive rods are common inhabitants of the human skin and have occasionally been isolated from dental plaque. They are distinguished by the production of large amounts of propionic acid from glucose. As with *Arachnia*, they may be difficult to identify unless their acid end-products are known. The significance of finding propionibacteria in the mouth is not known, and when detected they are often taken to be contaminants from the skin.

Rothia dentocariosa

This species is commonly present in plaque, producing typical large, rough, matt, ridged (cartwheel-type) colonies on aerobic blood agar plates. Under the microscope the cells are pleomorphic; large filamentous forms are seen, which may fragment to coccal forms at certain stages in the growth cycle. This organism was formerly call *Nocardia salivae*, and it does have a number of morphological factors resembling a true *Nocardia*. Notwithstanding the specific epithet 'dentocariosa', this organism is not currently considered to play an important role in caries, although the original isolates were obtained from carious teeth.

Bacterionema maturchotii

This is another pleomorphic, Gram-positive filamentous species, which typically produces raised, rough colonies. It is usually a facultative anaerobe, and although strictly anaerobic varieties have been described, isolations are more commonly made after aerobic incubation. Microscopically, the long filaments commonly have a thickened, rod-like end, giving rise to the characteristic 'whip-handle' morphology. Recent chemical and taxonomic studies indicate that *Bacterionema* may be closely related to the genus *Corynebacterium*.[89]

This species is fairly common in plaque samples, but usually in low numbers. It has no known association with caries, but has been considered to be of significance in the formation of calculus, since cultures of *B. matruchotti* will calcify under appropriate experimental conditions. Recent work indicates that this species occupies the central, filamentous position in the structures referred to as 'corn-cobs'[90].

Eubacterium

Although there are a number of recognisable genera and species among the Gram-positive rods found in dental plaque, as described briefly above, there remain other isolates, usually anaerobic, which cannot easily be identified at present. Some of these are probably varieties of *Eubacterium*, a rather ill-defined genus which includes a number of anaerobic, non-sporing, Gram-positive rods that generally produce gas from glucose. This is an area where further work

is required before clear statements can be made as to the identity of these particular anaerobes. Fortunately they do not usually represent a numerically important proportion of the plaque flora, as far as is known, but presumptive *Eubacteria*, including *E. alactolyticum*, have been isolated from the advancing front of carious dentine.

4.8.3 *Gram-negative cocci*

Aerobic

Several species of aerobic, catalase- and oxidase-positive, Gram-negative cocci belonging to the genus *Neisseria* are commonly isolated from plaque. The taxonomy of this group of organisms is very confused at present, and there is an abundance of names in use which are difficult to define (for example, *N. flava, subflava, per-flava, sicca*, etc.). One species, *N. catarrhalis*, has been transferred to a new genus, *Branhamella*.

Preliminary studies indicate that the *Neisseria* species from the mouth can be divided conveniently into four groups

(1) Saccharolytic, polysaccharide producers.
(2) Saccharolytic, non-polysaccharide producers.
(3) Asaccharolytic, polysaccharide producers.
(4) Asaccharolytic, non-polysaccharide producers.

The most common varieties in plaque appear to belong to group (1). However, further work is required before strains isolated from dental plaque can be identified with confidence.

It has been shown that neisseriae may play a significant role in the colonisation of teeth[30], and approximal plaque samples usually contain relatively large numbers of these organisms. The extracellular polysaccharides produced by some species may be of significance in the ecology of plaque, possibly providing a substrate which can be utilised by other bacteria, or by contributing towards the bulk of the plaque matrix.

Anaerobic

Small anaerobic Gram-negative cocci belong to the genus *Veillonella*, the two species found being *V. alkalescens* and *V. parvula*, are almost invariably present in plaque often in high numbers. These organisms do not provide any great problems for isolation or identification. Metabolically they are interesting in that they can utilise lactic acid, which is an end-product of many of the other bacteria present in plaque. Studies on mixed cultures of *Veillonella* with various other organisms, such as streptococci, have been reported by Dutch workers[74]. It is possible that the presence of lactate-utilising bacteria in plaque might modify the potentially damaging effects of lactic acid produced by streptococci or lactobacilli (chapter 5).

4.8.4   Gram-negative rods and filaments

Bacteroides

Anaerobic Gram-negative rods belonging to the genus *Bacteroides* are commonly present in plaque, particularly near the gingival crevice. Black pigmented varieties have been studied more than non-pigmented ones, probably because they are easier to recognise and isolate from primary isolation plates. Three subspecies of *Bacteroides melaninogenicus* have been described, ss. *intermedius*, ss. *asaccharolyticus* and ss. *melaninogenicus*, and all have been reported from the mouth. Recent taxonomic studies indicate that despite their similar colonial and microscopic appearance, these organism should be divided into at least two separate species[81]. There have been suggestions in the literature that *B. melaninogenicus*, which produces a collagenase, may be of significance in destruction of periodontal tissues in periodontitis.

The non-pigmented *Bacteroides* strains, which include *B. oralis*, are not very well understood at present, and further work on these is required. The common intestinal inhabitant, *B. fragilis*, which is frequently implicated in anaerobic infections all over the body, does not appear to be a prominent member of the flora of dental plaque, if present at all. However further studies are needed to confirm this impression and to establish the identity of the fairly high numbers of non-pigmented, Gram-negative rods found in plaque.

Fusobacterium

Long, spindle-shaped, filamentous rods of the genus *Fusobacterium* are also commonly isolated from plaque, and usually can be recognised on the basis of their colonial and microscopic morphology. The diagnosis is readily confirmed by showing that they produce butyric acid as a major end-product of glucose utilisation. These organisms have frequently been implicated, together with spirochaetes, in acute ulcerative gingivitis (Vincent's gingivitis).

Other Gram-negative microorganisms

Leptotrichia buccalis   This is another anaerobic filamentous rod which sometimes resembles fusobacteria microscopically. In young cultures it may appear to be slightly Gram-positive, but has been shown to possess a cell wall composition more typical of Gram-negative organisms. This species produces characteristic rhizoid colonies on culture plates.

Although isolated quite commonly from plaque samples, *L. buccalis* is usually only present in low numbers and its significance, either in plaque ecology or disease processes, is unknown at present.

Aerobic or facultative Gram-negative rods are also recovered from plaque. *Haemophilus* species are probably present much more commonly than most people have hitherto realised[75,79]. It is likely that their presence in plaque has often been obscured by overgrowth of other bacteria on non-selective media, but suitable selective media (for example, chocolate agar containing 10 units/ml bacitracin and 5 μg/ml. cloxacillin) can be used to demonstrate them.

Curved, motile, anaerobic rods are present in plaque and these have been described as *Vibrio* or

Campylobacter species. In addition, small protozoa called *Selenomonas sputigenum* are also found. All of these, and other types which often defy precise identification, are commonly isolated in small numbers from dental plaque, and their numbers are greater in samples from the gingival crevice[80].

Spirochaetes

Several morphologically different types of spirochaetes can be demonstrated in dark-field preparations of plaque, particularly from gingival areas or periodontal pockets. The small spirochaetes have been differentiated into three species, *Treponema denticola*, *T. macredentium* and *T. oralis*[76]. The large spirochaetes include *Borrelia vincentii*. Special techniques are required for isolation and characterisation of these strictly anaerobic organisms, and they are not seen on routine culture plates such as blood agar. They can be isolated from dental plaque by inoculating material on to a membrane filter which is laid on the surface of a serum-enriched agar plate. After incubation, the spirochaetes grow through the filter into the agar beneath, while the other bacteria are confined to the upper surface of the filter. Subcultures can be made from the 'haze' of spirochaetal growth in the agar.

Purification and maintenance of cultures of spirochaetes is extremely difficult and is usually only carried out in a few specialist laboratories.

Other microorganisms

From time to time, bacteria other than those described above are isolated from dental plaque, although often these are transient inhabitants. In addition to bacteria, it is sometimes possible to demonstrate the presence of yeasts, mycoplasmas and also several types of protozoa, including amoebae and trichomonads.

Morphological examination of dental plaque, either at the light-microscopic level using dark-ground or phase contrast illumination, or at the electron-microscopic level, frequently shows the presence of microorganisms which are not normally, if ever, cultivated in the laboratory. It is clear that more sophisticated methods are required to isolate the very fastidious organisms, and particular attention must be paid to achieve appropriate conditions for strict anaerobes. As laboratory techniques improve, it is likely that other microorganisms, hitherto unrecognised, will be discovered to play a significant role in dental plaque.

Further reading

Bowden, G. H. and Hardie J. M. (1978). Oral pleomorphic (coryneform) Gram-positive rods. In *Coryneform Bacteria* (Ed. I. J. Bousefield and A. G. Cally), Special Publications of the Society for General Microbiology No. 1, Academic Press, London, New York and San Francisco, pp. 235–63

Hardie, J. M. and Marsh, P. D. (1978). Streptococci and the human oral flora. In *Streptococci* (Ed. F. A. Skinner and L. B. Quesnel), Society for Applied Bacteriology Symposium Series No. 7, Academic Press, London, New York and San Francisco, pp. 157–206

Melcher, A. H. and Zarb, G. A. (Eds) (1976). Preventive dentistry. Nature, pathogenicity and clinical control of plaque. *Oral Sciences Reviews*, 9, Munksgaard, Copenhagen

Nolte, W. A. (Ed.). *Oral Microbiology*. Mosby, St. Louis

Parker, M. T. (Ed.) *Pathogenic Streptococci*. Reedbooks Ltd., Chertsey, Surrey

Skinner, F. A. and Carr, J. G. (Eds). *The Normal Microbial Flora of Man*. Society for Applied Bacteriology Symposium Series, No. 3, Academic Press, London and New York

References

1. McHugh, W. D. (Ed.) (1970). *Dental Plaque*, E. and S. Livingstone, Edinburgh and London

2. James, P. M. C. and Beal, J. F. (1974). Dental epidemiology and survey procedures, in '*Dental Public Health. An Introduction to Community Dentistry*' (Ed. Slack, G. L.), John Wright, Bristol

3. Mandel, I. D. (1974). Indices for measurement of soft accumulations in clinical studies of oral hygiene and periodontal disease. *Journal of Periodontal Research*, **9**, suppl. 14, 7–30

4. Greene, J. C. and Vermillion, J. R. (1960). The Oral Hygiene Index: a method for classifying oral hygiene status. *Journal of the American Dental Association*, **61**, 172–9

5. Loe, H. (1967). The Gingival Index, the Plaque Index and the Retention Index. *Journal of Periodontology*, **38**, 610–17

6. Loe, H. and Silness, J. (1963). Periodontal disease in pregnancy. *Acta Odontologica Scandinavica*, **21**, 533–51

7. Chilton, N. W. (Ed.) (1974). International conference on clinical trials of agents used in the prevention/treatment of periodontal diseases. *Journal of Periodontol Research*, **9**, Suppl. 14

8. Egelberg, J. (1970). A review of the development of dental plaque, in *Dental Plaque* (Ed. McHugh, W. D.), E. and S. Livingstone, Edinburgh and London

9. Lindhe, J. and Wicén, P–O (1969). The effects on the gingivae of chewing fibrous foods. *Journal of Periodontal Research*, **14**, 193–201

10. Longhurst, P. and Berman, D. S. (1973). Apples and gingival health. Report of a feasibility study. *British Dental Journal*, **134**, 475–9

11. Loesche, W. J. (1968). Importance of nutrition in gingival crevice microbial ecology. *Periodontics*, **6**, 245–9

12. Egelberg, J. (1965). Local effect of diet on plaque formation and development of gingivitis in dogs. 2. Effect of frequency of meals and tube feeding. *Odontologisk Revy*, **16**, 50

13. Carlsson, J. and Egelberg, J. (1965). Effect of diet on early plaque formation in man.

Odontologisk Revy, **16**, 112

14. Staat, R. H., Gawronsky, T. H., Cressey, D. E., Harris, R. S. and Folke, L. E. A. (1975). Effects of dietary sucrose levels on the quantity and microbial composition of human dental plaque. *Journal of Dental Research*, **74**, 872–80.

15. Gibbons R. J. and Houte, J. van. (1973). On the formation of dental plaques. *Journal of Periodontology*, **44**, 347–60

16. Gibbons, R. J. (1972). Ecology and cariogenic potential of oral streptococci, in *Streptococci and Streptococcal Diseases* (Ed. Wannamaker, L. W. and Matsen, J. M.), Academic Press, New York and London

17. Houte, J. van, Gibbons, R. J. and Pulkkinen, A. J. (1971).Adherence as an ecological determinant for streptococci in the human mouth. *Archives of Oral Biology*, **16**, 1131–41

18. Hay, D. J. (1967). The adsorption of salivary proteins by hydroxyapatite and enamel. *Archives of Oral Biology*, **12**, 937–46

19. Saxton, C. A. (1975). The formation of human dental plaque *M.Phil. Thesis*, Univ. of London

20. Frank, R. M. and Brendel, A. (1966). Ultrastructure of the approximal dental plaque and the underlying normal and carious enamel. *Archives of Oral Biology*, **11**, 883–912

21. Meckel, A. H. (1965). The formation and properties of organic films on teeth. *Archives of Oral Biology*, **10**, 585–97

22. Leach, S. A. and Saxton, C. A. (1966). An electron microscopic study of the acquired pellicle and plaque formation on the enamel of human incisors. *Archives of Oral Biology*, **11**, 1081–94

23. Lenz, H. and Muhlemann, H. R. (1963). Repair of etched enamel exposed to the oral environment. *Helvetica Odontologica Acta*, **7**, 47–49

24. Armstrong, W. G. and Hayward, A. F. (1968). Acquired organic integuments of human enamel: a comparison of analytical studies with optical, phase-contrast and

electron microscope examinations. *Caries Research*, **2**, 294–305

25. Sonju, T. and Rolla, G. (1973). Chemical analysis of the acquired pellicle formed in two hours on cleaned human teeth *in vivo*. *Caries Research*, **7**, 30–8

26. Armstrong, W. G. (1968). Origin and nature of the acquired pellicle. *Proceedings of the Royal Society of Medicine*, **61**, 923–30

27. Lie, T. (1975). Pellicle formation on hydroxyapatite splints attached to the human dentition: morphologic confirmation of the concept of adsorption. *Archives of Oral Biology*, **20**, 739–42

28. Socransky, S. S. and Manganiello, A. D. (1971). The oral microbiota of man from birth to senility. *Journal of Periodontology*, **42**, 485–96

29. Saxton, C. A. (1973). Scanning electron microscopic study of the formation of dental plaque. *Caries Research*, **7**, 102–19

30. Ritz, H. L. (1970). The role of aerobic Neisseriae in the initial formation of dental plaque, in *Dental Plaque* (Ed. McHugh, W. D.), E. and S. Livingstone, Edinburgh and London

31. Ritz, H. L. (1967). Microbial population shifts in developing human dental plaque. *Archives of Oral Biology*, **12**, 1561–8

32. Slack, G. L. and Bowden, G. H. (1965). Preliminary studies of experimental dental plaque *in vivo*. *Advances in Fluoride Research and Dental Caries Prevention*, **3**, 193–215

33. Kenney, E. B. and Ash, M. M. (1969). Oxidation–reduction potential of developing plaque, periodontal pockets and gingival sulci. *Journal of Periodontology*, **40**, 630–3

34. Leach, S. A. (1970). A review of the biochemistry of dental plaque, in *Dental Plaque* (Ed. McHugh, W. D.), E. and S. Livingstone, Edinburgh and London

35. Guggenheim, B. (1970). Extracellular polysaccharides and microbial plaque. *International Dental Journal*, **20**, 657–78

36. Carlsson, J. Newbrun, E and Krasse, B.

(1969). Purification and properties of dextransucrase from *Streptococcus sanguis*. *Archives of Oral Biology*, **14**, 469–78

37. Newbrun, E. (1971). Dextransucrase from *Streptococcus sanguis*, Further characterization. *Caries Research*, **5**, 124–34

38. Hotz, P., Guggenheim, B and Schmid, R. (1972). Carbohydrates in pooled dental plaque. *Caries Research*, **6**, 103–21

39. Bowden, G. H. (1969). The components of the cell wall and extracellular slime of four strains of *Staphylococcus salivarius* isolated from human dental plaque. *Archives of Oral Biology*, **14**, 685–97

40. McDougall, W. A. (1963). Studies on the dental plaque 2. The histology of the developing interproximal plaque. *Australian Dental Journal*, **8**, 398–407

41. Listgarten, M. A. Mayo, H. E. and Tremblay, R. (1975). Development of dental plaque on epoxy resin crowns in man. A light and electron microscopic study. *Journal of Periodontology*, **46**, 10–26

42. Listgarten, M. A. Mayo, H. E. and Amsterdam, M. (1973). Ultrastructure of the attachment device between coccal and filamentous microorganisms in 'corn-cob' formations of dental plaque. *Archives of Oral Biology*, **18**, 651

43. Newman, H. N. and Poole, D. F. G. (1974). Structural and ecological aspects of dental plaque, in *The Normal Microbial Flora of Man* (Ed. Skinner, F. A. and Carr, J. G.), Academic Press, New York and London

44. Schroeder, H. E. and De Boever, J. (1970). The structure of microbial dental plaque, in *Dental Plaque* (Ed. McHugh, W. D.), E. and S. Livingstone, Edinburgh and London

45. Critchley, P., Saxton, C. A. and Kolendo, A. B. (1968). The histology and histochemistry of dental plaque. *Caries Research*, **2**, 115–29

46. Bowden, G. H., Hardie, J. M. and Slack, G. L. (1975). Microbial variations in approximal dental plaque. *Caries Research*, **9**, 253–77

47. Gibbons, R. J., Socransky, S. S., Araujo, W. C. de and Houte, J. van (1964). Studies of the predominant cultivable microflora of dental plaque. *Archives of Oral Biology*, **9**, 365–70

48. Handelman, S. L. and Hess, C. (1966). Bacterial populations of selected tooth surface sites. *Journal of Dental Research*, **48**, 67–70

49. Socransky, S. S., Gibbons, R. J., Dale, A. C. Bortnick, L., Rosenthal, E. and MacDonald, J. B. (1963). The microbiota of the gingival crevice area of man. 1. Total microscopic and viable counts of specific organisms. *Archives of Oral Biology*, **8**, 275–80

50. Syed, S. A. and Loesche, W. J. (1973). Efficiency of various growth media in recovering oral bacteria flora from human dental plaque. *Applied Microbiology*, **26**, 459–65

51. Gordon, D. F. Stutman, M. and Loesche, W. J. (1971). Improved isolation of anaerobic bacteria from the gingival crevice area of man. *Applied Microbiology*, **21**, 1046–50

52. Gilmour, M. N. and Poole, A. E. (1970). Growth stimulation of the mixed microbial flora of human dental plaques by haemin. *Archives of Oral Biology*, **15**, 1343–53

53. Poole, A. E. and Gilmour, M. N. (1971). The variability of unstandardized plaques obtained from single or multiple subjects. *Archives of Oral Biology*, **16**, 681–7

54. Loesche, W. J., Hockett, R. N. and Syed, S. A. (1972). The predominant cultivable flora of tooth surface plaque removed from institutionalized subjects. *Archives of Oral Biology*, **17**, 1311–25

55. Loesche, W. J. and Green, E. (1972). Comparison of various plaque parameters in individuals with poor oral hygiene. *Journal of Periodontal Research*, **7**, 173–9

56. Hardie, J. M. and Bowden, G. H. (1974). The normal microbial flora of the mouth, in *The Normal Microbial Flora of Man* (Ed. Skinner, F. A. and Carr, J. G.), Academic Press, New York and London

57. Hardie, J. M. and Bowden, G. H. (1975). Bacterial flora of dental plaque. *British Medical Bulletin*, **31**, 131–6

58. Loesche, W. J. and Syed, S. A. (1973). The predominant cultivable flora of carious plaque and carious dentine. *Caries Research*, **7**, 201–16

59. Gibbons, R. J., Socransky, S. S., Araujo, W. C. de and Houte, J. van (1964). Studies on the predominant cultivable microflora of dental plaque. *Archives of Oral Biology*, **9**, 365

60. Howell, A., Rizzo, A. and Paul, F. (1965). Cultivable bacteria in developing and mature dental calculus. *Archives of Oral Biology*, **10**, 307–13

61. Donoghue, H. D. (1974). Composition of dental plaque obtained from eight sites in the mouth of a ten-year-old girl. *Journal of Dental Research*, **53**, 1289–93

62. Gibbons, R. J., Depaola, P. F., Spinell, D. M. and Skobe, Z. (1974). Interdental localization of *Streptococcus mutans* as related to dental caries experience. *Infection and Immunity*, **9**, 481–8

63. Bowden, G. H. and Hardie, J. M. (1973). Commensal and pathogenic *Actinomyces* species in man, in *Actinomycetales: Characteristics and Practical Importance*, Society of Applied Bacteriological, Symposium Series No. 2

64. Bowden, G. H., Hardie, J. M. and Fillery, E. D. (1976). Antigens from *Actinomyces* species and their value in identification, *Journal of Dental Research*, **55**, Special Issue A, A192–A204

65. Colman, G and Williams, R. E. O. (1972). Taxonomy of some human viridans streptococci, in *Streptococci and Streptococcal Diseases* (Ed. Wannamaker, L. W. and Matsen, J. M.), Academic Press, New York and London

66. Carlsson, J. (1968). A numerical taxonomic study of human oral streptococci. *Odontologisk Revy*, **19**, 137–60

67. Hardie, J. M. and Bowden, G. H. (1976).

Physiological classification of oral viridans streptococci. *Journal of Dental Research,* **55**, Special Issue A, A166–A176

68. Clarke, J. K. (1924). On the bacterial factor in the aetiology of dental caries. *British Journal of Experimental Pathology*, **5**, 141–7

69. Bratthall, D. (1970). Demonstration of five serological groups of streptococcal strains resembling *Streptococcus mutans. Odontologisk Revy,* **21**, 143–52

70. Perch, B., Kjems, E and Ravn, T. (1974). Biochemical and serological properties of *Streptococcus mutans* from various human and animal sources. *Acta Pathologica et Microbiologica Scandinavica, Section B,* **82**, 357–70

71. Coykendall, A. L. (1974). Four types of *Streptococcus mutans* based on their genetic, antigenic and biochemical characteristics. *Journal of General Microbiology,* **83**, 327–38

72. Mejare, B. and Edwardsson, S. (1975). *Streptoccus milleri* (Guthof); an indigenous organism of the human oral cavity. *Archives of Oral Biology,* **20**, 757–62

73. Loesche, W. J., Paunio, K. U., Woolfolk, M. P. and Hockett, R. N. (1974). Collagenolytic activity of dental plaque associated with periodontal pathology. *Infection and Immunity*, **9**, 329–36

74. Mikx, F. H. M. and Van der Hoeven, J. S. (1975). Symbiosis of *Streptococcus mutans* and *Veillonella alcalescens* in mixed continuous cultures. *Archives of Oral Biology,* **20**, 407–10

75. Tuyau, J. E. and Sims, W. (1975). Occurrence of haemophili in dental plaque and their association with neuraminidase activity. *Journal of Dental Research,* **54**, 737–9

76. Socransky, S. S., Listgarten, M., Hubersak, C., Cotmore, J. and Clark, A. (1969). Morphological and biochemical differentiation of three types of small oral spirochaete. *Journal of Bacteriology,* **98**, 878–82

77. Guggenheim, B. and Schroeder, H. (1967). Biochemical and morphological aspects of extracellular polysaccharides produced by cariogenic streptococci. *Helvetica Odontologica Acta,* **11**, 131–52

78. Linzer, R. (1976). Serotype polysaccharide antigens of *Streptococcus mutans*: composition and serological cross-reactions, in *Immunologic Aspects of Dental Caries* (Ed. Bowen, W. H. Genco, R. J., and O'Brian, T. C., Information Retrieval Inc., Washington DC and London

79. Kilian, M. and Schiott, C. R. (1975). Haemophili and related bacteria in the human oral cavity. *Archives of Oral Biology,* **20**, 791–6

80. Van Palenstein Helderman, W. H. (1975). Total viable count and differential count of *Vibrio (Campylobacter) sputorum, Fusobacterium nucleatum, Selenomona sputigena, Bacteroides ochraceus* and *Veillonella* in the inflamed human gingival crevice. *Journal of Periodontal Research,* **10**, 294–305

81. Shah, H. N. Williams, R. A. D., Bowden, G. H. and Hardie, J. M. (1976). Comparison of the biochemical properties of *Bacteroides melaninogenicus* from dental plaque and other sites. *Journal of Applied Bacteriology,* **41**, 473–92

82. Mitchell, R. (1976). Mechanism of attachment of micro-organisms to surfaces. In *Microbial Aspects of Dental Caries.* (Ed. H. M. Stiles, W. J. Loesche and T. C. O'Brien). A Special Supplement of Microbiology Abstracts, Vol. 1., 47–53. Information Retrieval Inc., Washington DC and London

83. Rutter, P. R. and Abbott, A. (1978). A study of the interaction between oral streptococci and hard surfaces. *Journal of General Microbiology,* **105**, 219–226

84. Loesche, W. J. (1975). Bacterial succession in dental plaque: role in dental disease. *Microbiology*, 1975, 132–136.

85. Österberg, S. K-A, Sudo, S. Z. and Folke, L. E. A. (1976). Microbial succession in subgingival plaque of man. *Journal of*

Periodontal Research, **11**, 243–55

86. Ronström, A., Edwardsson, S. and Attström, R. (1977). *Streptococcus sanguis* and *Streptococcus salivarius* in early plaque formation on plastic films. *Journal of Periodontal Research*, **12**, 331–9.

87. Socransky, S. S., Manganiello, A. D., Propas, D., Oram, V. and Van Houte, J. (1977). Bacteriological studies of developing supragingival dental plaque. *Journal of Periodontal Research*, **12**, 107–19

89. Alshamaony, L., Goodfellow, M.,

Minnikin, D. E., Bowden, G. H. and Hardie, J. M. (1977). Fatty and mycolic acid composition of *Bacterionema matruchotii* and related organisms. *Journal of General Microbiology*, **98**, 205–13

90. Mouton, C., Reynolds, H. and Genco, R. J. (1977). Combined micromanipulation, culture and immunofluorescent techniques for isolation of the coccal organisms comprising the 'corn-cob' configuration of human dental plaque. *Journal Biology Buccale*, **5**, 321–32

Chapter 5

Biochemical Events in Dental Plaque

5.1   Introduction

The objective of this chapter is to outline the significance of some of the biochemical processes of dental plaque. Energy metabolism is of central importance for bacteria, which are able to use various materials as energy sources, and produce characteristic end-products from them. The impact of these end-products, and also materials produced by extracellular hydrolyses and decarboxylations, are briefly described together with the role of salivary buffers, and the consumption of a strong acid in plaque. Reference is made to the unlikely role of complexing agents in the dissolution of enamel mineral.

The central role of glycogen as an intracellular store of energy is emphasised, although polyphosphate may act as a sink for phosphate within the cells of plaque bacteria.

Extracellular polymers make a contribution to the bulk of plaque and its ability to retain acids at the tooth surface.

Finally, the occurrence of the inorganic components of plaque that are likely to affect tooth mineral solubility (calcium, phosphate and fluoride) are summarised, and the classical theories of caries are reviewed in the light of the biochemistry of plaque.

5.2   Metabolism of Substrates by Plaque Bacteria

Metabolism is the term given to all the biochemical reactions of an organism. *Catabolism* is that part of the metabolism which involves degradation of organic starting materials, called *substrates*, to form a number of end-products (called *metabolites* or *catabolites*). Thus, foodstuffs are converted to waste products by catabolism, and in the process energy is released for use by the organism concerned. The other major aspect of metabolism is called *anabolism*, which comprises all the synthetic processes and which uses much of the energy produced in catabolism.

Strains of bacteria are found in dental plaque which are aerobic (requiring oxygen), facul-

tatively anaerobic (able to live with or without oxygen), and obligately anaerobic (unable to tolerate oxygen). The two types of anaerobes predominate in plaque, especially as the layer thickens and oxygen penetration into the depths of the plaque is reduced. Anaerobic catabolism of substrates involves no use of oxygen, and the end-products therefore have the same empirical formula as the starting material. Such anaerobic metabolic transformations are called *fermentations*. For example, glucose catabolism by lactic acid bacteria may be summarised:

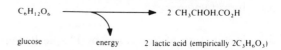

$$C_6H_{12}O_6 \longrightarrow 2\ CH_3CHOH.CO_2H$$

glucose   energy   2 lactic acid (empirically $2C_3H_6O_3$)

Fermentations are therefore molecular rearrangements in which a certain amount of energy is made available to the bacterium. In a process such as lactic acid fermentation, end-products other than lactic acid may account for 10 per cent of the glucose used. An accurate picture of the process is thus not obtained by a simple equation such as that given above, and a fermentation balance table (for example, table 5.3) is to be preferred, especially for the more complex fermentations where no single end-product predominates. Carbohydrates are the preferred fermentation substrates for many bacteria, but amino acids may be used by some species as alternatives to carbohydrates, while other organisms may be unable to use carbohydrates and depend upon amino acids. Some bacteria can use the fermentation products of other species as substrates, and examples of this are found in dental plaque. Fermentation of nucleic acid bases is rare, and fats seem not to be good substrates for fermentative metabolism; hence these two groups of compounds will not be considered here.

Whatever the type of substrate used for fermentation it should be emphasised that the process of fermentation is energy-supplying. Besides needing a supply of energy for growth, oral bacteria also need a series of structural components in order to synthesise cell material. Oral bacteria are often quite demanding in their requirements for growth; for example, strains of *Streptococcus sanguis* have been shown to need nine amino acids and vitamins, in addition to mineral salts and a carbohydrate fermentation substrate for energy.

5.2.1 Catabolism of carbohydrates

Dental plaque contains bacteria capable of using many different carbohydrates as substrates. Use is made of this fact in the identification and classification of bacteria, but many of these substrates are sugars which occur at a very low concentration, if at all, in the human diet and in saliva, and are therefore not significant in the nutrition of plaque bacteria.

The total carbohydrate content of the diet varies from country to country, and is lowest in the richer western nations (table 5.1). The majority of carbohydrate foods are supplied by starchy plant products. Sucrose (cane or beet sugar) consumption is highest in the richer countries where total carbohydrate intake is lowest. It has been estimated that the average

Table 5.1 Composition of the average diet in selected countries 1954–56 (from FAO (UN) Food Balance Sheets)

Country	Protein	Per cent calories from fat	Carbohydrate
Japan	12	8	80
India	11	12	77
Italy	12	22	66
France	14	29	57
Belgium	12	35	53
UK	11	38	51
USA	12	39	49

American and Briton eats sucrose equivalent to 500 cal per day, amounting to over one-third of his total carbohydrate consumption. As outlined in chapter 1, sucrose has a special role in the production of dental caries, and this will be emphasised in this chapter and also chapter 9. Sucrose is a disaccharide, its two sugar components being βD-fructose and αD-glucose. They are linked from carbon atom 1 of glucose to carbon atom 2 of fructose by a bond which has a free energy of hydrolysis similar to that of adenosine triphosphate (ATP):

* 1–6 are the numbers of the carbon atoms in each ring

The starch which comprises much of the carbohydrate we eat consists of αD-glucose molecules linked in chains by bonds between carbon atom 1 of one glucose and carbon 4 of another:

This linear soluble polymer called amylose, commonly 250–300 glucose units long, accounts for 20–30 per cent of native starches. Glycogen, which we eat in meats and in liver, is a branched polymer of glucose, containing up to 30 000 glucose units per molecule, in which the main chains are of the amylose type, but with a branch point every 10–14 glucose units. Such branches are provided by bonds between carbon 1 and carbon 6 of two glucose molecules:

Amylopectin, which comprises 70–80 per cent of starch, has a similar structure to glycogen, but is less branched and has a smaller molecular weight. Digestion of starch and glycogen begins in the mouth, where hydrolysis by salivary amylase produces lower-molecular-weight saccharides including glucose and maltose. Such hydrolysis products are suitable fermentation substrates for many plaque bacteria (table 5.2). Glucose, galactose and fructose are isomers which are metabolised by the glycolytic and analogous pathways in bacteria. They are equivalent as sources of energy. Metabolism leads to a mixture of fermentation end-products. Minor differences in the proportions of metabolic end-products are found for different strains of bacteria grown on glucose (e.g. a cariogenic strain of streptococcus and a non-cariogenic strain, table 5.3). The differences between these types are no greater than that found between two non-cariogenic strains, and such differences are not significant in the caries-producing potential of the strains.

Table 5.2   Dietary sugars significant as substrates for plaque bacteria

Sugar	Occurrence
MONOSACCHARIDES	
Glucose	Small amounts in many foods and beverages, minor end-product of oral starch digestion, occurs in equal amounts with fructose in 'golden syrup' (partially hydrolysed sucrose syrup) and with maltose and higher saccharides in 'liquid glucose' (hydrolysed starch used in confectionery)
Fructose	Small amounts in some foods particularly fruits, 'golden syrup' (above), becoming more common due to use of increasing amounts of glucose isomerase-treated corn syrup, particularly in North America. Fructose polymers occur as storage compounds in some plants
Others	Free pentose sugars occur in fruits, particularly berries
DISACCHARIDES	
Maltose	Small amounts free in honey and other foods, major end-product of starch digestion, also found in 'liquid glucose'
Sucrose	Widely used in manufactured foods, may be one-third of the total carbohydrate in diets in Western countries; also in honey, treacle, molasses and 'golden syrup'
Lactose	Glucose-galactose disaccharide, occurs in milk (4–8 % w/v)

The majority of lactic acid bacteria ferment sugars producing at least 90 per cent of lactic acid (e.g. streptococci, table 5.3, and many lactobacilli) when growing rapidly. Such bacteria are called 'homofermenters' or 'homolactic' strains, but the proportion of lactic acid formed may be altered markedly by the growth conditions. Some species of lactobacilli produce 40 per cent or more of metabolites other than lactic acid according to a simplified linear formula that approximates to:

$$C_6H_{12}O_6 \longrightarrow CH_3.CHOH.CO_2H + CO_2 + CH_3CH_2OH$$

glucose   lactic acid   ethanol

Heterofermentative lactobacilli probably account for 10–25 per cent of the total lactobacilli of plaque, and they may form a rather higher proportion of the lactobacillus population in carious dentine and enamel. The total lactobacillus count in saliva or plaque is low, and the carious lesion, once formed, seems to provide them with a favourable environment for growth, probably because of their tolerance towards acidic conditions.

When bacteria are grown anaerobically on carbohydrates in the presence of all the nutrients they require, the glucose is fermented completely. Incorporation of glucose carbon into the components of the cell is negligible and glucose is thus used entirely as an energy source, not for the synthesis of new cell material. In glycolysis, the pathway by which homofermentative lactic acid bacteria (such as the streptococci) metabolise glucose, 2 mol of the 'energy-coinage' material adenosine triphosphate (ATP) are synthesised per mol of glucose. Because all bacterial cells contain the same types of structural components in about the same quantities, it takes the same amount of energy to produce a fixed weight of any type of cell from growth requisites such as amino acids. Any bacterium using glycolysis obeys the following relationship: 1 mol glucose

(180 g) will produce 2 mol ATP sufficient for the growth of 20 g (dry weight) of cells. Homofermenters will produce approaching 180 g of lactic acid in the process (2 mol). Therefore, such

Table 5.3 Fermentation balances of cariogenic and non-cariogenic streptococci (from Jordan[1]).

Product	Cariogenic strain	Non-cariogenic strain
	(mol Product per 100 mol Glucose)	
Lactic acid $CH_3.CHOH.CO_2H$	181.09	184.54
Acetic acid $CH_3.CO_2H$	9.18	9.52
CO_2	8.31	10.96
Ethanol $CH_3.CH_2OH$	2.77	5.75
Formic acid $H.CO_2H$	3.42	4.52
Acetoin $CH_3.CO.CHOH.CH_3$	0.60	0.20
Diacetyl $CH_3.CO.CO.CH_3$	0.01	0.01
Total recovery	96.98 %	100.08 %

bacteria may produce nine times their own dry weight of lactic acid during growth, and the significance of this will be discussed in section 5.3.1 with respect to the acid produced by dental plaque.

Recent work has demonstrated the biochemical basis of the departure from homolactic fermentation with differing growth conditions[2, 3]. There are two alternative fates for pyruvate, the well-known reduction to lactate, and splitting into formate and acetyl CoA by pyruvate formate lyase (PFL):

$$CH_3.CO.CO_2H + CoASH \rightarrow CH_3.CO\text{-}SCoA + HCO_2H$$

pyruvate   acetyl CoA   formate

followed by the conversion of acetyl CoA into acetate and ethanol. Lactate dehydrogenase (LDH) of *Streptococcus mutans* is stimulated by the high concentration of fructose diphosphate in cells exposed to plentiful carbohydrate, while PFL is simultaneously inhibited by the high concentration of glyceraldehyde-3-phosphate

(G3P):

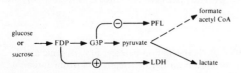

This explains the plentiful production of lactic acid when high concentrations of sugars are present in plaque, or when the bacteria are grown rapidly under cultural conditions in which carbohydrate is not the growth-limiting factor.

By contrast, when fermentable carbohydrate is not available in high concentration, or when bacteria are grown in conditions where carbohydrate is growth-limiting, the lower intracellular concentration of FDP and G3P release the stimulation of LDH and the inhibition of PFL, respectively. At the same time, such cells have an induced synthesis of PFL and therefore form much more acetate ethanol and formate and less lactate.

5.2.2 Catabolism of amino acids

Although carbohydrates are the preferred substrates of most oral bacteria, some strains use amino acids as alternative sources, and others catabolise amino acids but not carbohydrates.

Amino acids are found in low concentrations in saliva, in foods, and in the fluid that oozes from the gingiva in gingivitis. The lysis (breakdown) of both host cells and plaque bacteria releases further small quantities. Much greater amounts of amino acids occur combined in the proteins of foodstuffs, saliva, the host cells and the oral bacteria, but combined amino acids are not available for catabolism until the protein molecules which contain them are hydrolysed by proteolytic enzymes. Proteolysis occurs in human digestion, but proteases are not secreted in the saliva. The limited availability of nutrients such as amino acids contributes to the low growth rate of bacteria in dental plaque, which is

much less than in excess nutrient concentration. However, some oral bacteria produce proteases which release amino acids that are available to all bacteria in the vicinity. These proteases have been implicated in damage to the gingival tissues.

Degradation of amino acids by oral bacteria is not as well studied as the catabolism of carbohydrates, and in many cases the energy yield and the pathway of metabolism is unknown. The fermentation of arginine by certain oral streptococci and lactobacilli is, however, well known:

$$\begin{array}{ccc}
NH_2 & & NH_3 \\
| & & + \\
C{=\!\!=}NH & \xrightarrow[\substack{\text{arginine} \\ \text{dihydrolase} \\ \text{(two enzymes} \\ \text{are involved)}}]{} & CO_2 + NH_3 \\
| & +2H_2O & + \\
NH & & NH_2 \\
| & & | \\
(CH_2)_3 & & (CH_2)_3 \\
| & & | \\
CH{-\!\!-}NH_2 & & CH{-\!\!-}NH_2 \\
| & & | \\
CO_2H & & CO_2H \\
\text{arginine} & & \text{ornithine}
\end{array}$$

This simple fermentation comprises the hydrolysis of the guanido group of arginine, producing the shorter amino acid ornithine together with carbon dioxide and two moles of ammonia. One mole of ATP is synthesised for each mole of arginine, compared with glycolysis in which two moles of ATP are produced for each mole of glucose. Bacteria which possess the arginine dihydrolase system can grow on arginine as an alternative to carbohydrates, and it is noteworthy that the metabolic end-products are basic rather than acidic. The fermentation of arginine by streptococci and lactobacilli is unusual as these bacteria are primarily fermenters of carbohydrates. In other groups of bacteria, however, amino acid fermentation is more significant in the overall plan of energy production. Several *Bacteroides* grow well on media containing hydrolysed proteins but no carbohydrate, and produce a mixture of volatile organic acids as catabolic end-products. Many amino acids can be fermented, so it is worth emphasising that not all acids produced in dental plaque are derived from carbohydrate fermentation. The acids formed by catabolism of amino acids include acetic, propionic, butyric and valeric acids, but the proportions of these vary with the strain, and with the mixture of amino acids present. These acids are easily demonstrated in dental plaque, but are weaker than lactic acid. A second important consideration is that amino acid fermentations usually produce a net excess of acid. In this respect, arginine is exceptional as it contains a higher proportion of nitrogen to carbon than any other amino acid, and its fermentation produces a net excess of base.

Other degradative processes which involve amino acids, but which are not concerned with energy production, include deamination and decarboxylation. These reactions, which are not fermentations, are brought about by enzymes which are extracellular, or located at the cell surface, and are described in section 5.3.2.

5.2.3 Catabolism of the products of other bacteria

Bacteria in dental plaque are continually dying and lysing (breaking open) and in so doing release their components, as nutrients for other bacteria. The phenomenon of 'regrowth', 'cannibalism' or 'syntrophism' ensures that some bacteria in plaque survive at the expense of others. However, besides this re-use of the structural components of dead cells, some bacteria specialise in the utilisation of the catabolic end-products of other strains, and the most significant genus in this respect is *Veillonella*. Many strains use the products of others as growth-stimulating factors, but *Veillonella* species use three carbon substrates, such as lactic acid, as an energy source.

When plaque is allowed to develop over a period of 9 days[4] the *Veillonella* strains increase in numbers only after the initial colonisation by the lactic acid bacteria. *Veillonella* cannot use carbohydrate because they lack key enzymes of glycolysis[5] and the hexose monophosphate pathway[6]. Lactic acid is metabolised by them in a fermentative process which approximates to:

$$2CH_3.CHOH.CO_2H \longrightarrow CH_3.CH_2.CO_2H + CH_3.CO_2H$$
$$\text{lactic acid} \qquad \text{propionic acid} \qquad \text{acetic acid}$$
$$+ CO_2 + H_2$$

This process provides the energy for the growth of *Veillonella*. The significance of the conversion of one acid into two others in terms of the acid-base relationships of plaque is described in section 5.3.4. The dependence of *Veillonella* on lactic acid bacteria has been demonstrated by growing a strain together with *Streptococcus mutans* in a chemostat[7] and in gnotobiotic rats[8].

5.3 Acid-Base Phenomena in Plaque

From the above discussion it is evident that dental plaque may produce acid or base according to the types of bacteria present and the substrate molecules available to it. The extent of both of these processes and the balance between them is explored in this section.

5.3.1 Acid production in plaque

In all living organisms the metabolic pathways leading from substrates (for example, glucose) to end-products (for example, lactic acid) are linked to energy-generating systems. As we have seen (section 5.2.1) the relationship between glucose fermentation and growth of cells is fixed for bacteria using glycolysis. Because many of the bacteria of plaque use this metabolic process, it is possible to estimate the order of magnitude of lactic acid production by plaque as a consequence of growth on carbohydrate. Given the composition of mixed dental plaque as far as it is presently known, it is reasonable to assume that plaque will have produced approximately its own weight of acid during growth. This is likely to be an overestimate because of the operation of the PFL system (page 107–8) at low growth rates. Although carbohydrates from foodstuffs are available only intermittently to plaque bacteria, many oral bacteria store glycogen for use later, and some extracellular carbohydrates, and carbohydrates from salivary glycoproteins, may also be used*.

Therefore, carbohydrate fermentation is possible in plaque most of the time, although the magnitude of the process is obviously greatest when fermentable carbohydrates are ingested. The amount of plaque per day that can be scraped from the mouth of an individual who is observing standard oral hygiene procedures varies from 1 mg to 50 mg or more. Therefore, the quantity of lactic acid likely to be produced per day is of the same magnitude. The impact which this quantity of acid may have on the pH of the saliva and plaque is discussed in section 5.3.3. It may be argued that some plaque bacteria obtain their energy by fermentation of amino acids rather than of carbohydrates, and this is true. However, as we have seen (section 5.2.2), the fermentation of individual amino acids only rarely produces net base, and fermentation of mixed amino acids by plaque bacteria generally causes a fall in pH. Therefore, amino acid fermentation does not counteract the acid production of carbohydrate fermentation, although amino acid decarboxylation may.

So far, we have considered the chronic production of acid by plaque as it grows. As was explained in chapter 1, the most dramatic pH effects are observed in acute acid production, when fermentable carbohydrate is ingested. The pH of plaque may fall from close to 6 to around 4 in a matter of minutes, and this sharp fall in pH, followed by a slow return to the resting pH when the fermentable carbohydrate is exhausted, is called the 'Stephan curve' (figure 5.1). Stephan[9] noted that the drop in pH was progressively more pronounced in individuals in whom caries was active at the time of the test. The curve was recorded by placing an antimony electrode in

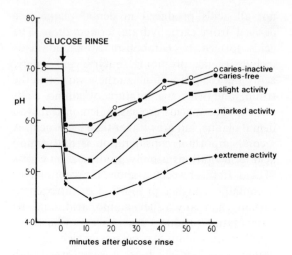

Figure 5.1 The fall in pH of plaque after a rinse with 10 per cent glucose solution in individuals scored for caries activity (after Stephan, 1944[9])

contact with the plaque, and a reference electrode in the saliva in the floor of the mouth. After recording the resting level of pH in an individual at least 1 h after the last meal, on a day during which no fermentable carbohydrates were consumed, the mouth was rinsed for 2 min with 25 ml of 10 per cent glucose. After a further 2 min the pH was recorded again, and at 10-min intervals thereafter. Stephan found that the shape of the curve was the same in all cases, but that both the resting pH value, and the minimum pH value, which occurred at 12 min after the rinse, were lower in individuals with active dental caries. The pH values plotted (figure 5.1) were the means for the number of individuals in each group. If another low-molecular-weight carbohydrate that is readily fermented by plaque bacteria (such as sucrose or fructose) is used instead of glucose, a similar curve is obtained. Low-molecular-weight substances which diffuse into dental plaque, but which are not fermented rapidly in plaque (such as sorbitol, mannitol and xylitol),

---

* If 1.5 l of saliva are formed per day, and this contains 8–10 per cent hexoses (as well as 10–12 per cent of other carbohydrates) in salivary glycoprotein, which is present at a total concentration of 300 mg/100 ml, then the day's flow of saliva contains over 400 mg of hexose component and more than this amount of other sugar molecules. If the hexose component were completely used for fermentation in the presence of adequate other nutrients, it would support the growth of over 200 mg of plaque. Clearly, the utilisation of sugars from glycoprotein is incomplete in the mouth (partly because it is polymeric, partly because much of the hexose is not glucose), but the quantity of carbohydrate potentially available is considerable!

do not produce a large pH drop or perhaps none at all (see section 9.3.2). Furthermore, little or no pH drop is observed with high-molecular-weight polysaccharides such as starch. This may be for one, or both, of the following reasons:

(1)   The starch molecules are long and do not penetrate into the packed mass of the plaque.
(2)   Starch must be hydrolysed to glucose and/or maltose before it can be fermented by plaque bacteria.

Starch hydrolysis can be effected by salivary amylase, but the extent to which this occurs in the mouth is negligible if the starch is soluble and rapidly cleared from the mouth. If the physical form of the starch favours its retention in proximity to the plaque, the production of diffusable and fermentable sugars from it will be facilitated. The effect of frequently consuming fermentable carbohydrate is to produce a series of Stephan curves. If the pH drop due to one ingestion of carbohydrate occurs before the plaque pH has returned to resting level after the previous ingestion, a summation of curves may occur which results in decalcifying pH values being maintained in the plaque for prolonged periods of time.

Recent results indicate that despite the emphasis on the importance of lactic acid in caries, there are considerable concentrations of other acids in plaque[10, 11]. In earlier sections we have seen how volatile acids can be formed from carbohydrates at low concentrations and also from amino acids. The actual concentration ranges of the various acid anions in dental plaque were $1-110$ mmol/l formate, $21-81$ mmol/l acetate, $3-208$ mmol/l lactate, $1-16$ mmol/l propionate, and $1.5-75$ mmol/l butyrate. Variation within these ranges was particularly due to variation in plaque mass and availability of sucrose. The light thin plaques tended to have higher formate and butyrate together with a lower propionate than heavy plaques. This was considered to be due more to the limitation of substrate availability in heavy plaque rather than to differences in the microflora. The glycolytic

process, which gives rise mainly to lactic acid when homolactic bacteria are exposed to excess glucose (table 5.3), may produce large proportions of other acids when fermentable carbohydrates are not plentiful (section 5.2.1).

5.3.2   Ammonia and base production in plaque

Fermentation (energy-yielding transformation) of amino acids rarely produces more moles of base than of acid (section 5.2.2), but dental plaque can become alkaline, a circumstance favouring calculus formation (the mineralisation of plaque). This may be achieved by two mechanisms which do not yield energy for use by the cells concerned. These are the hydrolysis of urea by urease:

$$\begin{array}{c} NH_2 \\ | \\ C=O \\ | \\ NH_2 \end{array} + H_2O \longrightarrow \begin{array}{c} NH_3 \\ \\ \\ NH_3 \end{array} + CO_2$$

and the decarboxylation of amino acids to produce carbon dioxide and a primary amine:

$$R \begin{array}{c} NH_2 \\ | \\ -C- \\ | \\ H \end{array} CO_2H \longrightarrow R.CH_2.NH_2 + CO_2$$

In this last reaction, the amine is much less volatile than the carbon dioxide. Both of these enzymes probably play a part in the production of alkaline conditions in the plaque. Urease is a widespread enzyme among plaque bacteria, and decarboxylases for a number of amino acids have been demonstrated in mixed human plaque[12]. Decarboxylase enzymes require the coenzyme pyridoxal phosphate in order to function. However, adding pyridoxine to the sugar fed to experimental animals does not increase the decarboxylase activity of their plaque, and unfortunately does not reduce their caries score[13], nor is there a decrease in the net acid production caused by adding sugar solutions. Probably the decarboxylases produced by plaque bacteria are fully saturated with pyridoxal phosphate which is firmly bound to the enzyme protein.

It seems likely that urea provides most of the base formed in plaque because of the widespread occurrence of urease, and the large quantity of urea available in the saliva*. Statements are commonly made to the effect that ammonia from urea causes alkaline plaque pH values, but few attempts have been made to measure the activity of urease in plaque. According to Stephan[14], 0.1 per cent urea abolished the net acid production caused in homogenised plaque by 6 per cent glucose; during a 4–5 h period the pH remained between 8.0 and 7.1, while the pH of the control sample had fallen to 4.9. Biswas and Kleinberg[15] have shown that 0.17 per cent urea caused the pH of 'suspended salivary sediment' (SSS) to rise from 7.5 to close to 9.0 within an hour. Some of the ammonia formed from urea is used in amino acid synthesis, but this is only a small proportion of the total. Dentifrices containing urea have not been successful in reducing caries, probably because of the intermittent application of urea involved, and the fact that urea is available for base formation at times other than at mealtimes when the formation of acid mainly occurs. Preliminary studies of caries incidence in patients receiving dialysis treatment because of renal failure, show that they have markedly less dental caries than would be expected for adults residing in the same area. Such patients have abnormally high concentrations of urea in their plasma, and therefore in their saliva[16], and these conditions prevail for prolonged periods. This low caries activity occurs with diets that are deliberately low in protein in order to minimise urea formation, but high in carbohydrate and, in particular, intermittent consumption of sweets is

permitted *ad libitum*. Such dietary regimes might be expected to produce rampant caries in non-uraemic individuals[17].

5.3.3   Buffering in saliva and plaque

The complete removal of the salivary glands of hamsters fed on a high-sucrose diet causes a sixfold increase in caries compared to unoperated animals[18]. Such a drastic procedure would be expected to have its effect on the composition of dental plaque, the retention of food in the mouth, and the duration of eating, as well as to deny salivary buffers to the plaque. However, increased caries has also been related to reduced salivary flow (xerostomia) in several pathological states in man. In correlations between salivary composition and caries score, the most significant relationship was with the buffer capacity of the saliva[19].

Saliva was reported to be ineffective as a buffer after dialysis to remove the small molecular components. Two inorganic buffer systems which participate in buffering the plasma also occur in saliva, namely the carbonate buffers (HCO_3^-/H_2CO_3, $pK_a' = 6.1$ at 25°C) and the phosphate system ($HPO_4^{2-}/H_2PO_4^-$, $pK_a^- = 7.2$ at 25°C). The concentration of the carbonate buffers (expressed as volumes CO_2 that can be displaced from 100 ml) lies between 5.5 vol % for resting saliva and as high as 80 vol% for stimulated saliva. This latter figure is higher than the mean value for whole blood (60 vol%), in which the carbonate system is the most significant buffer. Because of its low concentration, inorganic phosphate is a relatively unimportant buffer in plasma (3.36 mg phosphorus/100 ml, range 2.56–4.16), and in whole blood (2.9 mg phosphorus/100 ml, range 2.1–3.8). The concentration of inorganic phosphorus is higher in saliva (14.9 mg phosphorus/100 ml, range 8.1–

---

*   If 1.5 l of saliva are formed per day and the urea concentration is approximately 20 mg/100 ml the total flow of urea into the mouth is 300 mg. If completely hydrolysed by urease this would produce 212 mg of ammonia, more than 10 times the amount that would be needed to neutralise the 50 mg of lactic acid formed during the growth of 50 mg of plaque. Again, hydrolysis by plaque bacteria can account for only a small amount of the urea which flows into the mouth, but the potential capacity of this base-forming mechanism is enormous.

21.7) than in blood or plasma. By contrast with blood, where proteins are the second most important buffers, the proteins of saliva are not considered to contribute greatly to the total buffer capacity[20]. The only significant amino acid residue capable of buffering between pH 5 and 8 is histidine. This amino acid is not uncommon in salivary proteins; indeed, a protein with a very high histidine content (18 per cent)[21] and basic peptides with as much as 26 per cent histidine have been isolated from saliva[22]. However, the total protein content of whole blood is of the order of 100 times higher than that of saliva, and it is undoubtedly this high concentration which makes protein such a significant buffer in blood. There is no doubt that the diffusion of inorganic buffers from the saliva into dental plaque plays a part in reducing the effect of acids produced by plaque bacteria. However, plaque contains proteins (both of bacterial origin and from degraded salivary glycoprotein) in much higher concentration than the saliva and therefore buffering by proteins may be expected to be more significant in plaque than in saliva. A third component of plaque buffers will comprise the salts of weak organic acids (such as acetic and propionic) formed by bacterial metabolism, and neutralised by salivary cations.

Despite these buffering systems, it is clear that the acid-forming potential of plaque is such that when confronted with sufficient fermentable carbohydrate the buffers are 'broken' within minutes, as the pH is observed to fall dramatically in the Stephan curve.

As we have seen, plaque is likely to have formed of the order of its own weight of acid during growth. This acid will diffuse from the plaque as it is formed, at a rate that depends on the rate of acid production, the thickness of plaque and the diffusion-limiting properties of plaque itself. If the acid likely to be formed during the growth of plaque in a day could be dispersed into the 1.5 l of saliva formed per day, the pH of the saliva would be unaltered. The buffer capacity of saliva is enormous relative to this amount of acid. However, the Stephan curve

shows us that plaques do become acid rapidly when presented with fermentable carbohydrate. The damage done to the tooth surface is caused by the intense local production of acid which 'breaks' the buffers of the plaque itself, and is only slowly neutralised by the diffusion of acid into saliva, the diffusion of salivary buffer into plaque, and the dissolution of tooth mineral. Plaque appears to act as a membrane which obeys the laws of diffusion, and its ability to restrict diffusion of small molecules varies as the square of the plaque thickness. It therefore seems logical to clean the teeth to reduce plaque thickness (if not remove it altogether) before a meal, rather than afterwards!

5.3.4 Utilisation of lactic acid by *Veillonella*

The dependence of members of the anaerobic genus *Veillonella* upon lactic acid as an energy source was described above (5.3.1). Although no reduction in the total number of acid molecules occurs as a result of the *Veillonella* fermentation, the substrate, lactic acid, is very much stronger than the products, acetic and propionic acids. This is indicated by the lower pK_a for lactic acid (pK_a is equal to the pH at which an acid is half-dissociated, table 5.4). A millimolar (mmol/l) [conc. wt/vol millimoles per litre] solution of lactic acid in water has a pH of 3.0 (91 per cent dissociated), whereas the corresponding values for acetic and propionic acids are around pH 3.9 (12–13 per cent dissociated). Hence, the effect of *Veillonella* fermentation is to tend to reduce the pH of the plaque.

Table 5.4 Strength of acids concerned in fermentation by *Veillonella*

Acid	Formula	$pK_a(25°)$
Lactic	$CH_3.CHOH.CO_2H$	3.08
Acetic	$CH_3.CO_2H$	4.75
Propionic	$CH_3.CH_2.CO_2H$	4.87

5.4 Bacterial Products as Complexing Agents

A sparingly soluble inorganic salt, such as the calcium phosphate of tooth mineral, will dissolve in water until a saturated solution is formed. If one of a number of organic 'complexing agents' are added, the quantity of undissolved solid will be reduced, but the extra salt (or more strictly its cations) concerned will not be in solution as ions, but bound to the organic molecules. Complexing agents usually have electron pairs which they share with cations, but they may also release protons in exchange for the bound cations. In spite of this proton release the binding agents themselves need not be strong acids. For example, if a neutral solution of magnesium sulphate is shaken with the complexing agent 8-hydroxy-quinoline (figure 5.2) in chloroform, the latter binds magnesium ions into the organic phase and ejects protons in their place. Thus the aqueous solution becomes acid and can be titrated with sodium hydroxide. Organic compounds such as this, which bind metal ions with electron pairs on several sites within each complexing molecule, are called 'chelating agents' (*chele*—from the Greek claw).

One of the best-known and most powerful chelating agents is ethylenediamine tetra-acetic acid (EDTA, 'Versene'):

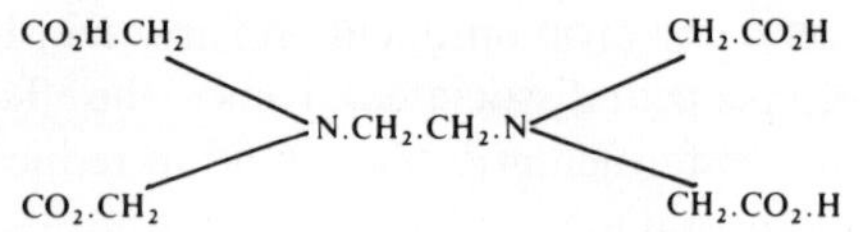

$$CO_2H.CH_2 \qquad\qquad CH_2.CO_2H$$
$$N.CH_2.CH_2.N$$
$$CO_2.CH_2 \qquad\qquad CH_2.CO_2.H$$

This molecule is a strong acid, but its ability to dissolve calcium salts is not due solely to its acidity, although some dissolution of calcium salts will be due to the neutralisation of EDTA free acid. However, a neutral solution of the sodium salt of EDTA is a powerful complexing agent for calcium salts. The complexing power of a number of agents is listed in table 5.5. The higher the value of the log_{10} of the stability constant of the calcium complex, the more

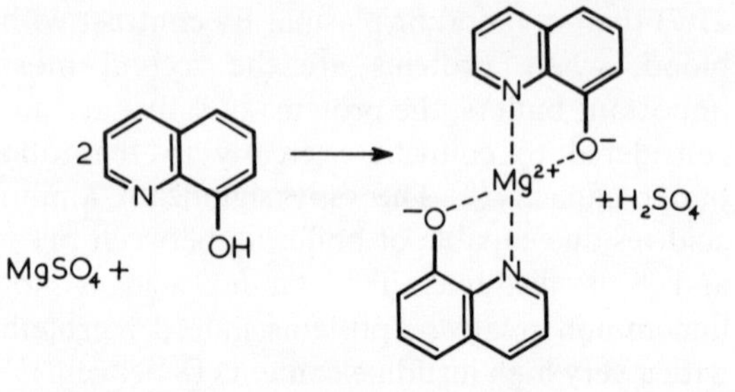

Figure 5.2 The chelation of a divalent ion by 8-hydroxyquinoline

powerful the complexing agent. It has been shown that 0.1 mol/l solutions of the trisodium salt (pH 8.22) and tetrasodium salt (pH 11.32) of EDTA can decalcify human enamel[25]. However, EDTA is a powerful chelater which does not occur in plaque or saliva. Citrate is a significant chelating agent for calcium and is a constituent of mineralised tissue[26], but it is not an important component of plaque or saliva. The organic molecule which is both quantitatively significant in plaque, and a moderate chelating agent, is

Table 5.5 Stability constants of calcium complexes (from Sillen and Martell[23])

Complexing agent	log_{10} stability constant of calcium complex
Butyrate	0.5
Acetate	0.6
$H_2PO_4^-$	0.7*
Propionate	0.7
Lactate	about 1
H_2 citrate$^-$	1.1
Glycine	1.4
Aspartate	1.6
Albumin	2.2
Globulin	2.2
HPO_4^{2-}	2.4*
H citrate^{2-}	3.1
Citrate^{3-}	4.7
Pyrophosphate	5.0
Polyphosphate	about 6
EDTA^{4-}	10.8

* Value from Gregory, Moreno and Brown[24].

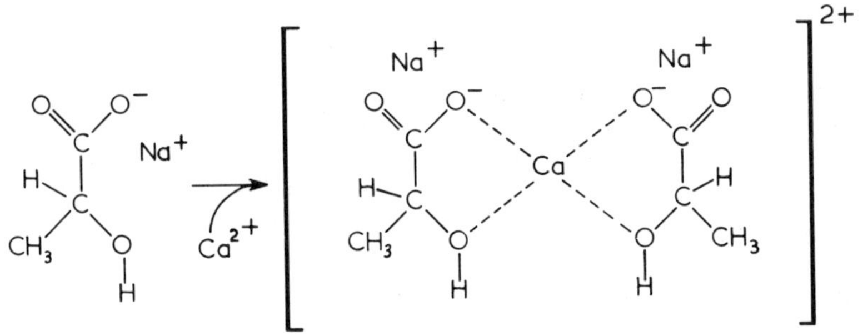

Figure 5.3 The chelation of a calcium ion by the sodium salt of lactic acid

lactic acid. It should be re-emphasised that chelating agents which are also acids may form the calcium salts of their acid radicals. However, the neutral salts of these acids also solubilise calcium phosphates (figure 5.3). There is some evidence that the sodium salt of lactic acid can dissolve tooth mineral when high concentrations (for example, 0.5 mol/ℓ) are used[25]. These experiments differ from the situation in plaque in two significant ways; first, rather high concentrations of lactate were used, and secondly the enamel was the only source of calcium to be complexed. Plaque itself contains high concentrations of calcium (section 5.8), and saliva is supersaturated with calcium. It therefore seems likely that, as plaque develops, any chelating agents which accumulate in it will complex the readily available salivary calcium. This would partly explain the high calcium content of plaque.

The situation in which chelaters are likely to have the greatest impact is that of rapid formation of complexing agents by a thick layer of plaque. The only significant complexing agent likely to be formed as a metabolic end-product in relatively high concentrations is lactic acid. The factors that limit the neutralisation of a local accumulation of acid in plaque will be parallelled by similar factors limiting the satisfaction of its calcium chelating capacity. These will include limitation of the rate of diffusion of calcium into the plaque and of the rate of diffusion of lactate out of the plaque, and the utilisation of lactate by

Veillonella. Thus, there might be a role for chelation in the dissolution of tooth mineral by lactic acid produced in carbohydrate catabolism. Lactic acid is the strongest of the organic acids but only a moderate chelating agent (millimolar lactic acid in water has a pH close to 3, whereas the experiments that demonstrate chelation by sodium lactate involved 500 mmol concentrations). Although it is difficult to evaluate the relative contributions of the two mechanisms of calcium phosphate dissolution, the major factor definitely seems to be acidity. Therefore, the theories of caries aetiology involving chelation (chapter 1) are not considered significant. In any event, the two mechanisms are the result of a single process, carbohydrate fermentation.

5.5 Formation and Functions of Intracellular Storage Polymers in Bacteria

Bacteria, like other cells, contain the biopolymers essential for life. These include nucleic acids (concerned with the storage of genetic information and its use in the cell) and proteins, which are quantitatively the most important, and mediate all the cell reactions. Other structural components include carbohydrates, lipids and complex molecules containing these macromolecules combined together, and with proteins. In addition, bacteria also polymerise within their cells storage materials for the identification of which Wilkinson[27] has established three criteria:

(1) The accumulation of the reserve substance when exogenous energy sources are in excess of the immediate requirement for growth of cells.

(2) The utilisation of the reserve when exogenous energy sources are insufficient for maintenance of viability, and for growth (if other nutrients permit this).

(3) The degradation of the reserve to produce energy in a form utilisable by the cells, thus conferring an advantage over cells which do not possess such a compound.

Storage compounds are important in the survival of bacteria, and in the competition between them in mixed cultures such as dental plaque[28].

5.5.1 Storage polysaccharides

The most common storage polysaccharide is glycogen (section 5.2.1), which is readily formed by many bacteria when the external concentration of fermentable carbohydrate is in excess of that required by the immediate energy demands of growth.

The mechanism of synthesis and degradation of bacterial glycogen is similar to that in mammalian systems except that the substrate for glycogen synthetase is ADP-glucose instead of UDP-glucose[29]. The plaque bacterium *Streptococcus mitis* can accumulate a highly branched glycogen to the extent of 37 per cent of the dry weight of the cells[30]. When this streptococcus was inoculated into medium containing 0.1 per cent glucose, glycogen storage commenced immediately (figure 5.4). Over the first 3h growth occurred (indicated by the increase in cell nitrogen per ml), and glycogen synthesis also took place (shown by the increase in carbohydrate to nitrogen (CH_2O/N) ratio) in the cells. At this point growth ceased due to exhaustion of glucose, and polysaccharide degradation began. The turbidity of the culture fell during this phase due to the loss of cell mass as the carbohydrate to nitrogen ratio fell. However, no lysis took place,

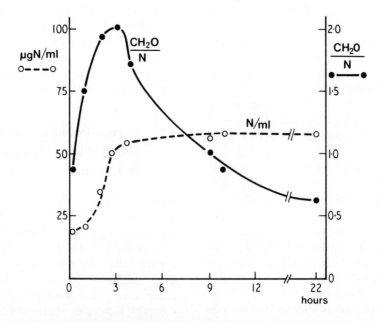

Figure 5.4 The growth and storage of glycogen by a streptococcus. Growth is indicated by increase in cellular nitrogen (N/ml) and glycogen storage by the carbohydrate to nitrogen ratio CH_2O:N (after Gibbons and Kapsimalis[30])

as indicated by the constant total bacterial nitrogen graph; therefore, the cells were not dying while the glycogen store was available. Washed cells of polysaccharide-rich streptococci packed to a depth of 2 mm in a chamber 10 mm in diameter were shown to produce lactic acid from their glycogen stores (figure 5.5). When the surface of the packed cells was constantly rinsed with 67 mmol phosphate buffer 7.0 at 0.1 ml/min, the pH at the bottom of the layer was

was only 0.01 per cent. This emphasises the value of glycogen in the survival of plaque streptococci.

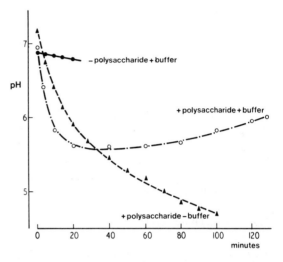

Figure 5.6 The pH of packed cells of streptococci with and without glycogen stores when irrigated with phosphate buffer or with water (after Gibbons and Kapsimalis[30])

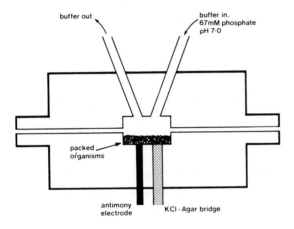

Figure 5.5 Apparatus for testing the acid production by packed cells of streptococci (after Gibbons and Kapsimalis[30])

between 5.7 and 6.0 over a period of 2h (figure 5.6). If water was used instead of buffer the pH dropped continuously to reach 4.7 in 100 min. When cells without polysaccharide were treated in the same way the pH remained above 6.8. This experimental design mimics dental plaque in a tooth rinsed with saliva, and reveals how stored glycogen can extend the period of acid production at a tooth surface beyond the time when exogenous carbohydrate is available.

Van Houte and Jansen[31] have shown that glycogen-rich cells of *Streptococcus mitis* suspended in phosphate-buffered saline pH 6.5 at 37°C, survived well during glycogen degradation, and were 60 per cent viable at the end of 16 h. At this time the residual viability of glycogen-free cells

Although some serological types of S. *mutans* do not form prolific intracellular polysaccharide, and are nevertheless able to cause caries in experimental animals, the formation of intracellular polysaccharide does appear to be a factor in the virulence of other strains. Mutants of two strains of S. *mutans* serological group Ic with impaired ability to form and utilise this type of reserve, were able to colonise the tooth surface and persist as prominent members of the oral flora of rats, but with loss of cariogenic potential[32].

5.5.2 Storage lipid

Most of the lipids in bacteria are not reserve materials, and the triglyceride stores of higher organisms do not appear to be formed in microorganisms. There is, however, one reserve lipid exclusive to bacteria, which is the polyester of β-hydroxybutyric acid.

CH₃—CHOH—CH₂—CO₂H structure *β-hydroxybutyric acid* and poly *β-hydroxybutyrate* structure

β-hydroxybutyric acid   *poly β-hydroxybutyrate*

This substance is found in bacilli, where it may comprise a substantial proportion of the cell mass under appropriate physiological conditions. Analyses by the author (unpublished) failed to detect this material in a collection of oral bacteria including strains of streptococci, lactobacilli, fusobacteria and actinomyces.

5.5.3 Polyphosphate

Many microorganisms possess stainable intracellular granules ('volutin'), which consist largely of polyphosphate in association with RNA, lipid and protein. Some microorganisms can use polyphosphate to generate ATP and others use it as a source of phosphorus for the synthesis of nucleic acids and phospholipids. The only instance in which polyphosphate has been studied in a plaque bacterium appears to be in the caries-conducive streptococcus SL1[33]. This strain produced a small polyphosphate of 10–20 units ($n = 8-18$):

linear polyphosphate

There is no indication of the possible role of polyphosphate in such bacteria at present.

However, it may act as a 'sink' for phosphate derived from the saliva and the teeth in the presence of an energy source. The source of phosphate for plaque bacteria is more likely to be saliva than the tooth, for reasons described below (5.8). It is also possible that polyphosphates may be involved in the accumulation of fluoride by plaque.

In summarising this section on storage polymers of bacteria we are led to conclude that glycogen is the only storage material of proven significance to the bacteria of plaque, although there is some evidence that RNA (which has an essential role in protein synthesis) also decreases in starving cells. This seems more likely to be the run-down of a component at an unnecessarily high concentration, rather than the consumption of a reserve material. The role of polyphosphate is uncertain in the metabolism of plaque bacteria.

5.6   Formation and Function of Extracellular Polymers by Plaque Bacteria

Polysaccharides are the most common extracellular polymers. Some bacteria do form extracellular polypeptides (which are of quite different composition to proteins, being polymers of a single amino acid, for example, polyglutamic acid), but such products have not been detected in dental plaque. Most is known about the polysaccharides which are polymers of one type of carbohydrate subunit (for example, glucose), the homopolysaccharides. However, plaque bacteria have also been shown to produce extracellular heteropolysaccharides containing several different carbohydrates.

5.6.1   Glucans

Polymers of glucose of all types including starch, glycogen and cellulose are called glucans. The structures of glucose, sucrose, and glycogen were illustrated earlier (section 5.2.1) and it was noted that glycogen monomers are linked together by $\alpha 1:4$ bonds in chains which branch by means of

$\alpha 1:6$ bonds. Other glucans, in which the $\alpha 1:6$ link predominates, have been called dextrans (after dextrose—an old name for glucose). The simplest dextran is that formed by *Leuconostoc mesenteroides*, which does not occur in dental plaque, but is important as a spoilage organism in sugar refining. Sucrose readily gives rise to extracellular polysaccharides because the bond between the fructose and glucose has sufficient energy to support the synthesis of a polysaccharide bond without another energy source. Therefore, polysaccharide synthesis can be achieved by mixing sucrose with a single enzyme, dextransucrase (synonym $\alpha 1:6$ glucan:D-fructose glucosyltransferase):

Some authors claim that a primer dextran molecule is needed to accept glucose residues from sucrose, but there is good evidence that such a primer is not absolutely essential for dextran synthesis, but does increase the rate of synthesis, and may also protect dextransucrase against inactivation[34]. Similar polymers are made by living bacteria, causing the liquid in which the cells are growing to become slimy and viscous. The fate of the two components of the sucrose molecule is therefore quite different. The glucose molecule is polymerised externally to the cell, but the fructose molecule is taken up by the cell and metabolised. Extraction of dental plaque with water and cold dilute alkali has produced mixtures of polysaccharides in which glucans predominate. Some authors use the term 'dextran' for all such polymers in which α1:6 links predominate irrespective of whether branching occurs or the type of branch link. Thus Jeanes described three groups of 'dextrans' from several strains of bacteria[35]. Type A had up to 2 per cent 1:3 linkages, type B 3–6 per cent of 1:3 linkages and type C had over 6 per cent of 1:3 linkages. Others prefer to retain the name dextran strictly for the linear 1:6 linked polymer, and use the more general term glucan for all glucose polymers, but the new trivial name 'mutan' for the branched, insoluble, polymers of plaque.

Unlike the situation with glycogen synthesis, separate enzymes are not required to synthesise the branching structure. Linear dextran is attached to the enzyme by the reducing end, and glucose units from sucrose are inserted between the enzyme and the existing dextran chain. It seems that the dextran chain can also be transferred on to the 3'-hydroxyl of other dextran chains by the dextransucrase enzyme[36].

Extracellular polysaccharides are often produced by bacteria that might otherwise be washed away from their ecological niche. They help the bacteria to adhere to each other and to solid surfaces. If this adherence were reduced significantly, a large contribution would be made to the prevention of dental disease. The mechanism of adherence is under investigation at present and is likely to be multifactorial. Contributions are expected to be made by physical forces[37], by ionic bridges formed by calcium ions between negative charges on the enamel pellicle and the bacterial surface, and by hydrogen bonding or other interactions between extracellular polysaccharides and the pellicle[38]. Bacterial adherence in oral biology has been reviewed by Gibbons and van Houte[39]. It is clear that, in some cases, extracellular polysaccharides favour adherence and coherence of oral bacteria, and the loss of ability to synthesise such polymers in mutants of *Streptococcus mutans* is associated with loss of virulence. However, in a (non-oral) strain of *Leuconostoc*, production of copious quantities of

soluble dextran from sucrose inhibits aggregation such as is found in dextran-free cells grown on glucose[40]. Clearly, the chemical structure and quantity of the polysaccharide is significant in adherence and coherence phenomena. In the dental context the highly hydrated polysaccharides do not present a great barrier to the diffusion of ions and small molecules. The bacteria themselves, with their selective surface membranes, are less penetrable to small molecules diffusing through a layer. However, the production of voluminous polysaccharide in plaque thickens the plaque layer, spacing out the bacteria cells in the gel that they form, and this thickness of the plaque layer has its diffusion-limiting effect as diffusion varies with the square of the length of the diffusion path.

5.6.2   Levans

Polymers of fructose (old name: laevulose) called levans are produced extracellularly from glucose by plaque bacteria. Dextrans are more plentiful in plaque matrix, but after sucrose consumption levans form a significant secondary component of the polysaccharide[40a]. However, levan is utilised quite rapidly by plaque bacteria (by comparison with dextran) and is a substrate for acid production after sucrose has been cleared from the mouth[40b]. Levan production has been ascribed to *Streptococcus salivarius*, *Streptococcus mutans* and *Actinomyces viscosus*.

A levansucrose (fructosyl transferase) capable of forming the classical linear β2:6 linked levan has been purified from *Streptococcus mutans*[40c]. The levan from *Streptococcus salivarius* has a linear structure of this type with β2:1 branch points and has a molecular weight of up to 3×10^7 daltons[40d]. However, the levan produced by *Streptococcus mutans* has been recently described as predominantly β2:1 linked[40e]. Different polymeric variations of the levan structure may be formed by different strains; it has been shown that some strains of *Streptococcus mutans* form virtually no levan from sucrose while other strains may produce levan as 30 per

Sucrose (*n* mol)

cent of the total extracellular polysaccharide[40f].

5.6.3   Heteropolysaccharides

Few studies have been carried out on the more complex polysaccharides formed by plaque bacteria. An acidic heteropolymer was first detected as Alcian Blue-positive material around cocci subsequently identified as *Staphylococcus salivarius*. This material, which was detected in 50 per cent of experimental dental plaque samples tested, contained glucose, mannose, rhamnose, amino sugars and possibly, uronic acid residues, although the reason for its acidic nature was not established. Also present in the material, which was firmly adherent to the cells as a slime layer, were traces of other sugars and amino acids that might be derived from the cell wall. The ineffectiveness of dextranase against such polymers was recognised as a factor that might limit the usefulness of the enzyme as an agent against plaque[40g].

Heteropolysaccharides have also been isolated from strains of *Actinomyces viscosus* containing *N*-acetyl glucosamine as the predominant component (60–62 per cent) with glucose, galactose, uronic acid and lesser amounts of other sugars and glycerol[40h, 40i].

5.7   Calcium and Phosphorus Turnover in Plaque

At the pH of freshly secreted saliva, the calcium and phosphate concentrations are sufficient for the fluid to be supersaturated. Spontaneous dissolution of enamel mineral does not therefore occur. In the mouth, saliva loses CO_2 derived from dissolved bicarbonate, and the pH rise which results causes calcium phosphate to precipitate. Salivary protein appears to assist this precipitation which can occur when little or no plaque is present[41]. The calcium and phosphorus concentrations of dental plaque specimens are considerably higher than those of saliva. Plaque from the lower incisor teeth has a higher calcium content than that from around the maxillary molars[42]. It is also more prone to form calculus, because it is irrigated with saliva from the submaxillary glands, which has approximately twice the calcium concentration of parotid saliva.

The pH of plaque is the key factor determining whether calcium phosphates will tend to dissolve, or to precipitate within it. Figure 5.7 is a schematic plot of pH versus calcium and phosphate concentrations, which illustrates the relative roles of these factors[43]. The ionic product of solution will be taken as the concentration of calcium multiplied by the phosphate concentration (species of phosphate not specified). At any pH, the maximum value of the ionic product in a saturated solution is the solubility product. Under neutral, basic and mildly acid conditions the solid line representing the solubility product falls below the broken line representing the ionic product of saliva. Therefore, the enamel mineral will not dissolve and there will be a tendency for saliva mineral to precipitate. The stippled area bounded by the solubility product line, a second solid line and the broken ionic product line represents the metastable zone of supersaturation where there is a tendency to precipitation, favoured by fall in pH and by the presence of salivary protein, but in which precipitation may nevertheless be slow and incomplete. At more basic pH values, spontaneous deposition of mineral occurs extensively, mineralising the plaque to form calculus. Under acid conditions, the solid line intersects the broken line at a point known as the critical point, beyond which mineral begins to dissolve. The solubility product line rises sharply with fall in pH beyond that critical point.

Figure 5.7 is drawn in terms of saliva, and the critical point for a plaque sample will be set by the ionic product of that plaque specimen. Critical pH values are commonly accepted to be in the region of pH 5.5. Under conditions more acid than the critical point the solubility product required for saturation of the fluid phase is higher than the actual ionic product of the fluid, and mineral will therefore tend to dissolve. When acid is produced in plaque, presumably mineral crystals within the plaque will tend to dissolve more readily than the enamel mineral beneath. Thus a high calcium and phosphate content of plaque acts as a buffer towards enamel dissolution.

In view of the relative stability of salivary calcium concentration compared to salivary phosphate concentration, and its high concentration in plaque (perhaps 20 times that of saliva), it seems unlikely that variation in calcium concentration could affect the susceptibility of the teeth to caries. However, Luoma has shown that salivary phosphate is much more variable[44], and it is well known that bacteria require phosphate for growth. Inorganic phosphate is used by plaque bacteria for synthesis of phosphate esters of intermediary metabolism, for example during glycolysis, and for the synthesis of nucleic acids

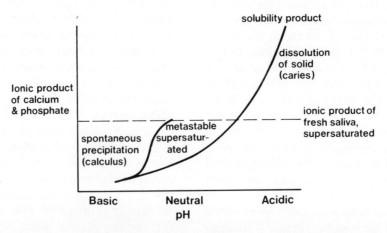

Figure 5.7 Idealised solubility product curves for calcium phosphate in basic, neutral and alkaline conditions (after Kleinberg[43])

and phospholipids. Therefore, bacteria growing in the plaque will take up some phosphate from the plaque fluid, and may therefore facilitate the dissolution of mineral caused by their metabolic end-products. Luoma estimated that phosphorus uptake by dental plaque bacteria was maximal at pH 6.8–7.0, and that uptake became progressively less at lower pH values[44]. This reflects the preference of the predominant plaque bacteria for neutral, or moderately acid, conditions for growth. At higher acid concentration the bacterial cells of plaque may release phosphate rather than taking it up. In this way plaque may actually protect the enamel surface from acid beverages. A further component in this protective effect may be the diffusion-limiting properties of plaque[45], which may restrict the access of acid beverages to the enamel surface. However, the erosion of teeth by acid beverages is much more readily prevented (by voluntary restriction of consumption of such drinks) than is dental caries, and any possible beneficial effect of plaque is likely to be much less significant in dental health than the cariogenic effect.

5.8   Effects of fluoride in plaque

Dental plaque contains a surprisingly high concentration of fluoride, estimated at between 6 and 179 p.p.m.* in a group of 81 people, with a mean of 54.8 p.p.m.[46]. The concentration of fluoride in plaque may be increased by rinsing with 0.2 per cent sodium fluoride, but remains higher than controls rinsed with sodium chloride for only 24 h or less[47]. The fall in plaque fluoride concentration after a fluoride rinse is probably due mainly to the growth of new plaque bacteria and the accretion of new matrix. There is little doubt that the majority of the plaque fluoride is not present as free anions. The concentration of

ionic fluoride in human dental plaque has been estimated to be only 1–2 p.p.m.[48]. Nevertheless, this concentration is still higher than that in saliva (commonly 0.1 p.p.m.[49]), or in plasma (0.14–0.19 p.p.m. in people using water with up to 2.5 p.p.m. of fluoride, and slightly raised at 0.26 p.p.m. in people whose drinking water contains 5.4 p.p.m. of fluoride[50]). Dental plaque may be expected to be saturated with calcium phosphate, and several species of oral bacteria have been shown to calcify when exposed to such saturated solutions in pure culture[51, 52]. Extensively mineralised plaque (calculus) has been shown to contain both hydroxyapatite and brushite[53], and although frank mineralisation is not often observable in soft plaque, the occurrence of microcrystals within and between the cells cannot be discounted. Early mineralisation of plaque appears to begin in the intercellular matrix[54]. It seems likely that the fluoride bound in dental plaque is extensively in the form of fluorapatite[55]. It has been suggested that plaque bacteria 'concentrate' fluoride. Clearly any apatite or other phosphates that crystallise within bacteria will be available as a 'sink' for fluoride. It is also possible that intracellular proteins bind fluoride.

What is less clear is whether non-mineralising bacteria take up fluoride to a higher concentration than that of their environment. In a series of determinations of the permeability of streptococci to fluoride at 8.5 p.p.m., fluoride entered the cells but cellular concentration was rather less than the extracellular concentration[56]. In these experiments, an indirect assay of cellular concentration was used because of the ease with which fluoride could be washed from the cells which were not mineralised. Streptococci grown on nutrient agar medium[48] (a medium that would not be considered conducive to mineralisation) containing 0.8 to 5 p.p.m. apparently

---

*   It is customary to express fluoride concentration in parts per million (p.p.m.) a measure which is used for trace elements (1 p.p.m. = 1 mg/l–1 μg/ml). This concentration refers to fluoride irrespective of its compound. Thus, the concentration of fluoride (at. wt. 19) in 0.1 per cent sodium fluoride (mol. wt. = 42) solution is 452 p.p.m., but that in 0.1 per cent potassium fluoride (mol. wt. 58) solution is 328 p.p.m. The use of molarity obviates the difficulty presented by percentages. 1 m mol (0.001 mol) fluoride is always equal to 19 p.p.m. whatever cation is present.

concentrated the fluoride 26 to 34-fold, and the fluoride was reported not to be removed by washing the cells. If the cells had been mineralising these findings could be rationalised (fluoride is not readily washed from plaque, which contains much calcium phosphate).

The general theory of permeability of cells to weak acids[57,58] presumes that the undissociated acid HF is the permeating species, that the process is one of passive diffusion, and that the internal cell concentration will be governed by Donnan equilibrium, in which the chief factors are the external concentration, and the external and internal pH values, but this does not take account of any fluoride binding components inside the cells. Other workers have suggested that plaque fluoride is not bound to plaque bacteria, or to the macromolecules that surround them[59]. Ultrafilterable cations from the saliva can play a significant part in binding fluoride, perhaps to the plaque matrix[60], which lends support to mineralisation as a fluoride-binding factor.

Recent work, which may well resolve these conflicting views, indicates that fluoride may be driven into bacteria by a pH gradient. At pH 5.5 in *Streptococcus sanguis* with an initial external concentration of 1.0 p.p.m., the cells accumulated 9.1 p.p.m. total fluoride of which almost 70 per cent was tightly bound, principally to cytoplasmic components[61]. In a strain of *S.mutans* the accumulation of fluoride was dependent on the pH gradient between the medium and the cells[62]. The accumulation of fluoride was greatest when the washed cells were suspended in more acid buffers and measurement made at short time intervals. On prolonged incubation the fluoride tended to return to the extracellular compartment, so that at pH 4 a cellular to extracellular ratio of almost 7 at 1.5 min became a ratio of 3.47 at 5 min. If the cells were pre-equilibrated with the buffer before fluoride was added, this accumulation was abolished so that at pH 4 the above ratio was 1.04 at 1.5 min and 1.07 at 5 min. When the external medium is more acid than the cells, HF enters the cells and ionises facilitating further entry of HF. As the pH gradient is abolished the

current of fluoride is reversed. This effect may explain the very different results of various workers who have studied this problem.

In summary then, plaque contains a high concentration of fluoride, but there is some doubt about its distribution and its form. What is certain is that relatively little of it is in the form of the soluble fluoride ions and undissociated acid that are significant inhibitors of enzymes. It now remains to speculate about the interaction between this plaque fluoride and the bacterial metabolism within the plaque. Before doing so, however, it should be stated that there is no doubt that 1 p.p.m. of ionic fluoride in solution in the plaque fluid will have a marked effect in reducing the solubility of enamel mineral[63], and promoting remineralisation of incipient caries lesions[64].

The question of the likely effects of fluoride in plaque is not easy to answer, and for the purposes of discussion will be divided into two aspects, posed as questions. Consideration will be given to the effects of fluoride that has accumulated in plaque from sources such as drinking water, the normal diet and fluoridated dentifrices. Topical application of fluoride in gels and washes that produce temporary high concentrations of plaque fluoride, which subsequently revert to the more normal levels within 24 h, is a quite different circumstance akin to acute poisoning, and will be discussed later. The two questions then are:

(1) Is it likely that the fluoride in plaque inhibits the enzymes of plaque bacteria, and hence their growth and production of metabolic end-products?

(2) Is it likely that the bacteria in plaque, being constantly exposed to fluoride at the prevailing concentrations of plaque over countless generations, are optimally adapted to minimise the likely inhibitory effects of that fluoride?

The anti-enzyme theory of fluoride action is based on the fact that fluoride is known to inhibit many enzymes including phosphatases, catalase, peroxidase and cytochrome oxidase[65], hexokinase[66], phosphoglucomutase[67], enolase[68] and succinate dehydrogenase[69]. Most of these studies are of isolated enzymes examined in vitro, and interpretation of these results in terms of whole cells, where the enzymes are compartmentalised and, in many cases, coupled in metabolic sequence, is highly problematical.

The only biochemical analysis of the effects of fluoride in moderate concentration upon an oral microorganism has been carried out on *Streptococcus salivarius*. Fluoride at 9 p.p.m. completely blocked the synthesis of glycogen when non-growing cells were incubated anaerobically with glucose at pH 7.0. Inhibition of glycogen synthesis was 15 per cent at 1 p.p.m. fluoride, and 50 per cent at 2–3 p.p.m. Degradation of glycogen was nowhere near as sensitive as glycogen synthesis, and 135 p.p.m. fluoride were required to inhibit glycogenolysis by 50 per cent[70]. The sensitivity of glycogen synthesis in vivo was not paralleled by the sensitivity of the enzymes of glycogen synthesis in vitro. This indicates a highly fluoride-sensitive site in glucose absorption and phosphorylation. The degradation of endogenous glycogen was negligibly reduced by 36 p.p.m. fluoride, a concentration that completely suppressed the metabolism of exogenous glucose[71]. This discounts a major effect of fluoride upon enzymic processes common to glycogenolysis and the glycolysis of glucose (for example, phosphoglucomutase and enolase) and indicates a significant inhibition prior to the formation of glucose-6-phosphate. In *S. salivarius* and many other bacteria, glucose is transported into the cells and phosphorylated to glucose-6-phosphate by phosphoenolpyruvate phosphotransferase (PEP-PT) rather than by hexokinase[72]:

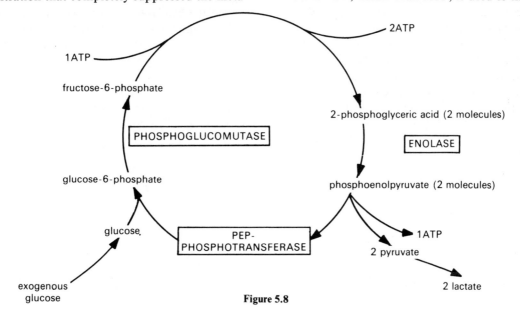

phosphoenol pyruvate   glucose   pyruvate   glucose-6-phosphate

The addition of 46 p.p.m. fluoride to cells incubated anaerobically with glucose at pH 7.2 caused a rapid drop in intracellular concentrations of both glucose-6-phosphate and ATP. Figure 5.8 shows the circular nature of glycolysis in bacteria using the PEP-PT system for phosphorylating glucose.

Since PEP, rather than ATP, is used to make

Figure 5.8

glucose-6-phosphate, the fall in ATP concentration is consequent upon the fall in glucose-6-phosphate, and PEP phosphotransferase is the major site of inhibition. Evidence is accumulating for an effect of fluoride upon membrane function. In *Escherichia coli* fluoride does not affect the phosphorylation of glucose by PEP-PT but did affect its translocation into the cell. Luoma and Tuompo have shown that fluoride affects the cellular potassium concentration in *S.mutans* and that inhibition of glucose uptake by fluoride can be partly alleviated by extracellular potassium[73].

Fluoride treatment of the *S.salivarius* cells does appear to inhibit enolase to some extent, as the concentration of 2PGA does rise somewhat and the concentration of PEP falls[74]. Such changes have also been found in streptococci made resistant to fluoride[75], and are to be expected in view of the finding that fluoride behaves as a competitive inhibitor to enolase[76]. As fluoride competes with 2PGA for the enolase molecules, 2PGA would be expected to rise to a new equilibrium concentration in the same way that the water in a reservoir would rise if height were added to a dam. Thereafter, conversion of 2PGA to PEP (flow over the dam) may be resumed. Thus it can be calculated from the data of Cimasoni[76] that enolase has the same velocity in the presence of 7 p.p.m. fluoride with 3.5 mM 2PGA as it has in the absence of fluoride if the concentration of 2PGA is 0.7 mM. It should be noted, however, that although the 2PGA pool size increases somewhat, it does not accumulate as an end-product in the way that lactic acid

does[77], nor could it possibly do so for fundamental biochemical reasons.

The concentration of fluoride in plaque therefore seems sufficient to inhibit uptake and phosphorylation of glucose. Whether it actually does so in plaque depends on the pH, and the proportion of fluoride sequestered as inactive calcium salts. A fall in pH increases the activity of a given amount of fluoride, probably by increasing the conversion of F to undissociated HF[57] which can then cross cell membranes. However, a fall in pH also favours the uptake of fluoride by the enamel[78], and thus reduces the quantity of fluoride available for inhibition.

There is little direct evidence for an inhibitory effect of fluoride under conditions resembling those of plaque. Many experiments have been carried out with saliva or salivary sediment and are of dubious applicability to plaque because of the differences in the flora. Furthermore, the concentration of cells in saliva is much less than in plaque, and the ratio of fluoride to sensitive enzyme system much higher. Therefore, a given concentration of fluoride in saliva, or any other dilute suspension of cells, would be expected to be more effective as an inhibitor than it would be in plaque. A second shortcoming of the saliva experiments is that there is no enamel surface to deplete the available fluoride. On balance, the evidence that the fluoride in plaque significantly inhibits bacterial metabolism within plaque is weak, and the point must be considered unproven.

The second point to be considered is whether plaque bacteria, being constantly exposed to

2-phosphoglyceric acid (2PGA)   phosphoenolpyruvate (PEP)

fluoride, are resistant to its inhibition. Several strains of streptococci have been rendered fluoride resistant by successive daily transfers in media containing 38, 190, 627 and 1900 p.p.m. fluoride[79]. Similar results have been obtained with other streptococci using either exposure to 6 p.p.m. fluoride, or to ultraviolet radiation (a general mutagen)[80]. These fluoride-resistant strains were able to take up glucose and synthesise glycogen in the presence of 46 p.p.m. or 91 p.p.m. fluoride which normal fluoride-sensitive cells were unable to do[79]. They were also able to metabolise glucose at a rate of 56–86 per cent of controls in the presence of 46 p.p.m. fluoride and 24–70 per cent of the control rate in the presence of 91 p.p.m. fluoride[71]. It is important to realise that in these experiments resistant cells were being tested in the presence of fluoride, but the controls were normal sensitive cells in the absence of fluoride. This demonstrates the extent to which these fluoride-resistant streptococci are able to ignore high concentrations of fluoride, and metabolise glucose at high velocities in its presence. Normal sensitive cells exposed to 46 p.p.m. or 91 p.p.m. fluoride would barely metabolise glucose at all. It is clear that streptococci in the plaque with its high fluoride content are not resistant to fluoride in the way that strains have been rendered resistant in vitro. It therefore seems that the same factors that minimise the inhibitory effect of fluoride also minimise the selective pressure that would cause resistant bacteria to colonise the plaque. The non-occurrence of fluoride-resistant forms of bacteria in plaque therefore seems to provide a degree of proof that plaque fluoride does not significantly inhibit the metabolism of plaque bacteria.

Evidence that the fluoride available from fluoridated water alters the microbial population of dental plaque is fragmentary and unconvincing, although the effect upon caries is marked. The lower concentration of *S.mutans* in plaque from selected sites in the mouths of children drinking 1.1 p.p.m. fluoride than those drinking 0.1 p.p.m. fluoride was not statistically significant[81]. Bowen found that 2 p.p.m. fluoride administered to a small group of monkeys over 5 years reduced the caries and also reduced the extracellular polysaccharide producing streptococci[82]. The plaque also contained less soluble hexose but more insoluble ketohexose. This finding may be related to the reduction of adsorption of proteins and bacteria to hydroxyapatite by low concentrations of fluoride (1–5 p.p.m.)[83].

Topical application of fluoride to the tooth surface reduces caries but the effect seems not to depend upon the concentration of fluoride achieved in the enamel[84]. The mechanism of action may be by altering the metabolism of plaque[85], by reducing the plaque population on the tooth surfaces[86], or by specifically reducing the concentration of potentially cariogenic bacteria such as *S.mutans*[87,88]. The selective effect against *S.mutans* has been reported in some groups drinking fluoridated water as described above. By contrast other workers failed to find any such selective effect with topical fluoride treatments[89,90]. The significance of such discrimination against particular bacteria is therefore open to question. Nevertheless, the possible mechanisms of action of topical fluoride treatment seem to include an antimicrobial component, whereas the evidence points to changes in physical chemistry of the enamel mineral as the significant mechanism of action of dietary fluoride which gives rise to plaque concentrations of 50 p.p.m. fluoride.

References

1. Jordan, H. V. (1965). Bacteriological aspects of experimental dental caries. *Annals of the New York Academy of Sciences*, **131**, 905–12

2. Yamada, T. and Carlsson, J. (1975). Regulation of lactate dehydrogenase and change of fermentation products in streptococci. *Journal of Bacteriology*, **124**, 55–61

3. Yamada, T. and Carlsson, J. (1975). The role of pyruvate formate lyase in glucose metabolism of *Streptococcus mutans*, in *Microbial Aspects of Dental Caries* (Eds

Stiles, H. M., Loesche, W. J. and O'Brien, T. C.), *Sp. Supp. Microbiology Abstracts*, vol. III, pp. 809–19

4. Ritz, H. L. (1967). Microbial population shifts in developing human dental plaque. *Archives of Oral Biology*, **12**, 1561–8

5. Michaud, R. N. and Delwiche, E. A. (1970). Multiple impairment of glycolysis in *Veillonella alcalescens*. *Journal of Bacteriology*, **101**, 138–40

6. Michaud, R. N., Carrow, J. A. and Delwiche, E. A. (1970). Non-oxidative pentose phosphate pathway in *Veillonella alcalescens*. *Journal of Bacteriology*, **101**, 141–4

7. Mikx, F. H. M. and van der Hoeven, J.S. (1975). Symbiosis of *Streptococcus mutans* and *Veillonella alcalescens* in mixed continuous cultures. *Archives of Oral Biology*, **20**, 407–10

8. van der Hoeven, J. S., Toorop, A. I. and Mikx, F. H. M. (1978). Symbiotic relationship of *Veillonella alcalescens* and *Streptococcus mutans* in dental plaque in gnotobiotic rats. *Caries Research*, **12**, 142–7

9. Stephan, R. M. (1944). Intra-oral hydrogen-ion concentrations associated with dental caries activity. *Journal of Dental Research*, **23**, 257–66

10. Geddes, D. A. M. (1975). Acids produced by human dental plaque metabolism *in situ*. *Caries Research*, **9**, 98–109

11. Gilmour, M. N., Green, G. C., Zahn, L. M., Sparmann, C. D. and Pearlman, J. (1976). The C_1–C_4 monocarboxylic and lactic acids in dental plaques before and after exposure to sucrose *in vivo*, in *Microbial Aspects of Dental Caries* (Eds Stiles, H. M., Loesche, W. J. and O'Brien, T. C.), *Sp. Supp. Microbiology Abstracts*, vol. II, pp. 539–56

12. Hayes, M. L. and Hyatt, A. T. (1974). The decarboxylation of amino acids by bacteria derived from human dental plaque. *Archives of Oral Biology*, **19**, 361–9

13. Cole, M. F., Curtis, M. A. and Bowen, W. H. (1977). Ornithine decarboxylase activity in tooth surface plaque from monkeys (*Macaca fascicularis*) fed pyridoxine, phytate and invert sugar. *Archives of Oral Biology*, **22**, 503–6

14. Stephan, R. M. (1943). Effect of urea in counteracting the influence of carbohydrates on the pH of dental plaques. *Journal of Dental Research*, **22**, 63–71

15. Biswas, S. D. and Kleinberg, I. (1971). Effect of urea concentration on its utilisation, on the pH and the formation of ammonia and carbon dioxide in a human salivary sediment system. *Archives of Oral Biology*, **16**, 759–80

16. Shannon, I. L., Feller, R. P., Ekhoyan, G. and Suddick, R. P. (1977). Human parotid saliva urea in renal failure and during dialysis. *Archives of Oral Biology*, **22**, 83–6

17. Renson, C. E. and Mercer, C. E. (1973). The dental needs of a group of haemodialysis and renal transplant patients. *Journal of Dental Research*, **52**, 966

18. Finn, S. B., Klapper, C. E. and Volker, J. F. (1955). Intra-oral effects upon experimental hamster caries, in *Advances in Experimental Caries Research* (Ed. Sognnaes, R. F.), American Association for Advancement of Science, Washington DC, pp. 152–68

19. Ericsson, Y. (1962). Salivary and food factors in dental caries development. *International Dental Journal*, **12**, 476–95

20. Lilienthal, B. (1955). An analysis of the buffer system in saliva. *Journal of Dental Research*, **34**, 516–30

21. Jackson, P. and Armstrong, W. G. (1974). Isolation of a histidine-rich protein from human parotid saliva. *Journal of Dental Research*, **53**, 1050

22. Holbrook, I. B. and Molan, P. C. (1975). The identification of a peptide in human parotid saliva particularly active in enhancing the glycolytic activity of the salivary microorganisms. *Biochemical Journal*, **149**, 489–92

23. Sillen, L. G. and Martell, A. E. (1964). Stability constants of metal–ion complexes. *Chemical Society Special Publication No. 17*, London

24. Gregory, T. M., Moreno, E. C. and Brown, W. E. (1970). Solubility of $CaHPO_4 2H_2O$ in the system $Ca(OH)_2$-H_3PO_4-H_2O at 5, 15, 25 and 37.5°C. *Journal of the National Bureau of Standards*, **74A**, 461–75

25. Ravnik, C., Sand, H. F. and Morch, T. (1962). Enamel lesions produced *in vitro* by solutions of EDTA and EDTA-sodium salts. *Acta Odontologica Scandinavica*, **20**, 349–58

26. Neuman, W. F. and Neuman, M. W. (1968). *The Chemical Dynamics of Bone Mineral*, University of Chicago Press, Chicago, pp. 142–3

27. Wilkinson, J. F. (1958). The extracellular polysaccharides of bacteria. *Bacteriological Reviews*, **22**, 46–73

28. Dawes, E. A. and Senior, P. J. (1973). The role and regulation of energy reserve polymers in microorganisms, in *Advances in Microbial Physiology*, vol. 10 (Eds Rose, A. H. and Tempest, D. W.), Academic Press, London, pp. 136–266

29. Greenberg, E. and Preiss, J. (1965). Biosynthesis of bacterial glycogen. II. Purification and properties of the adenosine diphosphoglucose: glycogen transglucosylase of Arthrobacter Species NRRL B 1973. *Journal of Biological Chemistry*, **240**, 2341–8

30. Gibbons, R. J. and Kapsimalis, B. (1963). Synthesis of intracellular iodophilic polysaccharide by *Streptococcus mitis*. *Archives of Oral Biology*, **8**, 319–29

31. van Houte, J. and Jansen, H. M. (1970). Role of glycogen in survival of *Streptococcus mitis*. *Journal of Bacteriology*, **101**, 1083–5

32. Tanzer, J. M., Freedman, M. L., Woodiel, F. N., Eifert, R. L. and Rinehimer, L. A. (1976). Association of *Streptococcus mutans* virulence with synthesis of intracellular polysaccharide, in *Microbial Aspects of Dental Caries* (Eds Stiles, H. M., Loesche, W. J. and O'Brien, T. C.), *Sp. Supp. Microbiology Abstracts*, vol. III, pp. 597–616

33. Tanzer, J. M. and Krichevsky, M. I. (1970). Polyphosphate formation by caries conducive streptococcus SL_1. *Biochimica et Biophysica Acta*, **215**, 368–76

34. Robyt, J. F. and Corrigan, A. J. (1977). The mechanism of dextransucrase action. Activation of dextransucrase from *Streptococcus mutans* OMZ 176 by dextran and modified dextran and the non-existence of the primer requirement for the synthesis of dextran. *Archives of Biochemistry and Biophysics*, **183**, 726–31

35. Jeanes, A., Haynes, W. C., Wilham, C. A., Rankin, J. C., Melvin, E. H., Austin, K. J., Clusky, J. E., Fisher, B. E., Tsuchiya, H. W. and Rist, E. E. (1954). Characterisation and classification of dextrans from ninety-six strains of bacteria. *Journal of the American Chemical Society*, **76**, 5041–52

36. Robyt, J. F. and Taniguchi; H. (1976). The mechanism of dextransucrase action. Biosynthesis of branch links by acceptor reactions with dextran. *Archives of Biochemistry and Biophysics*, **174**, 129–35

37. Rutter, P. R. and Abbott, A. (1978). A study of the interaction between oral streptococci and hard surfaces. *Journal of General Microbiology*, **105**, 219–26

38. Rölla, G. (1976). Inhibition of adsorption—general considerations, in *Microbial Aspects of Dental Caries* (Eds Stiles, H. M., Loesche, W. J. and O'Brien, T. C.), *Sp. Supp. Microbiology Abstracts*, vol. II, pp. 309–24

39. Gibbons, R. J. and van Houte, J. (1975). Bacterial adherence in oral microbial ecology. *Annual Review of Microbiology*, **29**, 19–44

40. Harris, R. H. and Mitchell, R. (1973). The role of polymers in microbial aggregation. *Annual Review of Microbiology*, **27**, 27–50

40a. McDougall, W. A. (1964). Studies on the dental plaque. IV. Levans and the dental plaque. *Australian Dental Journal*, **9**, 1–5

40b. Wood, J. M. (1967). The amount, distribution and metabolism of soluble polysaccharides in human dental plaque. *Archives of Oral Biology*, **12**, 849–58

40c. Carlsson, J. (1970). A levansucrase from *Streptococcus mutans*. *Caries Research*, **4**, 97–113

40d. Stivala, S. S., Bahary, N. S., Long, L.W., Ehrlich, J. and Newbrun, E. (1975). Levans. II. Light scattering and sedimentation data of *Streptococcus salivarius* levan in water. *Biopolymers*, **14**, 1283–92

40e. Baird, J. K., Longyear, V. M. C. and Ellwood, D. C. (1973). Water insoluble and soluble glucans produced by extracellular glycosyltransferases from *Streptococcus mutans*. *Microbios*, **8**, 143–50

40f. Robrish, S. A., Reid, W. and Krichevsky, M. I. (1972). Distribution of enzymes forming polysaccharide from sucrose and the composition of extracellular polysaccharide synthesised by *Streptococcus mutans*. *Applied Microbiology*, **24**, 184–90

40g. Bowden, G. H. (1969). The components of the cell walls and extracellular slime of four strains of *Staphylococcus salivarius* isolated from human dental plaque. *Archives of Oral Biology*, **14**, 685–97

40h. Rosan, B. and Hammond, B. F. (1974). Extracellular polysaccharides of *Actinomyces viscosus*. *Infection and Immunity*, **10**, 304–8

40i. Van der Hoeven, J. S. (1974) A slime-producing microorganism in dental plaque of rats, selected by glucose feeding. Chemical composition of extracellular slime elaborated by *Actinomyces viscosus* strain Nyl. *Caries Research*, **8**, 193–210

41. Baer, P. N. and Newton, W. L. (1959). The occurrence of periodontal disease in germ-free mice. *Journal of Dental Research*, **38**, 1238

42. Dawes, C. and Jenkins, G. N. (1962). Some inorganic constituents of dental plaque and their relationship to early calculus formation and caries. *Archives of Oral Biology*,

7, 161–72

43. Kleinberg, I. (1970). Biochemistry of the dental plaque, in *Advances in Oral Biology*, vol. 4 (Ed. Staple, P. H.), Academic Press, New York, pp. 43–90

44. Luoma, H. (1964). Lability of inorganic phosphate in dental plaque and saliva. *Acta Odontologica Scandinavica*, **22**, supplement 41

45. Huh, C., Blackwell, R. Q. and Fosdick, L. S. (1959). The diffusion of glucose through microbial plaques. *Journal of Dental Research*, **38**, 569–76

46. Hardwick, J. L. (1963). The mechanism of fluorides in lessening susceptibility of dental caries. *British Dental Journal*, **114**, 222–8

47. Birkeland, J. M., Jorkjent, L. and von der Fehr, F. R. (1971). The influence of fluoride rinses on the fluoride content of dental plaque in children. *Caries Research*, **5**, 169–79

48. Jenkins, G. N., Edgar, W. M. and Ferguson, D. B. (1969). The distribution and metabolic effects of human plaque fluorine. *Archives of Oral Biology*, **14**, 105–19

49. Hodge, H. C. and Smith, F. A. (1970). Minerals: Fluorine and dental caries, ch. 7 in *Dietary Chemicals versus Dental Caries* (Ed. Gould, R. F.), pp. 93–115, Advances in Chemistry Series, American Chemical Society

50. Armstrong, W. D., Blomquist, C. H., Singer, L., Pollock, M. E. and McLaren, L. C. (1965). Sodium fluoride and cell growth. *British Medical Journal*, 20 Feb., **1**, 486–8

51. Streckfuss, J. L., Smith, W. N., Brown, L. R. and Campbell, M. M. (1974). Calcification of selected strains of *Streptococcus mutans* and *Streptococcus sanguis*. *Journal of Bacteriology*, **120**, 502–6

52. Ennever, J., Vogel, J.-J. and Brown, L. R. (1972). Survey of microorganisms for calcification in a synthetic medium. *Journal of Dental Research*, **51**, 1483–6

53. Reithe, P. (1974). Dental calculus, its formation, structure and role in the pathogenesis of gingival and periodontal diseases, in *Metabolism and Cariogenicity of Dental Plaque*, Forum Medici, Zyma, Nyon, pp. 37–50

54. Schröder, H. E., Lenz, H. and Muhlemann, H. R. (1964). Microstructures and mineralisation of early dental calculus. *Helvetica Odontologica Acta*, **8**, 1–22

55. Gron, P., Yao, K. and Spinelli, M. (1969). A study of the inorganic constituents in dental plaque. *Journal of Dental Research, Supplement*, **48**, 799–805

56. Williams, R. A. D. (1968). Permeability of fluoride-trained streptococci to fluoride. *Archives of Oral Biology*, **13**, 1031–3

57. Simon, E. W. and Beevers, H. (1952). The effect of pH on the biological activities of weak acids and bases. I. The most usual relationship between pH and activity. *New Phytologist*, **51**, 163–89

58. Albert, A. (1965). *Selective Toxicity*, Methuen, London

59. Singer, L., Jarvey, B. A., Venkateswarlu, P. and Armstrong, W. D. (1970). Fluoride in plaque. *Journal of Dental Research*, **49**, 455

60. Birkeland, J. M. and Rölla, G. (1971). *In vitro* affinity of fluoride to proteins, dextrans, bacteria and salivary components. *Archives of Oral Biology*, **17**, 455–63

61. Kashket, S. and Rodriguez, V. M. (1976). Fluoride accumulation by a strain of human oral *Streptococcus sanguis*. *Archives of Oral Biology*, **21**, 459–64

62. Whitford, G. M., Schuster, G. S., Pashley, D. H. and Venkateswarlu, P. (1977). Fluoride uptake by *Streptococcus mutans* 6715. *Infection and Immunity*, **18**, 680–87

63. Birkeland, J. M. (1975). *In vitro* study on the mechanisms of action of fluoride in low concentrations. *Caries Research*, **9**, 110–18

64. Grøn, P. (1973). Remineralisation of enamel lesions *in vivo*. *Oral Sciences Reviews*, **3**, 84–98

65. Hewitt, E. J. and Nicholas, D. J. D. (1963). Cations and anions: inhibitors and interactions in metabolism and enzyme activity, in *Metabolic Inhibitors*, vol. III (Eds Hochster, R. M. and Quastel, J. H.), Academic Press, New York, pp. 311–436

66. Melchoir, N. C. and Melchoir, J. B. (1956). Inhibition of yeast hexokinase by fluoride ion. *Science*, **124**, 402–3

67. Nejjar, V. A. (1948). Isolation and properties of phosphoglucomutase. *Journal of Biological Chemistry*, **175**, 281

68. Cimasoni, G. (1972). The inhibition of enolase by fluoride *in vitro*. *Caries Research*, **6**, 93–102

69. Slater, E. C. and Bonner, W. D. (1952). The effect of fluoride on the succinic oxidase system. *Biochemical Journal*, **52**, 185–96

70. Hamilton, I. R. (1969). Studies with fluoride-sensitive and fluoride-resistant strains of *Streptococcus salivarius*. I. Inhibition of both intracellular polyglucose synthesis and degradation of fluoride. *Canadian Journal of Microbiology*, **15**, 1013–9

71. Hamilton, I. R. (1969). Studies with fluoride-sensitive and fluoride-resistant strains of *Streptococcus salivarius*. II. Fluoride inhibition of glucose metabolism. *Canadian Journal of Microbiology*, **15**, 1021–7

72. Kabak, H. R. (1970). Transport. *Annual Reviews of Biochemistry*, **39**, 561–98

73. Luoma, H. and Tuompo, H. (1975). The relationship between sugar metabolism and potassium translocation by caries-inducing streptococci and the inhibitory role of fluoride. *Archives of Oral Biology*, **20**, 749–55

74. Kanapka, J. and Hamilton, I. R. (1971). Fluoride inhibition of enolase activity *in vivo* and its relationship to the inhibition of glucose-6-P formation in *Streptococcus salivarius*. *Archives of Biochemistry and Biophysics*, **146**, 167–74

75. Williams, R. A. D. (1969). Glycolytic intermediates in 'fluoride-trained' and con-

trol cultures of an oral enterococcus. *Archives of Oral Biology*, **14**, 265–70

76. Cimasoni, G. (1972). The inhibition of enolase by fluoride *in vitro*. *Caries Research*, **6**, 93–102

77. Jenkins, G. N., Ferguson, D. B. and Edgar, W. M. (1967). Fluoride and the metabolism of salivary bacteria. *Helvetica Odontologica Acta*, **11**, 2–10

78. Leach, S. A. (1959). Reactions of fluoride with powdered enamel and dentine. *British Dental Journal*, **106**, 133–142

79. Williams, R. A. D. (1967). The growth of Lancefield Group D streptococci in the presence of sodium fluoride. *Archives of Oral Biology*, **12**, 109–17

80. Hamilton, I. R. (1969). Growth characteristics of adapted and ultra-violet induced mutants of *Streptococcus salivarius* resistant to fluoride. *Canadian Journal of Microbiology*, **15**, 287–95

81. De Stoppelaar, J. D., van Houte, J. and Backer Dirks, O. (1969). The relationship between extracellular polysaccharide-producing streptococci and smooth surface caries in 13-year-old children. *Caries Research*, **3**, 190–9

82. Bowen, W. H. (1972). The effect of fluoride and molybdate on caries activity and the composition of plaque in monkeys (*M. irus*). *Caries Research*, **6**, 254–5

83. Rölla, G. and Melsen, B. (1975). Desorption of protein and bacteria from hydroxyapatite by fluoride and monofluorophosphate. *Caries Research*, **9**, 66–73

84. Aasenden, R., De Paola, P. F. and Brudevold, F. (1972). Effects of daily rinsing and ingestion of fluoride solutions upon dental caries and enamel fluoride. *Archives of Oral Biology*, **17**, 1705–14

85. Woolley, L. H. and Rickles, N. H. (1971). Inhibition of acidogenesis in human dental plaque *in situ* following the use of topical sodium fluoride. *Archives of Oral Biology*, **16**, 1187–94

86. Birkeland, J. M. (1972). Effect of fluoride on the amount of dental plaque in children. *Scandinavian Journal of Dental Research*, **80**, 82–4

87. Loesche, W. J., Murray, R. J. and Mellberg, J. R. (1973). The effect of topical fluoride on percentages of *Streptococcus mutans* and *Streptococcus sanguis* in interproximal plaque. *Caries Research*, **7**, 283–96

88. Loesche, W. J., Syed, S. A., Murray, R. J. and Mellberg, J. R. (1975). Effect of topical acidulated phosphate fluoride on percentages of *Streptococcus mutans* and *Streptococcus sanguis* in plaque. *Caries Research*, **9**, 139–55

89. Jordan, H. V., Englander, H. R. and Lim, S. (1969). Potentially cariogenic streptococci in selected population groups in the Western Hemisphere. *Journal of the American Dental Association*, **78**, 1331–5

90. Edwardsson, S., Koch, G. and Öbrink, M. (1972). *Streptococcus sanguis, Streptococcus mutans* and *Streptococcus salivarius* in saliva. Prevalence and relation to caries increment and prophylactic measures. *Odontologisk Revy*, **23**, 279–96

Chapter 6

Enamel Caries

6.1   Macroscopic and Radiographic Appearance

The earliest macroscopic evidence of caries may be seen on an extracted tooth as a small opaque white region positioned on either one or both of the approximal surfaces. Similar opacities may also be seen supragingivally on facial or lingual surfaces; these will also be visible in the mouth if the tooth surface is clean and dry. The approximal surface will show a small oval flattened area of interdental attrition, the contact point. The small carious lesion is seen as an opaque white region, usually positioned at the cervical margin of the interdental facet. This 'white spot' lesion contrasts with the translucency of adjacent sound enamel (figure 6.1), and is best demonstrated when the specimen is dried thoroughly.

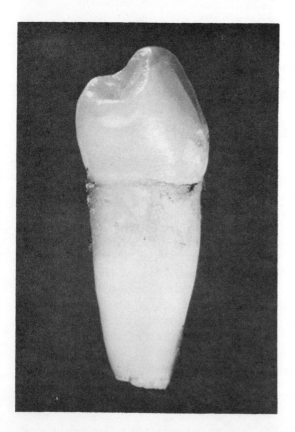

Figure 6.1   Premolar tooth showing a small white spot lesion on the approximal tooth surface

More advanced lesions still give the macroscopic appearance of white spots but are more extensive in outline, usually following the curvature of the cervical border of the interdental facet to give the lesion a kidney-shaped contour. The enamel surface overlying the white spot lesion is hard and shiny, and cannot be distinguished from the surface of adjacent sound enamel when examined with a sharp dental probe. When examined with reflected light, the perikymata can often be seen passing from the sound enamel, undisturbed over the surface of the lesion.

Intact surface lesions may also appear brownish in colour, whereupon they are described as 'brown spot' lesions. The extent of discoloration or staining is dependent upon the degree of exogenous material adsorbed by the porous enamel and it has often been stated that the degree of discoloration is related to the length of time the lesion has been present in the mouth. Thus, stained white spots have been assumed to be lesions of slow progress. However, factors such as smoking, and other habits, must influence the degree of staining of the original white spot lesion. If the lesion progresses, the enamel surface superficial to the lesion eventually fractures and a cavity is formed, although this can take anything from a few months to several years. Not all lesions, however, progress to cavitation.

Radiographic examination is an insensitive method of diagnosing the full extent of a carious lesion in both the permanent[1-4] and deciduous[5] dentition. When a lesion is first detected on a 'bite-wing' radiograph, appearing as a small radiolucent wedge in the outer enamel, histologically there is alteration of the underlying dentine. The enamel surface is still, however, intact so that it is important to emphasise that at this stage the dentine is not infected by bacteria; this can only occur after cavitation. Thus, small lesions detected by radiography need not be restored immediately. Restoration can be delayed or avoided if adequate preventive procedures are carried out (chapter 12). However, such teeth must be kept under constant review by radiography as well as by clinical examination. If there is evidence of progression of the lesion, it is advisable to insert a small restoration.

With control of the cariogenicity of the tooth environment, lesions may become arrested or even remineralize (chapter 12).

The enamel lesion on the smooth surface of a tooth is conical in shape, having its apex pointing towards the dentine. On reaching the enamel–dentine junction, spread of the carious process is usually rapid along this plane. In the case of smooth surface lesions, lateral spread along the enamel–dentine junction results in a broad base to the dentine lesion. In this manner the carious process undermines sound enamel (see figure 7.6, page 171).

With fissure caries, the enamel lesion broadens as it approaches the underlying dentine, since it is guided by prism direction. With lateral spread at the enamel–dentine junction, the area of involved dentine is larger than with smooth surface lesions. The lesion of fissure caries does not occur at the base of the fissure but bilaterally on the walls of the fissure, giving the appearance of two small smooth surface lesions[6] (figure 6.2). Eventually the lesions increase in size, coalescing at the base of the fissure. Clinically, fissure caries may be seen as an opaque border zone related to part or whole of the fissure periphery. Such regions may also take up stain to become discoloured. As the lesion increases in extent, more of the surrounding enamel will be undermined by spread of the carious process along the enamel–dentine junction. This is seen clinically as an extension of the opaque or stained region across the occlusal surface. Eventually, the surface enamel fractures to produce a cavity, by which time the underlying dentine will be stained (dark) brown.

The histological features of the small carious lesion in human dental enamel have been described by a number of workers. The small lesion has been divided into zones based upon its histological appearance when longitudinal ground sections are examined with the light microscope[6–20]. The number of zones described has varied from three[8] to seven[10], the larger subdivision probably being due to varying de-

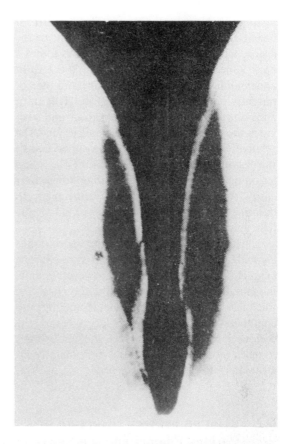

Figure 6.2 Microradiograph of a longitudinal ground section through an occlusal fissure showing a small carious lesion (× 40). The lesion does not commence at the base of the fissure, but occurs bilaterally on its walls

grees of overlap. The division of the lesion into zones is important in that it separates, at the histological level, different types as well as magnitudes of change in the tissue, some of which are extremely subtle. While this is a useful procedure in the classification and subsequent identification of various regions of a lesion, it must be emphasised that there is no sudden or dramatic change in the tissue from zone to zone. The entire lesion should be regarded as showing a gradual and progressive series of changes rather than one with changes occurring abruptly in a step-like manner.

It is most convenient to subdivide the small enamel lesion into four zones[19], each clearly distinguishable from the others. There is a translucent zone at the inner advancing front of the lesion, whereas just superficial to this is found a dark zone. The body of the lesion is the third zone and lies between the dark zone and the apparently undamaged enamel surface. This third zone shows marked demineralisation and provides the greater mass of the small lesion. The relatively unaffected surface zone superficial to the lesion is the fourth zone. Since the small lesion in enamel consists essentially of these four easily recognisable zones, it is convenient to describe the structure of carious enamel, at the light microscope level, on this basis.

The histological features of caries in deciduous enamel are essentially similar to those in the enamel of permanent teeth[20]. However, enamel in deciduous teeth is approximately half the thickness of that in permanent teeth and the pulp chambers are relatively much larger. Thus, the carious process needs to travel a shorter distance to reach the pulp in a deciduous molar relative to a molar from the permanent series.

6.2   Relation between Structure of Carious Enamel and the Image in Polarised Light

Mature human dental enamel consists largely of crystals of apatite which are packed closely together in the tissue and which are aligned approximately along the length of the prism in an orderly arrangement. Between the crystals, minute spaces are present which contain both the organic component of the tissue as well as an aqueous phase. The mineral component of enamel, like most biological structures and noncubic crystals, has the property of resolving a beam of plane polarised light into two rays which travel at different velocities. Such structures are termed 'birefringent'; that is, the structure has two refractive indices, related to the two planes of transmission within the crystal.

With non-cubic crystals, a sign of birefringence is given to the structure, determined by the path taken by the slower (+) and faster (−) rays in relation to the morphology of the crystal. Since in biological materials it is difficult to recognise crystal morphology, the sign of birefrigence is related arbitrarily to some morphological feature of structure which is approximately parallel to one of the vibration directions. In an enamel prism, the slower ray is found to vibrate at right-angles to the length of the prism, and therefore the sign of birefringence is described as negative with respect to prism length (the opposite to that found with protein fibres). This is said to be the 'intrinsic birefringence' of the tissue. Enamel thus has a negative intrinsic birefringence, relative to prism direction. The sign of birefringence of the organic component is positive with respect to prism length but its strength of birefrigence is very small, and can be disregarded for present purposes.

Apart from the mineral and organic constituents of enamel, there are minute 'spaces' in the tissue. During both development and carious dissolution there is an increase in the total volume of 'spaces' in enamel and these spaces, or pores, themselves give rise to an additional type of birefringence. A system of rod-shaped elements such as enamel crystals, separated from each other by spaces containing a medium having a different refractive index from that of the rods, constitutes a 'mixed body'[21]. A rodlet mixed body produces positive birefringence relative to the direction of orientation of the rods. This is known as 'form birefringence'. Therefore, form birefringence is produced when the spaces in the tissue contain a medium having a refractive index different from that of the enamel crystals (RI = 1.62). Whereas the intrinsic birefringence is negative, relative to prism length, form birefringence is positive in sign.

Therefore, carious enamel will show a negative intrinsic birefringence due to its orientated crystal component and positive form birefringence due to the intercrystal spaces. Thus the 'observed birefringence' is the sum of these two. Only when the spaces, or pores, are filled with a medium having the same refractive index as enamel, will the form birefringence be eliminated. Therefore, when enamel is examined in longitudinal ground section with the polarising microscope, the image formed depends on both the refractive index of the mounting medium and its degree of penetration into the tissue. The greater the difference between the refractive index of the mounting medium and the enamel, the more positive form birefringence will be produced. Similarly, as the internal pore volume increases (i.e. increasing demineralisation), the amount of form birefringence will also increase. The negative intrinsic birefringence of the tissue can therefore be either reduced, compensated or reversed depending on the amount of form birefringence produced. Thus, the observed birefringence, which is the sum of the negative intrinsic birefringence and positive form birefringence, may be seen as a reduction, a cancellation or a complete reversal of the original negative birefringence. Cancellation will be observed as absence of birefringence and this is referred to as pseudo-isotropy.

It is also possible to deduce the percentage volume of spaces present in carious enamel by measuring the observed birefringence of the enamel. This is carried out using a suitable optical compensator in conjunction with the polarising microscope. The degree of positive form birefringence can then be calculated from the observed birefringence, if the intrinsic birefringence of the tissue is known. The intrinsic birefringence can be measured directly provided that all of the pores in enamel are filled with a medium having the same refractive index as the enamel apatite, thus eliminating positive form birefringence. An aqueous medium must therefore be employed so as to penetrate freely all spaces in the tissue[8]. A suitable medium is Thoulet's solution[8], prepared from potassium mercuric iodide, and this can be diluted with distilled water to give any desired refractive index. Enamel examined in Thoulet's medium (RI = 1.62) will exhibit only the negative intrinsic birefringence of the tissue. The volume of spaces in enamel can then be calculated[8].

Quantitative imbibition studies with the polarising microscope, based on the foregoing considerations, can give accurate information relating to the sub-microscopic structure of carious enamel. Two types of imbibition media are generally used in an attempt to explore the internal pore volume of the tissue. Dilutions of potassium mercuric iodide (Thoulet's solution) form a series of aqueous media which are able to penetrate the pore structure completely. These media are usually prepared having refractive indices of 1.41, 1.47 and 1.62 which, together with water (RI = 1.33) and air (RI = 1.0), form a series of aqueous media employed by most workers in the field[7, 8, 15, 17]. The second type of medium employed consists of a series of 'non-aqueous' fluids. These are normal aliphatic alcohols, which are particularly useful as they ascend progressively, from methanol to octanol, in both refractive index and molecular size. Quinoline is placed in this group of imbibition media and is commonly used because its refractive index (1.62) is the same as that of enamel mineral. The observed birefringence at a specific point, or points, in a particular zone of the lesion is calculated from values of total path difference, which is measured directly using a suitable optical compensator in conjunction with the polarising microscope[12-17].

6.3 The Structure of Carious Enamel as Seen with the Light Microscope and by Microradiography

6.3.1 Zone 1: the translucent zone

Much of our knowledge of the structure of normal and carious enamel is based on the examination of ground sections, approximately 100 μm thick, examined in the ordinary and polarised light microscope, as described above. In addition, much useful information has been gained by the technique of microradiography, in which the ground section is placed in contact with a photographic emulsion and exposed to a parallel beam of X-rays. After development an X-ray absorption image, largely reflecting the amount and distribution of mineral present in the section, is obtained.

The translucent zone of enamel caries lies at the advancing front of the lesion and there is full agreement that, when present, this zone represents the first observable change in structure in the tissue. However, only approximately 50 per cent of lesions demonstrate a translucent zone at the advancing front of the lesion[16]. This zone is only seen when a longitudinal ground section is examined in a clearing agent, such as Canada balsam or quinoline, having a refractive index

The zone appears translucent because the spaces, or pores, created in the tissue in this first stage of enamel caries are located at prism boundaries, and other junctional sites. Therefore, when the pores are filled with a medium, such as quinoline, having the same refractive index as enamel, normal structural markings are no longer visible (figure 6.3).

Several workers have shown that the translucent zone is positioned deep to the region of visible radiolucency seen on microradiographs[8, 17]. From this it was assumed that there

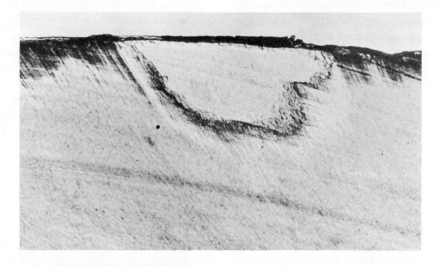

Figure 6.3 **Longitudinal ground section through a small enamel lesion. The section is examined in quinoline by transmitted light. The lesion shows a translucent zone over the entire advancing front, while superficial to this a dark zone can be seen, surrounding the body of the lesion. The striae of Retzius are enhanced in the body of the lesion (× 100)**

similar to that of the enamel (RI = 1.62). Canada balsam was the medium used by earlier histologists but quinoline is more suitable since its refractive index is identical to that of the enamel. When a ground section is examined in transmitted light after imbibition with quinoline, the translucent zone appears structureless, and well demarcated from the normal enamel on its deep aspect, in which structural markings such as prisms, cross-striations and striae of Retzius are visible, and from the dark zone (zone 2) on its superficial aspect (figure 6.3).

was no demineralisation in the translucent zone. Other workers claimed that the translucent zone was produced by a loss of soluble protein from enamel, but this work has not been substantiated. Using polarised light, it has been shown[8] that the translucent zone is more porous than sound enamel, having an imbibable pore volume of 1 per cent compared with about 0.1 per cent for sound enamel. Microradiographs of carious enamel have been examined using a sensitive two-dimensional microdensitometric technique[22]. Changes in density were recorded in the region of the translucent zone indicating, for the first time, that mineral loss had occurred in this region. The histological zones have also been micro-dissected from ground sections of enamel lesions and chemical studies have been carried out on the various regions[23]. The fluoride content of translucent zone enamel was found to be increased relative to adjacent sound enamel. No evidence of protein loss was found within this zone. The overall findings suggested that carious attack had preferentially removed magnesium and carbonate-rich mineral from the translucent zone. These studies provided direct evidence that the spaces created in the translucent zone were caused by the removal of mineral and not organic material.

6.3.2 Zone 2: the dark zone

The dark zone is the second zone of alteration from normal enamel and lies just superficial to the translucent zone. It appears dark brown in ground sections examined by transmitted light after imbibition with quinoline or Canada balsam (figure 6.4a). It is a more constant feature of the advancing front of the lesion than is the translucent zone, occurring in 90–95 per cent of lesions in permanent enamel[17], and 85 per cent of lesions in deciduous enamel[21]. Polarised light studies[8] have shown that the dark zone has a pore volume of 2–4 per cent of spaces. When examined with the polarising microscope after imbibition with quinoline, the dark zone shows positive birefringence in contrast to the negative birefringence of sound enamel, and a reduced negative birefringence of the rest of the lesion (plate 6.1a). Hence it is often also referred to as the 'positive' zone.

These effects were shown to be due to the presence of very small spaces, or pores, in the zone in addition to the relatively large pores which are present in the first stage, the translucent zone. Therefore, when a ground section is examined in a mounting medium such as quinoline or Canada balsam, the relatively large molecules of the medium are unable to penetrate the micropore system of the dark zone. This

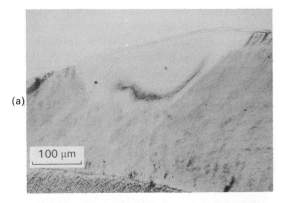

(a)

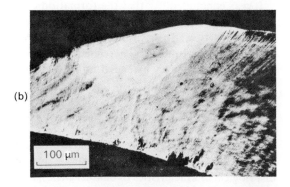

(b)

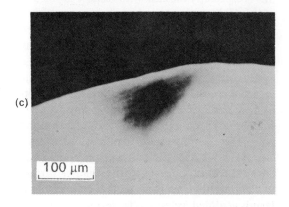

(c)

Figure 6.4 **(a) Longitudinal ground section of a small enamel lesion seen in quinoline with transmitted light (× 50). The advancing front of the lesion shows both a translucent zone and a dark zone. (b) When the section is examined in an aqueous medium having the same refractive index as enamel (1.62), the dark zone is no longer seen, since the micropore system has been completely penetrated by the medium. (c) Microradiograph of the section. The body of the lesion in the sub-surface enamel shows marked radiolucency in contrast to the surface zone, which remains well mineralised**

effect has been described as a 'molecular sieve'[12]. Since the micropores remain 'filled' with air or vapour, light is scattered on passing through the zone, causing the brown coloration of the dark zone (figure 6.3). In a similar manner, the presence of a medium of low refractive index within the micropores is responsible for the reversal of birefringence from negative to positive in the dark zone when examined in polarised light[8,19] (plate 6.1a). If the ground section is examined in an aqueous medium having small molecules which penetrate the micropores, the dark zone is no longer seen (figure 6.4b, plate 6.1b).

It was concluded[8,12] that the formation of a micropore system must be regarded as a result of demineralisation. This was consistent with evidence from microradiography, where the region of visible radiolucency extended into the region of the dark zone (figure 6.4c).

In vitro studies on the nature of the dark zone

Lesions created in human enamel *in vitro*, using dilute acid solutions, fail to demonstrate several histological characteristics of enamel caries, and this is especially the case with respect to the dark zone. Unlike the translucent zone, which is reproduced in enamel *in vitro* with no apparent difficulty[16], the dark zone is much more difficult to simulate. Using a technique consisting of hydroxyethyl cellulose acidified with lactic acid, *in vitro* lesions have been produced showing narrow dark zones at their advancing fronts in enamel[25]. However, from a histological standpoint, these lesions are not identical with those of natural caries since their advancing fronts maintain a direction parallel to the enamel surface, unlike the irregular fronts seen in enamel caries. Using acidified gelatin gels, lesions have been created in human enamel which appear indistinguishable from those of enamel caries when examined histologically with the polarising microscope[17,18]. Under these conditions, an exposure period of several months is required to create caries-like lesions. A dark zone was a constant feature of the advancing front of such lesions and appeared positively birefringent when examined in quinoline with the polarising microscope (plate 6.1a). As the concentration of the gel increased, so the prevalence and width of dark zones appearing in artificial lesions also increased, and the lesion appeared more caries-like[17,19].

It would seem from this work that the rate of attack on the enamel is an all-important criterion in producing tissue changes resembling those seen in caries. The concentration of the gel appeared to be the most critical single factor in determining rate of attack, there being an inverse relationship between concentration and rate. Quantitative imbibition studies with the polarising microscope showed that the dark zone in these artificial lesions behaved in an identical manner to the dark zone in caries. When the section was removed from quinoline and examined in an aqueous medium having an identical refractive index, the dark zone was no longer seen (plate 6.1b), indicating that its appearance was associated with a micropore system in the zone, which was again acting as a molecular sieve. On replacing the section into quinoline, the dark zone was observed once again. Thus, the appearance of the dark zone was related to a slow diffusion-controlled attack. These findings support other observations[15] on the relationship between speed of lesion formation and histological appearance.

In experimental studies on the 'remineralisation' of enamel caries[26,27], carious lesions and artificial caries-like lesions were exposed to either saliva or a synthetic calcifying fluid *in vitro*. After exposure, there was a significant reduction in pore volume throughout the lesions, resulting in the histological appearance of a much earlier stage in lesion formation than that existing prior to experiment. This occurred with both natural and artificial lesions and was found when either saliva or the calcifying fluid was employed. However, the synthetic calcifying fluid, which contained no organic material, was more effective in producing these changes than was saliva[27]. When examined in quinoline with polarised light, the most obvious change in the modified lesion was a significant broadening of

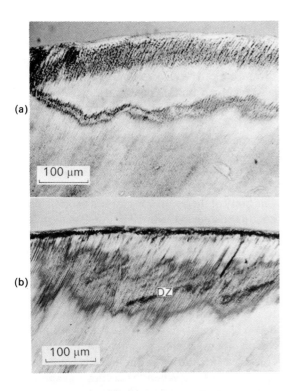

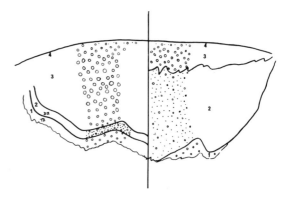

Figure 6.6 Diagrammatic representation of the lesion shown in figure 6.5. The left-hand side shows the pore-structure in the lesion before experiment (figure 6.5a). Zone 1 and 2 (translucent and dark zones) are seen at the advancing front of the lesion. The right-hand side shows the pore structure of the lesion after experiment (figure 6.5b), where the dark zone appears much broader, spreading back towards the enamel surface. For this to have occurred, a micropore system must have been created in an area that was previously the body of the lesion

Figure 6.5 (a) Longitudinal ground section of a small lesion examined in quinoline with polarised light before exposure to a calcifying fluid ($\times$ 100). The advancing front of the lesion shows a translucent zone and a positively birefringent dark zone. (b) Same section after exposure to a calcifying fluid *in vitro*, also examined in quinoline with polarised light ($\times$ 100). The dark zone is now seen to be much broader than in the control, extending back towards the enamel surface into the region previously identified as the body of the lesion

the dark zone as a consequence of its extension back towards the enamel surface (figure 6.5), into the region identified previously as the body of the lesion (figure 6.6). In addition, lesions which showed no evidence of a dark zone in quinoline were also exposed to the synthetic calcifying fluid. After experiment, many of the lesions demonstrated dark zones positioned at the 'correct' site between the translucent zone and the body of the lesion[19-27] when examined in quinoline. The imbibition behaviour of 'new' dark zones, and those which increased in width after experiment, was consistent with that of the dark zone proper. Thus part of the body of the lesion

(zone 3) had reverted to the histological characteristics of the dark zone (zone 2).

Prior to these findings, the dark zone at the advancing front of the lesion had been regarded as a breakdown stage successional to the translucent zone and preceding the body of the lesion. It has always been difficult to explain why in the first zone of enamel caries, the translucent zone, relatively large pores are found, whereas in the succeeding stage of breakdown, the dark zone, a smaller pore system is found in addition to the large pores. The micropores in the dark zone were explained as being due to demineralisation[12], or 'opening up' of specific sites in the tissue which were not attacked in the first zone of breakdown. However, in the experiments on remineralisation[26,27], an area previously identified as the body of the lesion had, after experiment, taken on the histological characteristics of the preceding stage, the dark zone. If some of the relatively large pores of the body of the lesion could, in effect, become the minute ones of the dark zone (figures 6.6 and 6.7) then this could indicate that the micropore system of the dark zone may not be formed by a simple process of

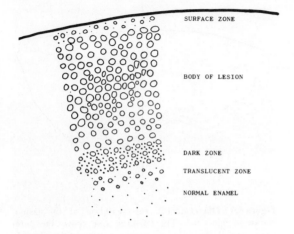

Figure 6.7 Diagram to show the pore structure of a carious lesion in human enamel. The translucent zone shows relatively large pores, numbers of which increase as the dark zone is approached. However, in the dark zone a micropore system is present in addition to the large pores. The body of the lesion shows an increased pore volume, with large pores which freely accept all imbibition media. The surface zone shows a low pore volume with a number of very small pores in addition to moderately sized ones, similar to those of the translucent zone

demineralisation. Thus, the dark zone may not simply be a stage in the sequential breakdown of the tissue as was previously thought, but the smaller micropores may be formed by 'remineralisation', whereby either the size or the accessibility of the large pores is reduced by the deposition of material. The results from *in vitro* studies suggest that mineral deposition could account for the 'closing down' of the original pores created as a result of demineralisation, although *in vivo* organic material might also contribute.

If this is the case, then this lends further support to the concept that the carious process in enamel is a dynamic one with phases of demineralisation alternating with phases of remineralisation, rather than a more simple process of continuing dissolution. In this way, the variation in distribution and width of the dark zone over the advancing front of the enamel lesion may be explained as functions of the efficacy of the 'remineralisation' process. Of significance in this respect are the observations[15]

that lesions of 'arrested' caries have wide, well-marked, dark zones. Additional support for the theory that remineralisation plays a role in the formation of the dark zone has arisen from the observation[28] that there was an apparent 'loss of structure and filling-in of the prism markings in the dark zone' when examined with the scanning electron microscope.

6.3.3   Zone 3: the body of the lesion

The body of the lesion is the largest proportion of carious enamel in the small lesion. It is the whole of the area positioned superficial to the dark zone and deep to the relatively unaffected surface layer of the lesion. When a longitudinal ground section is examined in quinoline with transmitted light, the body of the lesion appears relatively translucent compared with sound enamel (figure 6.3). However, the striae of Retzius within this region are well marked and therefore appear enhanced in contrast to the translucency of the area (figure 6.3). When the section is examined with the polarising microscope, the striae still appear as well-differentiated structures within the general translucency of the zone. After imbibition with water, the body of the lesion becomes positively birefringent, in contrast to the negative birefringence of the rest of the lesion and sound enamel (figure 6.8, plate 6.1c). This region shows a minimum pore volume of 5 per cent at its periphery, increasing to 25 per cent or greater in the centre of the small lesion. Within the body of the lesion, the striae of Retzius are seen to be enhanced when examined after imbibition with water, as they show a higher degree of positive birefringence relative to the intervening regions. The prism structure is also well marked within this region and shows a pattern of cross-striations.

When the lesion is examined by microradiography, the region of visible radiolucency corresponds almost exactly with the size and distribution of the body of the lesion (figure 6.4). However, when the microradiograph is examined in more detail with the light microscope, the advancing front of the radiolucent region is seen

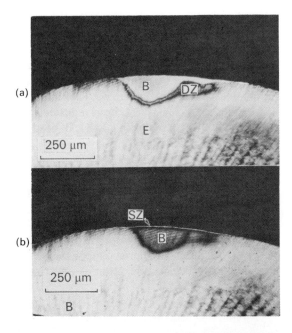

(a)

(b)

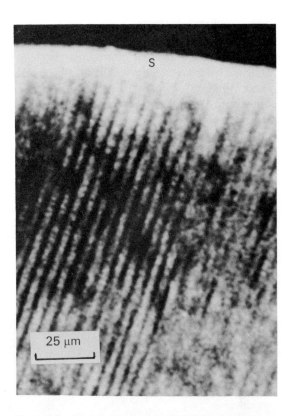

Figure 6.8 (a) Longitudinal ground section showing a small carious lesion examined in quinoline with polarised light (× 50). The dark zone (DZ) shows positive birefringence in contrast to the rest of the lesion (B) and the sound enamel (E) which appear negatively birefringent. (b) same section now examined in water with polarised light. The body of the lesion (B) shows positive birefringence in contrast to the relatively unaffected surface zone (SZ) which is negative in sign

Figure 6.9 Microradiograph of a longitudinal section through carious enamel (× 150). Radiolucent and radiopaque lines are seen almost at right-angles to the well-mineralised enamel surface (S). This indicates a pattern of demineralisation in relation to the long axes of the prisms

to extend beyond the body of the lesion, into the region of the dark zone. Superficially, the radiolucent region is limited by the presence of a well-mineralised, radiopaque layer at the surface of the lesion (figure 6.4c). Alternate radiolucent and radiopaque lines pass obliquely through the sub-surface region[8]. The radiolucent lines, showing an apparent preferential demineralisation, are spaced approximately 30 μm apart and are thought to be the striae of Retzius. The surrounding sound enamel shows no evidence of differential calcification of these structures. Within the radiolucent region, a pattern of alternating radiolucent and radiopaque lines is also observed running approximately at right-angles to the enamel surface (figure 6.9). These structures are spaced 6–8 μm apart and are parallel to prism structure. In addition, many

regions show a pattern of radiolucent lines passing at right-angles to prism direction. Since these are spaced at approximately 4 μm, they are thought to represent the cross-striations of the prisms. By varying the exposure time of the microradiographic plate to the source of CuK α-radiation, it is possible to highlight one or more of these structures exhibiting a so-called preferential attack.

These findings have also been recorded by other workers[6,10,11,15,29]. It was reasoned that the radiolucent lines passing to the enamel surface almost at right-angles were part of the prism structure, most probably the cores of the prisms[8]. Microradiographs of sections of carious enamel prepared in a direction transverse to prism structure showed a pattern of circles having radiolucent centres with narrow radio-opaque borders (figure 6.10). The radiolucent circles had a diameter of approximately 5 μm, while the outer opaque rim was 0.5–1.0 μm wide. These findings[8–30] were interpreted as demonstrating a preferential demineralisation of the prism cores.

Using the information gained from microradiography, together with observations in polarised light, the route along which the carious process spread through enamel was proposed. Entry of the carious process into the tissue was by way of the striae of Retzius at the enamel surface[8]. Demineralisation then progressed along the interprismatic 'substance', through the cross-striations of the prisms, to gain access to the prism cores which were subsequently de-

mineralised[8]. In contrast, it was also reported that dissolution of mineral started at the periphery of the prisms and then proceeded towards their centres[10,31]. However, not all workers agreed that the striae of Retzius were necessarily the channels along which there was a preferential demineralisation. It has also been reported that the striae of Retzius showed marked positive birefringence in the peripheral parts of the enamel lesion[15]. Since areas of positive birefringence seen in quinoline corresponded with regions of slow advance[15], the striae could represent pathways of resistance to the spread of the lesion rather than pathways of progress.

Quantitative microradiographic studies[32] suggested that the characteristic appearance of alternate radiolucent and radiopaque bands

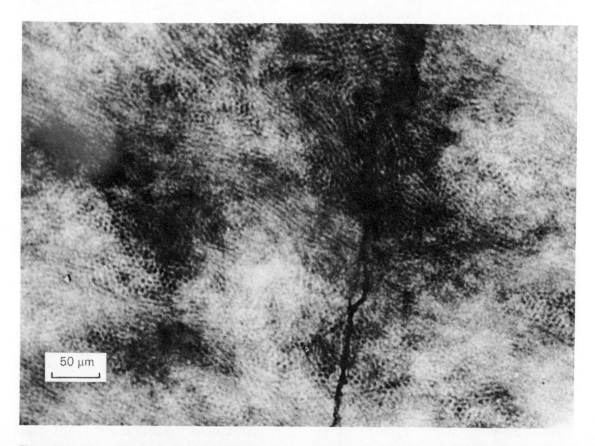

Figure 6.10   Microradiograph showing the body of the carious lesion from a section prepared in a direction transverse to the prisms (× 400). The prisms appear as circles having radiolucent centres with narrow radiopaque margins

parallel to the striae was not simply an indication of demineralisation proceeding along these planes. The appearances were explained on the basis that alternate bands were being demineralised in fixed proportions. The alternate incremental banding thus appeared to be only a reflection of an existing structural relationship 'unmasked' in predetermined proportions.

Several workers have described carious lesions in enamel which showed well-mineralised bands passing through the body of the lesion, giving the lesion a 'laminated' appearance[13, 15, 23]. Microradiographic examination of such lesions showed the presence of one or more radiopaque zones passing through the radiolucent subsurface region (figure 6.11). It has been suggested that these laminations may arise during a transient phase of the carious process and persist when the advance continued[13]. Laminated lesions were found in teeth of African and Indian origin[15]. The appearance of such lesions was thought to be more likely associated with variations in the local environment in the mouth, rather than the result of structural differences in the tissue. In a histological survey of 100 carious lesions in deciduous molars[21], 15 lesions showed relatively well-mineralised laminations passing through the body of the lesion. The laminations were less porous than the remainder of the body of the lesion. Examination of ground sections by microradiography showed that the bands of low porosity corresponded with the position of well-mineralised zones passing through the lesion (figure 6.11). The laminations were positioned with their greatest convexity towards the dentine and appeared to follow a contour similar in outline to that of the advancing front of the lesion. Therefore, each lamination might well have represented the advancing front of the lesion at an earlier point in time as suggested previously[13, 15, 23].

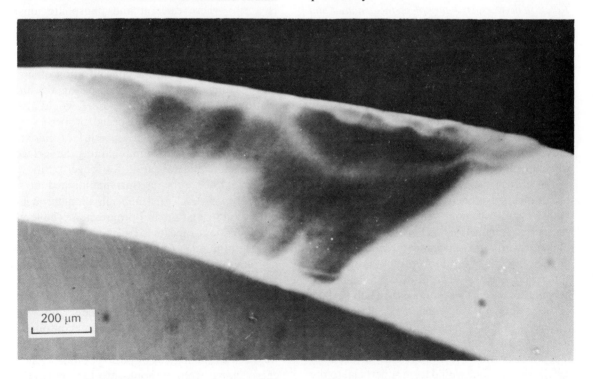

Figure 6.11 **Microradiograph of a longitudinal ground section through a carious deciduous molar (× 50). In addition to a relatively well-mineralised surface layer, there are several radiopaque bands or 'laminations' passing through the sub-surface body of the lesion (By courtesy of the *Journal of Dentistry for Children*: Silverstone, L. M., 1970, *37*, 17–27)**

6.3.4   Zone 4: the surface zone

One of the important characteristics of caries of human dental enamel is that the greatest degree of demineralisation occurs at a sub-surface level, so that the small lesion remains covered by a surface layer which appears relatively unaffected by the attack. When a small lesion of enamel caries is examined with the polarising microscope after imbibition with a medium having a refractive index remote from that of the enamel (e.g. water), although the porous sub-surface enamel is seen to be positively birefringent (figure 6.8), the surface zone retains a negative birefringence[18] (plate 6.1c). This relatively unaffected surface zone is also identifiable on microradiographs as a radiopaque surface layer, approximately 30 μm in depth, sharply demarcated from the underlying radiolucent sub-surface region of the lesion (figures 6.4c and 6.9).

Relation between structure of surface enamel and the presence of a surface zone superficial to a lesion

Many workers have suggested that the formation of a relatively unaffected surface layer overlying the small lesion of enamel caries is closely associated with the special properties of surface enamel. If the original enamel surface is removed, the remaining enamel is more susceptible to acid demineralisation. The greater resistance of the surface enamel to carious dissolution has been explained as being due, in part at least, to its higher degree of mineralisation compared with sub-surface enamel[33-35]. This, together with a higher fluoride and lead content[36], and perhaps a greater amount of insoluble protein in the most superficial layer of the surface enamel[8], may account for it being less soluble than sub-surface tissue as shown by acid-etching studies[37].

Several workers have removed part of the natural enamel surface prior to *in vitro* experiments with artificial caries systems, in order to see if a surface zone would form superficial to the lesion on the new enamel surface. It was shown by microradiography that when a tooth was abraded prior to exposure to various acid buffers, a lesion could be produced that still had a greater mineral content at the surface than at its sub-surface region both *in vitro*[28, 38] and *in vivo*[39]. Using an acidified gel technique, lesions were produced on artificially abraded enamel surfaces which had up to 500 μm of surface enamel cut away prior to experiment[18]. The lesions created on these surfaces still showed well-mineralised surface layers (figure 6.12). When examined in water with polarised light, a negatively birefringent surface zone was observed, overlying the more heavily demineralised sub-surface region.

These results suggest, therefore, that the 'special' physical and chemical properties of surface enamel, relative to sub-surface enamel, are not entirely responsible for the presence of a well-mineralised surface zone above the small carious lesion. An additional suggestion is that the surface zone remains well mineralised because it is a site where calcium and phosphate ions, released by sub-surface dissolution, or derived from the saturated solution in plaque (section 5.6), become re-precipitated into the surface enamel. The high fluoride concentration of surface enamel, presumably released at the initiation of solution of outer enamel, would also favour precipitation. The special properties of surface enamel relative to sub-surface enamel would be responsible for maintaining the surface zone from demineralisation for longer periods.

The surface zone is thus maintained at a relatively low level of demineralisation throughout lesion formation and progression. The level of mineral loss appears to be less than 5 per cent, in spite of a much greater degree of sub-surface dissolution. However, the well-mineralised surface zone is eventually demineralised. This attack upon the surface itself has been reported as being a late stage in the carious process and was observed to commence from the outer contour of the surface zone inwards[18]. Histologically, this was seen as small areas of positive birefringence encroaching, from without, into the negatively birefringent surface layer. When the surface was finally demineralised, it still appeared to have an

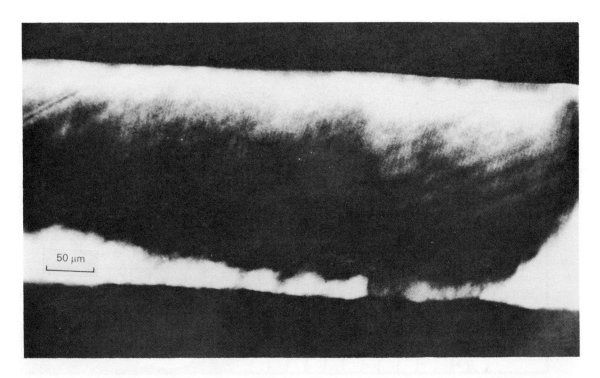

Figure 6.12 Microradiograph of an artificial caries-like lesion created on abraded enamel (× 100). Approximately 500μm of the original enamel was ground off the tooth surface prior to lesion formation. The lesion was produced in an acidified gelatin gel after an exposure time of 40 weeks. The lesion has penetrated the remaining enamel, showing marked demineralisation in the body of the lesion. However, the surface overlying the lesion shows a deep, well-mineralised, surface zone (By courtesy of the *British Dental Journal*: Silverstone, L. M., 1968, *125*, 145–57)

intact surface contour. *In vitro* studies have shown that when this occurred, the rate of lesion progression was significantly increased[18]. The surface enamel does, therefore, play a special role in the mechanisms involved in caries formation. The various integuments found in relation to the enamel surface, together with other parameters specific to the surface region, are shown diagrammatically in figure 6.13.

6.4   The effect of caries on the organic matrix of enamel

As developing enamel mineralises, much of its organic content disappears and that which remains in the fully mature tissue is not distributed evenly. Although much is known of the chemistry and structure of the protein matrices of developing and sound enamel, relatively little work has been carried out on the organic material within carious enamel.

It was shown in earlier studies[7] that demineralisation occurred before histological change could be demonstrated in the organic matrix. The time at which organic change in the matrix became histologically identifiable was only a short time before cavitation of the lesion occurred.

Two organic components of the enamel, one readily soluble in dilute acid and the other insoluble, have been described[40]. It was shown[41] that in the dissolution of powdered enamel by dilute acid, the first material to be dissolved was organic in nature and that its amount and nitrogen content was consistent with it being the soluble organic material[40]. The dissolution of mineral occurred later, followed by the loss of more organic material but still leaving an insoluble organic fraction. It has been reasoned[8]

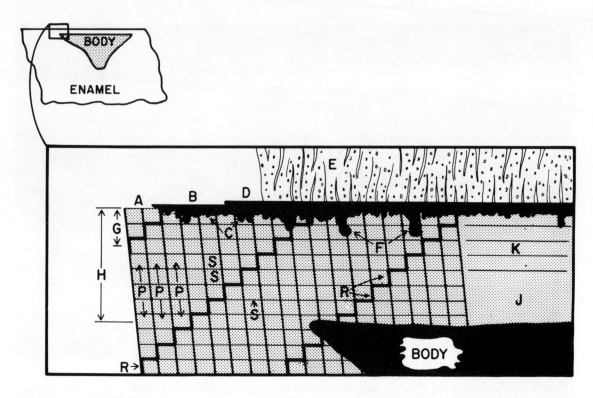

Figure 6.13   Diagram showing the various integuments found in relation to the enamel surface, together with other features specific to the surface layer of enamel

A.   *The enamel surface*: almost always covered by an organic film except immediately after a thorough dental prophylaxis.

B.   *Cuticle*: organic film on enamel surface derived mainly from salivary mucopolysaccharides and less than 1 μm in thickness.

C.   *Sub-surface pellicle*: exogenous organic material which penetrates 1–3 μm into the surface enamel, i.e. a sub-surface extension of the cuticle/pellicle.

D.   *Pellicle*: when the cuticle becomes 1 μm [and greater] in thickness it is called pellicle; a structureless organic film.

E.   *Plaque*

F.   *Wedge-shaped defects*: these are found at intervals along the enamel surface and filled with exogenous organic material

G.   *Fluoride-rich surface layer*: this is approximately 10 μm in depth.

H.   *The surface zone*: the fourth zone of enamel caries; approximately 30 μm in depth.

J.   *Prismless enamel*: enamel with no prismatic markings detectable by light microscopy.

K.   *Laminations*: laminations are often seen in prismless surface enamel running parallel to the enamel surface; thought by some to be comparable with the cross-striations of prisms.

P.   *Enamel prism*: structural unit of enamel having a 'keyhole' shape in transverse section and extending longitudinally from the enamel–dentine junction to the enamel surface; approximately 5 μm in diameter, those in the outer third of the enamel pass almost normal to the enamel surface whereas in the deeper enamel they follow more irregular courses.

R.   *Stria of Retzius*: developmentally, enamel is laid down in increments each separated by a stria of Retzius representing a period of quiescence during rhythmic deposition

S.   *Cross-striations*: these periodic markings traverse the prismatic structure at regular intervals of approximately 4 μm.
     Body: Body of the lesion; this is the third zone of the lesion of enamel caries and represents the greatest bulk of the small lesion.

that the mineral crystallites were embedded in, and coated by, the organic matrix. The soluble mineral structures, identified in the lesion by microradiography, had a matrix of soluble organic material. Similarly, the insoluble mineral component had an insoluble organic matrix. In this way the differential solubility of the tissue in caries was explained[8].

The appearance of the organic material in both normal and carious enamel is affected by the method of specimen preparation. It has been described as fibrillar or spongy in texture, or as a gel[42] which assumes different appearances depending on how it is fixed and demineralised. Likewise, its distribution has been considered to include condensations at the periphery of prisms—prism sheaths—or to spare these regions creating peripheral gaps.

Electron microscopic studies on the organic component of sound and carious enamel have been carried out[43-45]. In normal enamel these revealed a prism sheath type of structure having a double membrane of condensed filaments. Both prismatic and interprismatic areas were composed of a fine network of fibres. In areas of advanced caries, the basic morphology of the organic matrix was maintained and the sheath structure appeared to be quite resistant. The fibrillar network was less dense and less regular than in the sound tissue, frequently missing from the prisms and interprismatic areas. Many areas showed an apparent increase in organic material, and this confirmed previous reports[40, 46, 47].

Only two workers have directly supported the hypothesis that the initial attack in caries is on the organic matrix. Earlier studies[48] on artificially demineralised lesions suggested that proteolysis preceded demineralisation, since 'prism sheaths' were found to be damaged. Preferential proteolysis was also reported since the more soluble organic matrix was dissolved from prism cores allowing the crystallites to wash out[49-52]. This hypothesis was based on the findings of hollow prisms in electron micrographs of carious enamel. The claim that the removal of organic material by cold ethylenediamine produces changes in enamel *in vitro*, similar to those in the translucent zone of enamel caries[53], has not been confirmed. In fact, it has now been shown that mineral is lost from the translucent zone, with no evidence of change in the organic matrix[54].

There is widespread agreement that the organic content of carious enamel is greater than that of the sound tissue[25, 40, 43-47, 55, 56]. It is generally agreed that the additional organic material is amorphous in appearance and may be of bacterial, or mixed salivary and bacterial, origin. The outer layer of carious enamel has a higher organic content than deeper layers[57-59]. A thin 'surface cuticle' lying immediately upon the enamel surface has been described[57] (figure 6.13). Beneath this, extending into the enamel to a depth of $1-3\,\mu m$, was a dendritic network of fibrils, the 'sub-surface cuticle' (figures 6.13 and 6.22). This has been confirmed by several workers[58-60]. The presence of surface and sub-surface cuticles may play a significant role in the initiation and progress of the carious lesion by controlling the diffusion of ions into, and out of, the enamel. In addition to these organic membranes, many workers have reported the penetration of exogenous organic material into 'defects' in the surface enamel overlying the small carious lesion (figures 6.13 and 6.14). These plaque-filled defects are usually $4-5\,\mu m$ in width, penetrating the tooth surface to depths of $5-10\,\mu m$[59, 61] (figure 6.14).

After demineralisation of ultra-thin sections of carious enamel[59], the only structure remaining was a hyaline substance. This material, which filled the spaces between the crystals, appeared to be a mixture of organic matter and embedding material. Decalcified ultra-thin sections of carious enamel from the body of the lesion stage revealed, in both transverse and longitudinal sections of the prisms, a cellular network of organic material. The spaces within this cellular network were comparable in size and shape to the crystals in the sections before demineralisation (figure 6.15). This gave the impression that the organic network formed 'envelopes' which ensheathed the crystals[59]. Examination of ultra-thin sections of carious enamel which had been demineralised and stained specifically for carbohydrate gave a strongly positive histochemical reaction in dental plaque overlying the small lesion. Bacteria were stained intracellularly but the strongest reaction was related to the cell walls and polysaccharide capsules. Plaque matrix and surface pellicle stained moderately. The organic matrix of sound enamel stained faintly or not at all. In contrast, the organic residues of carious enamel showed a

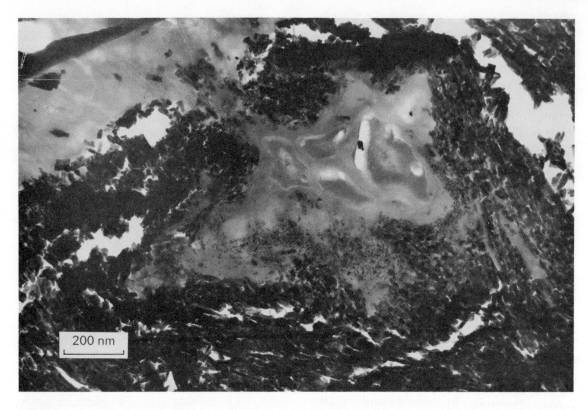

Figure 6.14   Electron micrograph showing the outer enamel from a small lesion demonstrating a typical surface defect 3–4 μm in diameter (× 31 500). This contains a few bacteria and is filled with hyaline material continuous with the surface pellicle. At the periphery of the defect, small residual fragments of extensively dissolved enamel crystallites can be seen (From Johnson[59]; courtesy of *Caries Research*)

reaction which was distinctly positive. The staining intensity was seen to decrease from the tooth surface inwards over a relatively short distance, but it was not possible to determine exactly how close to the advancing front of the lesion the positively staining matrix existed[59].

6.5   Electron Microscopic Studies of Carious Enamel

6.5.1   Scanning electron microscopy

The image capabilities of the scanning electron microscope enable simple and direct observations of the ultrastructure of dental tissues which are not possible by conventional trans-

mission electron microscopy. Whole tooth crowns or small blocks of tissue can be scanned at magnifications compared to those obtained with the light microscope, increasing to ultrastructural levels. The ease of specimen preparation, orientation of the field under examination, and its great depth of focus, makes the scanning electron microscope a valuable research tool. It is clear from the evidence of previous workers[7, 8, 31] that the carious process affects some structures in enamel more readily than others. However, as regards the location of sites of differential destruction, it has not always been easy to reconcile results obtained by different methods of examination.

In one study[62] small approximal carious lesions were examined with the scanning electron

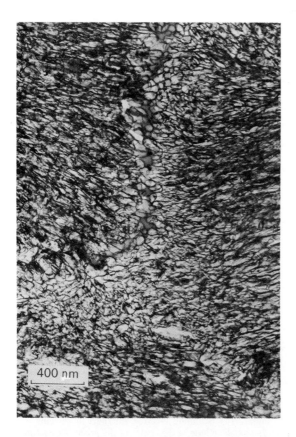

Figure 6.15 Electron micrograph showing the junction between three transversely sectioned prisms from a lesion (× 43 000). The section was demineralised on the grid with phosphotungstic acid; electron diffraction revealed no residual crystals. A cellular network remains, the spaces of which correspond in size and shape to that of the crystallites present before demineralisation. A band of hyaline material is present at one of the prism junctions and this corresponds to the junctional channels observed in the undemineralised section (From Johnson[66]; courtesy of *Archives of Oral Biology*)

microscope. Many of the carious surfaces possessed large cavities in which no structural features were visible since the carious tissue was covered with adherent organic material. However, in a number of cases surfaces covering white spot lesions had lost small flakes of enamel to depths of 100–300 μm. Micro-cavities such as these were quite free of organic debris because, apparently, they had been created traumatically during the process of tooth extraction (figure 6.16). Fractures tended to occur along structural planes which were identified as the striae of Retzius.

From the appearance of the fractured carious enamel it was stated that the crystals in the central part of the prism were often, but not always, loosened in such a manner that they were lost on fracture leaving shallow pits or occasional deep holes (figure 6.16), surrounded by walls of residual material. If a similar honeycomb is produced during the preparation of ground sections, it could account for the microradiographic image of sections of carious enamel cut in a plane perpendicular to prism direction, in which a so-called preferential demineralisation of prism cores is seen (figure 6.10). Despite the identification of a few deep pits of the order of 20 μm in depth, the results indicated that there was no general hollowing of the prisms into tube-like structures during caries, even in the body of the lesion stage. Nevertheless, there appears to be some property of the peripheral region of prisms enabling it to retain crystals more easily than the central region after both fracture of carious enamel and the acid-etching of sound enamel[63]. This property may be related to the structure at prism junctions where abrupt changes in crystal orientation occurs[64, 65] and where new crystal forms may arise during caries[43, 66, 67]. The arrangement of more parallel crystals with a lower organic content in the central part of the prism might make this region more liable to collapse than the periphery after loosening of the crystals has occurred.

In another study[28], the most striking feature was the appearance of the striae of Retzius which appeared to be less demineralised than the surrounding enamel. Gaps occurred between prisms which were thought to be the result of demineralisation. In more advanced lesions, loss of tissue from between the prisms and from the prism centres was reported. Evidence was presented showing that demineralisation of the surface zone occurred along the prism structure rather than along the striae of Retzius, as suggested previously[8]. However, *in vitro* studies with artificial caries have shown that deminerali-

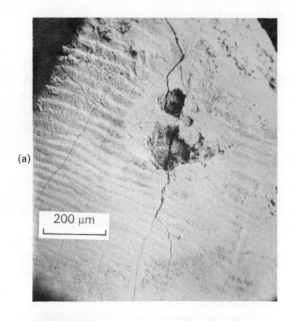

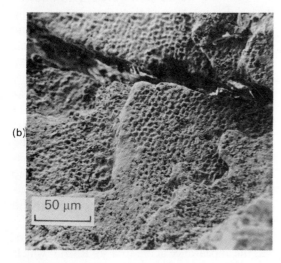

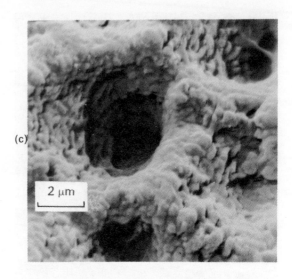

Figure 6.16   (a) Scanning electron micrograph of the approximal surface of a premolar tooth showing the interdental facet of attrition and surface perikymata. This surface showed a white spot lesion, from which flakes of enamel have fractured away to leave two small micro-cavities. (b) Scanning electron micrograph showing the detailed appearance of typical prism endings from the fracture plane seen in the previous figure. Prism centres show depressions which are shallow, varying in form from saucer-shaped to conical. The texture of the fractured surface is extremely granular. (c) Scanning electron micrograph showing an occasional deep hole in the centre of the prism. Around the wall of the hole is a suggestion of incremental rings. The texture of the carious enamel is again seen to be granular or lumpy in appearance. (By courtesy of *Archives of Oral Biology:* Poole, D. F. G and Silverstone, L. M., 1969, *14,* 1323–29).

sation could occur along either pathway in the surface zone[18].

6.5.2   Transmission electron microscopy

With the introduction of ultrastructural techniques in caries research, it was hoped that direct visualisation of the diseased tissue would help to resolve some of the problems of interpretation which have existed at the light microscope level.

However, progress has been slow mainly because of the technical difficulties involved in the preparation of ultra-thin sections from such a hard tissue. Much of the earlier ultrastructural work was carried out using replica techniques on fractured or acid-etched surfaces. Some workers claimed that their findings indicated that mineral loss preceded damage to the organic component of the tissue[68–70] whereas others[71] stated that it was the organic material which was preferentially lost.

Early work with ultra-thin sections, carried out on artificially demineralised enamel, could give no information on changes occurring to the crystals themselves. Some workers were able to prepare sections through advanced carious lesions which were soft enough to overcome many of the technical problems[45, 48, 72]. However, it was not possible to assess the initial changes which occurred during lesion formation when examining such extensively damaged tissue. In recent years, improved techniques have resulted in the sectioning of intact mature human dental enamel[64] and of small carious lesions[55, 59, 66, 73].

It is first relevant to clarify some aspects of the structure of sound enamel which have emerged as a result of the introduction of electron microscopy to dental research. In human dental enamel, three main types of prism shape and arrangement have been described[65]. In the most common of these patterns, the prism junctions are seen as arcade-shaped rows which are out of phase in successive layers, so that each prism appears to have a 'head' and a 'tail' region when cut in transverse section (figure 6.17). Such a 'keyhole'-shaped arrangement has also been described by others[64]. In this arrangement, termed type 3[65], the tails of the prisms in one row interdigitate with the heads of the prisms in the immediately cervical row. The relationship of the

prisms to each other is such that all parts of the tissue can be ascribed to a particular prism and there are no true interprismatic areas. The crystal orientation in the head region is predominantly parallel to the prism long-axis, but diverges from this in the tail. In the remaining patterns the relationship of prisms is such that parts of the tissue can be considered to be interprismatic. There is general agreement among electron microscopists that the basic structure of these two areas is identical, the only visible difference being one of crystal orientation. For this reason the term 'interprismatic enamel' is preferred to the previous term 'interprismatic substance'.

There are two major schools of thought concerning the pattern of destruction of enamel by caries. The first is that the 'prism sheaths' or the 'interprismatic substance' is destroyed before the prisms themselves. The second is that the prism is the more susceptible structure. Ultrastructural studies have supported both the former[25, 73] and the latter views[52, 68, 74]. In addition, it has also been proposed that all components are equally susceptible[66, 70]. Much evidence is available from the light microscope and microradiography to suggest that the initial breakdown in caries is dependent upon structure. However, the majority of ultrastructural studies of normal and carious enamel have failed to show several structural features which are readily observed with the light microscope.

It has been suggested that cross-striations of the prisms are due to periodic narrowing of the prisms[75], or periodic variations in the density of crystal packing[76]. In addition, localised changes in crystal orientation have been suggested as the reason for the appearance of the striae of Retzius[76]. However, neither of these structures can be identified unequivocally in routine ultrathin sections. Therefore, since these features are not observed at the ultrastructural level, it is difficult, if not impossible, to report on their significance in the initiation and spread of the carious lesion when using this technique.

The explanation, at the light microscope level, of differences in the degree of destruction of

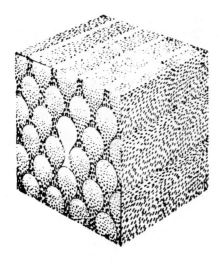

Figure 6.17 Diagrammatic representation of the structure of human dental enamel (By courtesy of Drs Meckel, Griebstein and Neal: *Archives of Oral Biology,* **10,** 775–83, 1965)

various regions of enamel, was related to the supposed differences in composition between the prisms, 'prism sheaths' and 'interprismatic substance'. However, as mentioned previously, there is now general agreement that the fundamental structure of the tissue between the prisms is identical with that inside, the only visible difference being one of crystal orientation.

One study[66] attempted to correlate the features of carious enamel seen with the electron microscope with the degree of breakdown of the lesion, as determined with the polarising microscope. This was carried out by measuring the pore volume in various regions of the lesion in a ground section prepared from the slice of tooth adjacent to that used for electron microscopy. The results from examining specimens cut transverse to prism direction suggested that obvious intercrystallite spacing, and damage to the crystals themselves, was not detectable unless the section came from areas having a pore volume of 10–25 per cent. Thus, the first region of identifiable change from a normal appearance, using transmission electron microscopy, was seen in the body of the lesion. No changes could be detected within the first two zones of the lesion as identified by polarised light microscopy.

At low magnification, carious tissue frequently appeared intact but examination at higher magnification revealed a diffuse demineralisation, with an increase in intercrystallite distance affecting all areas within the prisms and interprismatic enamel[66]. Many of the spaces between crystals were filled with a hyaline material which appeared to be a mixture of organic matter and embedding material, and was the only structure remaining after artificial demineralisation of the section. Narrow channels, 30–100nm wide, were seen partially surrounding the prisms in the carious tissue (figures 6.18 and 6.19) when examined in transverse section. These channels contained the embedding material and were therefore unlikely to have been sectioning artefacts. This breakdown of prism junctions with the development of narrow, sheath-like, structures could be ascribed to mechanical shaking apart of the prisms during the initial slitting of

the tooth. If this is true, they must be present in the average ground section and play a part in formation of the image seen with the light microscope and by microradiography. However, since these channels have not been identified in ultra-thin sections from sound enamel[64], it see-

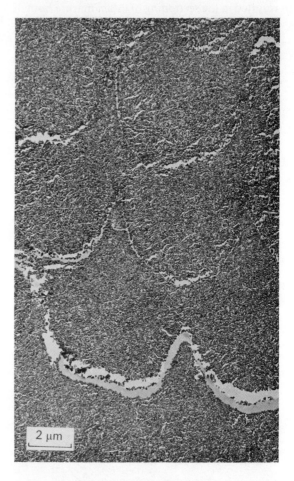

Figure 6.18   Electron micrograph through the body of a carious lesion cut transversely to prism direction (× 10 000). A large crack, filled with embedding material, crosses the field following the curved occlusal aspects of a few prism junctions. Prism junctions elsewhere are marked by the presence of narrow channels, which are sometimes due to tearing of the section but in which embedding material can frequently be seen, indicating that the channels existed before the enamel was embedded and sectioned. A diffuse demineralisation is present throughout the tissue, although it is difficult to detect. Intercrystallite spaces contain the embedding material (From Johnson[66]; *courtesy of Archives of Oral Biology*)

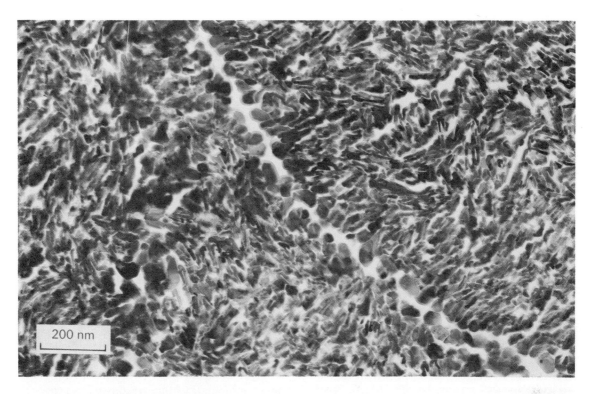

Figure 6.19 Electron micrograph showing parts of two transversely sectioned prisms from carious enamel. Intercrystallite space containing embedding material can be clearly differentiated from artefact. A double row of enlarged, polyhedral crystals is present at the prism junction lining a channel which is largely artefact, but which does contain Araldite. This is seen where it forms a halo to crystals. The majority of crystals are irregular flattened hexagons with central deficiencies (× 67 200) (From Johnson[66]; courtesy of *Archives of Oral Biology*)

med likely that they were produced as a result of the carious process.

The effects of caries on individual crystals in enamel appear to be of two main types. In order for the intercrystallite space to increase, mineral must be removed from the external surface of the crystals[59]. In general the crystals of outer enamel showed only slight etching, as evidenced by an irregularity of their margins (figure 6.20). However, large plaque-filled defects, up to 4 μm wide, commonly penetrated the enamel surface to depths up to 5 μm (figures 6.14 and 6.21). These contained a few bacteria and were surrounded by a layer of hyaline material continuous with the surface pellicle and plaque matrix. In the second type of attack on individual crystals, central defects are also found, the preferential loss of crystal centres resulting in the appearance of 'hairpin' or 'double rodlet' shapes when the

crystals are seen in longitudinal section (figure 6.20)[45, 55, 59]. In transverse section, the damaged crystals are seen as hollow hexagons or rectangles. A similar loss of structure in the centres of crystals has been reported when they are etched with acids *in vitro*[77] and this preferential loss of crystal centres appears to occur preferentially along the lattice c-axis[77] (crystal long axis).

In addition to damage to crystals in the carious process, several workers have also recorded the frequent finding of a different crystal form at prism borders when examining carious enamel in transverse section. These crystals at the prism periphery appear thicker and more electron dense than those elsewhere in the tissue (figure 6.19). Their average size appears to be 120–150 nm across[66], which is greater than the width of the crystals in sound enamel. Although often

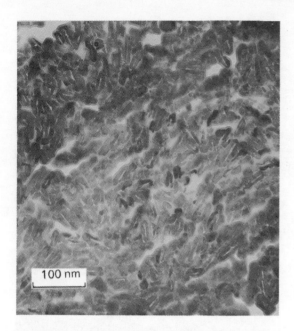

Figure 6.20 Electron micrograph showing details of transversely section crystals from the body of an intact surface carious lesion in enamel (× 106 250). The external outlines of the crystals are irregular, but the majority are basically hexagonal in outline, measuring 100–150 nm by 40–60 mm. Many crystals have central defects, from 5–15 nm wide. Evidence of embedding material infiltrating into the section is seen

angular, or even hexagonal, in outline, they are more isodiametric than either the remainder of the crystals in the carious tissue or those of normal enamel. These larger crystals are thought to be the result of recrystallisation or remineralisation rather than original crystals which have resisted dissolution.

Decalcified ultra-thin sections of carious enamel revealed a cellular network (figure 6.15), the spaces of which were comparable in size and shape to the crystals in the sections before demineralisation[59]. This created the impression that the membranes constituting this network formed the walls of 'envelopes' which had ensheathed the crystals. The narrowest of these membranes was 20–40 nm wide and was quite electron dense, particularly after treatment with phosphotungstic acid which appeared to enhance the contrast.

The finding that there is a preferential removal of magnesium-rich, and probably carbonate-rich, mineral from the translucent zone of enamel caries[54] suggests three possibilities for the first attack on the enamel at the ultrastructural level. First, crystal surfaces may be etched, as many workers believe that the enamel magnesium resides largely at, or near, the surface of apatite crystals. Evidence of surface etching occurring on individual crystals has already been presented. Secondly, the first attack may be a preferential dissolution of crystals containing relatively high concentrations of magnesium throughout their structure. Thirdly, the selective dissolution of a separate amorphous calcium phosphate phase, if present in enamel, may represent the initial attack.

Thus, experiments described by a number of electron microscopists indicate that carious destruction of human dental enamel may not be as dependent on the structural detail of the tissue as has previously been believed. However, such an interpretation must be viewed with caution, since many structural features readily visible with the light microscope cannot be identified by transmission electron microscopy. Indications are that tissue changes within the first two stages of enamel caries, as identified with the polarising microscope, cannot be distinguished from sound enamel by ultrastructural means. Such subtle changes, which are readily identified at the light microscope level, may never be observed by direct visualisation of the tissue with the electron microscope. Demineralisation of the bulk of the tissue appears to be diffuse, affecting both intra- and inter-prismatic enamel. The appearance of a so-called preferential demineralisation of certain regions of the prism, identified at the light microscope level and with the scanning electron microscope, may be due, in part at least, to damage caused by section preparation techniques. Prism junctions do appear to be sites where a preferential dissolution of tissue occurs, because narrow channels often develop between adjacent prisms, at the margins of which recrystallisation occurs. This results in the formation of crystals larger than those of the sound

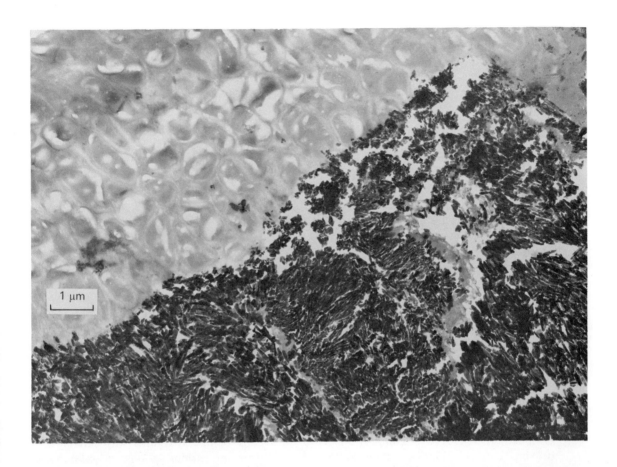

Figure 6.21   Electron micrograph of inner layers of plaque and outer enamel at the surface of a small enamel lesion (× 17150). Bacteria are seen in direct contact with the tooth surface and there is little plaque matrix. A large, wedge-shaped defect is present at the top of the field; elsewhere, narrow channels of organic material, 200 nm wide, can be seen penetrating the outer enamel. The channels of organic material are often located at prism junctions (From Johnson[59]; courtesy of *Caries Research*)

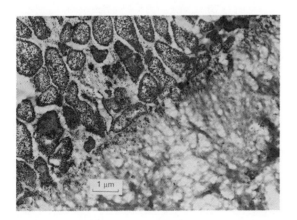

Figure 6.22   Electron micrograph showing plaque and outer enamel from a small lesion. The section, similar to that seen in figure 6.21, was demineralised with EDTA and stained by a modification of the Gomori silver hexamine technique for the identification of carbohydrates. Positive staining is demonstrated by the binding of discrete particles of metallic silver. A stronger reaction is seen in the bacterial cytoplasm and cell walls. All of the residual organic material within the lesion accepts the stain, but the greatest intensity is in the surface layer of enamel to a depth of approximately I μm, corresponding to the sub-surface cuticle (From Johnson[59]; courtesy of *Caries Research*)

tissue, and indicates the dynamic nature of the carious process in which phases of demineralisation alternate with phases of stasis, or of remineralisation.

Further reading

Schmidt, W. J. and Keil, A. (1971). *Polarizing Microscopy of Dental Tissues*, 1st Eng. edn (Eds Poole, D. F. G. and Darling, A. I.), Pergamon Press, Oxford

Stack, M. V. and Fearnhead, R. W. (1965). *Tooth Enamel*, Wright, Bristol

References

1. Darling, A. I. (1959). The pathology and prevention of caries. *British Dental Journal*, **107**, 287–96
2. Marthaler, T. M. and Germann, M. (1970). Radiographic and visual appearance of small smooth surface caries lesions studies on extracted teeth. *Caries Research*, **4**, 224–42
3. Gwinnett, A. J. (1971). A comparison of proximal carious lesions as seen by clinical radiography, contact microradiography and light microscopy. *Journal of the American Dental Association*, **83**, 1078–80
4. Silverstone, L. M. (1978). *Preventive Dentistry*, Update Books, London
5. Dwyer, D. M., Berman, D. S. and Silverstone, L. M. (1973). A study of approximal carious lesions in primary molars. *Journal of the International Association of Dentistry for Children*, **4**, 41–6
6. Mortimer, K. V. (1964). The histological features of caries in human dental enamel. *Ph.D. Thesis*, Univ. of Bristol
7. Darling, A. I. (1956). Studies of the early lesion of enamel caries with transmitted light, polarized light and microradiography. *British Dental Journal*, **101**, 289–97 and 329–41
8. Darling, A. I. (1958). Studies of the early lesion of enamel caries with transmitted light, polarized light and microradiography. Its nature, mode of spread, points of entry and its relation to enamel structure. *British Dental Journal*, **105**, 119–35
9. Darling, A. I. (1963). Resistance of the enamel to dental caries. *Journal of Dental Research*, **42**, 488–96
10. Gustafson, G. (1957). The histopathology of caries of human dental enamel, with special reference to the division of the lesion into zones. *Acta Odontologica Scandinavica*, **15**, 13–55
11. Soni, N. N. and Brudevold, F. (1959). Microradiographic and polarized light studies of initial carious lesions. *Journal of Dental Research*, **38**, 1187–94
12. Darling, A. I., Mortimer, K. V., Poole, D. F. G. and Ollis, W. D. (1961). Molecular sieve behaviour of normal and carious human dental enamel. *Archives of Oral Biology*, **5**, 251–73
13. Kostlan, J. (1962). Translucent zones in the central part of the carious lesions of enamel. *British Dental Journal*, **113**, 244–8
14. Carlstrom, D. (1963). Polarization microscopy of dental enamel with reference to incipient carious lesions, in *Advances in Oral Biology*, vol. 1, Academic Press, New York, pp. 255–96
15. Crabb, H. S. M. (1966). Enamel caries: observations on the histology and patterns of progress of the approximal lesion. *British Dental Journal*, **121**, 115–29 and 167–74
16. Silverstone, L. M. (1966). The primary translucent zone of enamel caries and of artificial caries-like lesions. *British Dental Journal*, **120**, 461–71
17. Silverstone, L. M. (1967). The histopathology of enamel lesions produced *in vitro* and their relation to enamel caries. *Ph.D. Thesis*, Univ. of Bristol
18. Silverstone, L. M. (1968). The surface zone in caries and in caries-like lesions produced *in vitro*. *British Dental Journal*, **125**, 145–57
19. Silverstone, L. M. (1973). Structure of

carious enamel including the early lesion, in *Oral Sciences Reviews: No. 3 Dental Enamel* (Eds Melcher, A. H. and Zarb, G. A.), Munksgaard, Copenhagen, pp. 100–160

20. Silverstone, L. M. (1970). The histopathology of early approximal caries in the enamel of primary teeth. *Journal of Dentistry for Children*, **37**, 17–27

21. Wiener, O. (1912). Theory of composite bodies. *Abh. sachs Ges. Wiss.*, **33**, 507

22. Crabb, H. S. M. and Mortimer, K. V. (1967). Two dimensional microdensitometry. A preliminary report. *British Dental Journal*, **122**, 337–43

23. Weatherell, J. A., Robinson, C. and Hallsworth, A. S. (1971). Micro-analytical studies on single sections of enamel, in *Tooth Enamel*, vol. 2 (Eds Stack, M. V. and Fearnhead, R. W.), Wright, Bristol, pp. 31–8

24. Poole, D. F. G., Mortimer, K. V., Darling, A. I. and Ollis, W. D. (1961). Molecular sieve behaviour of dental enamel. *Nature (London)*, **189**, 998–1000

25. Gray, J. A. and Francis, M. D. (1963). Physical chemistry of enamel dissolution, in *Mechanisms of Hard Tissue Destruction*, American Association for the Advancement of Science, Washington, publ. No. 75, p. 213

26. Silverstone, L. M. and Poole, D. F. G. (1968). Modification of the histological appearance of enamel caries after exposure to saliva and a calcifying fluid. *Caries Research*, **2**, 87–96

27. Silverstone, L. M. (1977). Remineralization phenomena. In *Cariostatic Mechanisms of Fluoride* (Eds Brown, W. E. and Konig, K. G.), *Caries Research*, **11** (Suppl. 1), 59–84

28. Mortimer, K. V. and Tranter, T. C. (1971). A scanning electron microscope study of carious enamel. *Caries Research*, **5**, 240–63

29. Bergman, G. and Lind, P. O. (1966). A quantitative microradiographic study of incipient enamel caries. *Journal of Dental Research*, **45**, 1477–84

30. Miller, J. (1958). Note on the early carious lesion in enamel. *British Dental Journal*, **105**, 135–6

31. Gustafson, G. and Gustafson, A. G. (1961). Human dental enamel in polarized light and contact microradiography. *Acta Odontologica Scandinavica*, **19**, 259–87

32. Crabb, H. S. M. (1972). Incremental bands in microradiographs of ground sections of a carious lesion in enamel. *Caries Research*, **6**, 169–82

33. Thewlis, J. (1940). The Structure of Teeth as Shown by X-ray Examination, Special Report Series 238, HMSO, London

34. Brudevold, F. (1948). A study of the phosphate solubility of the human enamel surface. *Journal of Dental Research*, **27**, 320–9

35. Hals, E., Morch, T. and Sand, H. F. (1955). Effect of lactate buffers on dental enamel *in vitro* observed in polarizing microscope. *Acta Odontologica Scandinavica*, **13**, 85–122

36. Isaac, S., Brudevold, F., Smith, F. A. and Gardner, D. E. (1958). Solubility rate and natural fluoride content of surface and subsurface enamel. *Journal of Dental Research*, **37**, 254–63

37. Sullivan, H. R. (1954). The formation of early carious lesions in dental enamel. *Journal of Dental Research*, **33**, 231–44

38. Sperber, G. H. and Buonocore, M. G. (1963). Enamel surface in white spot formation. *Journal of Dental Research*, **42**, 724–31

39. Fehr, F. R. von der (1967). A study of carious lesions produced *in vitro* in unabraded, abraded, exposed in F-treated human enamel surfaces with emphasis on the X-ray dense outer layer. *Archives of Oral Biology*, **12**, 797–814

40. Stack, M. V. (1954). The organic content of chalky enamel. *British Dental Journal*, **96**, 73–6

41. Rowles, S. L. and Little, K. (1955). Some observations on histological techniques. *Journal of Dental Research*, **34**, 778 (abst.)

42. Eastoe, J. E. (1966). The changing nature of

developing dental enamel. *British Dental Journal*, **121**, 451–4

43. Johansen, E. (1962). The nature of the carious lesion. *Dental Clinics of North America*, 305–20

44. Johansen, E. (1963). *Mechanisms of Hard Tissue Destruction* (Ed. Sognnaes, R. F.), American Association for the Advancement of Science, Washington, No. 75, pp. 187–211

45. Johansen, E. (1965). *Tooth Enamel* (Eds Stack, M. V. and Fearnhead, R. W.), Wright, Bristol, pp. 177–81

46. Hardwick, J. L. and Manley, E. B. (1952). Caries of the enamel and acidogenic caries. *British Dental Journal*, **92**, 225–36

47. Bhussry, B. R. (1958). Chemical and physical studies of enamel from human teeth. *Journal of Dental Research*, **37**, 1045–53

48. Frank, R. M. (1955). La carie dentaire au microscope electronique. *Schweitz Monatsschr Zahnheilkd*, **65**, 635–6

49. Little, K. (1957). The organic components of human dental enamel. *Journal of Dental Research*, **36**, 815 (abst.)

50. Little, K. (1959). Electron microscope studies on human dental enamel. *Journal of the Royal Microscopical Society*, **78**, 58–66

51. Little, K. (1961). The use of the electron microscope in the examination of pathological conditions affecting the connective and hard tissues. *Journal of the Royal Microscopical Society*, **80**, 35–45

52. Little, K. (1962). The matrix in caries resistant teeth. *Journal of the Royal Microscopical Society*, **80**, 199–208

53. Darling, A. I. and Mortimer, K. V. (1959). Further observations on the early lesion of enamel caries. *Journal of Dental Research*, **38**, 1226 (abst.)

54. Hallsworth, A. S., Robinson, C. and Weatherell, J. A. (1972). Mineral and magnesium distribution within the approximal carious lesion of dental enamel. *Caries Research*, **6**, 156–68

55. Frank, R. M. (1965). *Caries-Resistant Teeth* (Eds Wolstenholme, G. E. W. and O'Connor, M.), Churchill, London, pp. 169–84

56. Plackova, A. and Stepanek, J. (1965). Die submikroskopische struktur der braunen Schmelzflecken. *Deutsche Zahnarztliche Zeitschrift*, **20**, 925–30

57. Meckel, A. H. (1965). The formation and properties of organic films on teeth. *Archives of Oral Biology*, **10**, 585–97

58. Leach, S. A. and Saxton, C. A. (1966). An electron microscopic study of the acquired pellicle and plaque formed on the enamel of human incisors. *Archives of Oral Biology*, **11**, 1081–94

59. Johnson, N. W. (1967a). Transmission electron microscopy of early carious enamel. *Caries Research*, **1**, 356–69

60. Armstrong, W. G. (1968). Origin and nature of the acquired pellicle. *Proceedings of the Royal Society of Medicine*, **61**, 923–30

61. Silverstone, L. M. and Johnson, N. W. (1971). The effect on sound human enamel of exposure to calcifying fluids *in vitro*. *Caries Research*, **5**, 323–42

62. Poole, D. F. G. and Silverstone, L. M. (1969). Observations with the scanning electron microscope on trauma-induced micro-cavities in human enamel. *Archives of Oral Biology*, **14**, 1323–9

63. Poole, D. F. G. and Johnson, N. W. (1967). The effects of different demineralizing agents on human enamel surfaces studies by scanning electron microscopy. *Archives of Oral Biology*, **12**, 1621–34

64. Meckel, A. H., Griebstein, W. J. and Neal, R. J. (1965). Structure of mature human dental enamel as observed by electron microscopy. *Archives of Oral Biology*, **10**, 775–83

65. Boyde, A. (1965). *Tooth Enamel* (Eds Stack, M. V. and Fearnhead, R. W.), Wright, Bristol, pp. 163–67

66. Johnson, N. W. (1967). Some aspects of the ultrastructure of early human enamel caries seen with the electron microscope. *Archives of Oral Biology*, **12**, 1505–21

67. Silverstone, L. M. and Poole, D. F. G.

(1969). Histologic and ultra-structural features of 'remineralized' carious enamel. *Journal of Dental Research*, **48**, 766–70

68. Matsumiya, S., Takuma, S. and Tsuchikura, H. (1952). Etude au microscope electronique des surfaces dentaires lisses—carie de l'email dentaire humain. *Actualites Odontologica Stomatologic*, **6**, 409–19

69. Helmcke, J. G. (1955). Electronmikroskopische strukturuntersuchungen an gesunden und pathologischen zahn. *Schweitz Monatsschr Zahnheilkd*, **65**, 629–32

70. Awazawa, Y. (1964). Electron microscopy of enamel caries. *Journal of the Nihon University School of Dentistry*, **6**, 122–38

71. Frank, R. M. (1953). Etude de development en surface de la carie dentaire par la methode des repliques ombrees et par une technique d'usure inversee a la meule. *Schweitz Monatsschr Zahnheilkd*, **63**, 683–94

72. Scott, D. S. and Albright, J. T. (1954). Electron microscopy of carious enamel and dentine. *Journal of Oral Surgery*, **7**, 64–78

73. Vahl, J., Hohlung, H. J., Plackova, A. and Bures, H. (1966). Elektronenmikroskopische ultradunnschnittuntersuchungen an zahnen mit Schmelzflecken, herruhrend von initialer karies, artifizielles Karies und mineralisations storungen. *Deutsche Zahnarztliche Zeitschrift*, **21**, 983–9

74. Takuma, S. (1955). The electron microscopy of the enamel surfaces of teeth under various abnormal conditions. *Journal of Dental Research*, **34**, 152–63

75. Helmcke, J. G. (1963). New results of the electron microscope on shape structure of normal and pathologically changed teeth. *International Dental Journal*, **13**, 450–5

76. Hinrichsen, C. F. L. and Engel, M. B. (1966). Fine structure of partially demineralised enamel. *Archives of Oral Biology*, **11**, 65–93

77. Johnson, N. W. (1966). Differences in the shape of human enamel crystallites after partial destruction by caries, EDTA and various acids. *Archives of Oral Biology*, **11**, 1421–4

Chapter 7

The Caries Process in Dentine: The Response of Dentine and Pulp

Although caries of enamel is clearly a dynamic process, it is not a vital process in the sense that living, cellular reactions occur. Indeed, enamel is almost a unique tissue, because it is devoid of cells and cannot, therefore, respond to injury.

On the other hand, pulp and dentine must be considered as integral parts of the same living tissue. The odontoblast cell bodies lining the pulp chamber and their cytoplasmic extensions into dentinal tubules are just as much part of dentine as osteocytes and osteoblasts are part of living bone. The continued vitality of odontoblasts is dependent on the blood supply and lymphatic drainage of the pulp tissue itself. The dentine/pulp unit is thus a fully vital tissue capable of defending itself, and the progress of caries in dentine involves a fluctuating interplay between attacking forces and defence reactions. The state of the tissue at any time depends therefore on how these processes are balanced, so that a knowledge of the defence reactions of the pulp–dentine system is an essential prerequisite to understanding the nature of the caries process in dentine.

7.1   Defence Reactions of the Dentine–Pulp Unit

Caries attack is not the only form of injury to which the pulp–dentine system is subjected and the same defence reactions occur in response to a variety of stimuli of quite different nature. The more common stimuli may be grouped as follows:

(1)   Bacterial—for example, dental caries.

(2)   Mechanical—for example, trauma; tooth fracture; cavity preparation; attrition; abrasion.

(3)   Chemical—for example, penetration of oral fluids through root dentine following gingival recession; chemical erosion of enamel; medicaments, cements and dressings placed in cavities; dehydration of exposed dentine, particularly during the cutting of cavities.

(4)   Thermal—for example, excessive heat generated by rotary cutting instruments during cavity preparation; thermal shocks transmitted to dentine through large metal restorations from hot or cold foods.

The fundamental defence reactions of the pulp–dentine unit, irrespective of the nature of the stimulus, may be considered as developing at three levels within the tooth, namely in the substance of dentine, at the pulp/dentine interface and in the soft tissue of the pulp itself. These may be listed as: (a) within dentine—tubular sclerosis; (b) at the interface—reactionary dentine and atubular calcifications; (c) within the pulp—inflammation.

The phenomenon of *dead tract* formation is sometimes regarded as a defence reaction but, as explained below, this usually results from one of the first two processes listed above. Each of these processes will now be considered in detail.

7.1.1   Tubular sclerosis

This is a process in which mineral is deposited within the lumina of dentinal tubules. When examined by transmission electron microscopy[1] the tubules are partly or completely filled with crystals which are indistinguishable from those of normal peritubular dentine (figure 7.1a), and electron diffraction studies confirm that they are composed of apatite. Deposition begins on the walls of the tubules and appears to progress inwards in centripetal fashion[2] (figure 7.1a), so that the process of sclerosis is thought to be an acceleration of the normal mechanism of peritubular dentine formation. However, in demineralised ultra-thin sections, the organic matrix within the occluded tubules often appears denser and more homogeneous than that in normal peritubular dentine, and no characteristic collagen cross-banding can be seen (figure 7.1b). The process, therefore, may not be entirely analogous to that which happens during tooth formation. Nevertheless, microbiochemical assay of sclerotic dentine reveals a higher hydroxyproline content than that of sound tissue, indicating that its matrix is collagenous[3]. It is usually considered, therefore, that the process

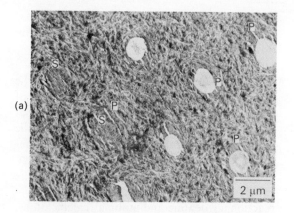

(a)

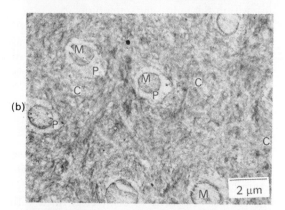

(b)

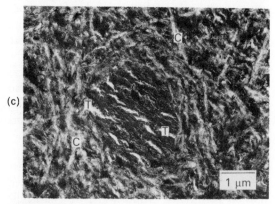

(c)

Figure 7.1 Electron micrographs of ultrathin sections of translucent (sclerosed) dentine, cut transverse to the long axis of the dentinal tubules. (a) The three tubules to the left are completely occluded (sclerosed, S) so that there is difficulty in distinguishing the zone of peri-tubular dentine (P). The four tubules to the right show much earlier stages of the process with a few fine intratubular aggregations of crystals growing predominantly from the tubule walls. Undecalcified section. (b) Similar section from translucent dentine, but decalcified and stained by treatment with phosphotungstic acid. Collagen fibres (C) with their characteristic cross-banding are seen coursing throughout the intertubular dentine. A network of fine non-banded fibres makes up the matrix of the peritubular dentine (P) and the original lumen contains a variable amount of fibrous or homogeneous organic matrix (M). (c) Enlargement of a sclerosed tubule similar to those seen in (a). Whereas the hydroxyapatite crystals of intertubular dentine are thin plates, appearing as denser needles when seen in edge-view, the crystals obliterating the tubule lumen are indistinguishable from those of normal peritubular dentine and are smaller and more rounded in outline. The spaces between the mineral in intertubular regions are occupied by organic matrix, principally collagen fibres (C), which are of low electron density because the section is unstained. Spaces between the mineral within the tubules are tears (T) produced during the sectioning process. (From Johnson *et al.*[1]; courtesy of *Caries Research.*)

requires the action of vital odontoblasts[1,4,5], and that it could not take place if the stimulus to the dentine and pulp was so severe as seriously to impair odontoblast function or to kill the odontoblasts in the area. Accordingly, this form of tubular sclerosis is best seen in response to relatively mild stimuli, for example as an age change in the apical third of roots of teeth[6,7], in the crowns of teeth beneath areas of attrition, and in response to a mild and discontinuous carious challenge[8] (see below). For the same reason, sclerosis tends to develop at the periphery of carious lesions in dentine, some distance away from the focus of injury. Sclerotic zones are an almost universal feature of the dentine and pulp response to caries, being present in 193 of 200 lesions surveyed by Levine[9].

Tubular sclerosis leads to translucency in tissue because the affected area is structurally more homogeneous: there is less scattering of light as it passes through the tissue and an area of dentine so affected is called a *translucent zone* or *sclerotic zone* (figure 7.2). Because of the increased mineral content, translucent zones appear more opaque than normal dentine in microradiographs[2], and it is important to realise that this is an essentially different type of translucent zone to that which appears in carious enamel (chapter 6), where it is produced by demineralisation.

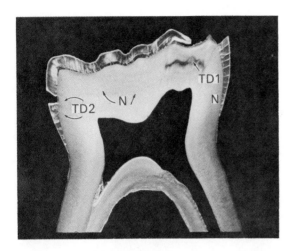

Figure 7.2 **Ground section of a deciduous molar placed on a dark background and photographed by reflected light so that areas of translucency appear black. A broad band of translucent or sclerosed dentine (TD1) has formed at the junction of the outer one-third and inner two-thirds of the coronal dentine beneath an occlusal carious cavity. A less pronounced, conical, translucent zone (TD2) has formed beneath a lesion on the opposite approximal surface. Note the well marked neonatal line in this specimen (N).**

Protection for the pulp and deeper dentine is presumably provided by the reduced permeability of translucent dentine, as has been demonstrated by isotope and dye diffusion studies[10]. In a carious lesion the penetration of acids and of bacterial toxins and enzymes towards the pulp would be inhibited, and there would be insulation against thermal and other stimuli.

7.1.2 Reactionary dentine and atubular calcifications at the pulp surface

Reactionary or reparative dentine is a layer of tubular dentine formed at the surface of the pulp chamber beneath, and as a reaction to, a stimulus acting further peripherally. Its distribution is thus limited to the area beneath which the stimulus is operating—for example, beneath a carious enamel fissure (figure 7.3a)—and is to be distinguished from primary dentine, formed prior to tooth eruption, and secondary dentine which forms all over the pulpal surface at a slow rate during the functional life of a tooth. Note,

however, that the term secondary dentine is commonly used in a loose fashion to refer to all types of post-eruptive dentine.

Reactionary dentine varies considerably in structure, or quality, from well-formed tissue with the appropriate number of evenly spaced tubules, indistinguishable from the adjacent normal primary and secondary dentine, through varying degrees of irregularity in the number, width and spacing of the tubules and in the degree of mineralisation, to severely dysplastic, (that is, abnormally formed) tissue in which there may be few tubules, numerous interglobular areas and possibly entrapped odontoblasts (figures 7.3b, c, d).

Regular reactionary dentine arises in response to a mild stimulus. With increasing degree of severity of stimulus there is increasing likelihood of damage to odontoblasts, with increasing dysplasia of the reactionary tissue formed. If the stimulus is overwhelming, causing death of large numbers of odontoblasts, no reactionary dentine may be formed. Under such circumstances a defence reaction may not be provided at the pulpal surface. Sometimes, however, other cells in the pulp differentiate to produce a layer of atubular calcified tissue, for which the word 'eburnoid' was coined by Sir Wilfred Fish many years ago, he being one of the first workers fully to appreciate the dynamic interplay between disease processes and the defence mechanisms of the tooth[11].

An important factor determining the ability of a tooth to respond to injury by the production of reactionary dentine is likely to be the blood supply to the pulp. Indeed, Corbett[12] showed that whereas reactionary dentine was present beneath the lesion in about three-quarters of carious deciduous teeth examined, it was present in less than half of the permanent teeth. This is possibly because deciduous teeth have wide apical foramena throughout much of their life cycle, since the completion of root formation is followed by root resorption provoked by development of the permanent successor tooth. Another factor influencing the presence or absence of reactionary dentine beneath caries is the

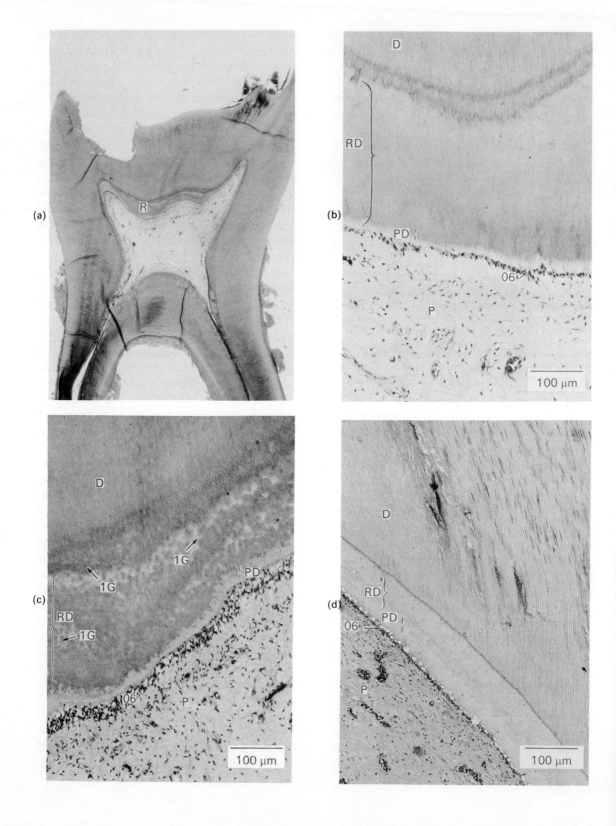

size and, by implication, the longevity of the lesion. In a survey of 200 teeth, Levine[9] showed that when the demineralised part of the lesion was limited to the outer third of the tissue, only 18 per cent had developed reactionary dentine, but this rose to 68 per cent by the time the lesion had reached the inner third. A slowly progressing lesion presumably provides the best opportunity for a wide, well-organised, reactionary dentine defence to develop.

When formed, reactionary dentine and eburnoid provide extra protection for the odontoblasts and other cells of the pulp by increasing the distance between them and injurious stimuli further peripherally.

7.1.3 Pulpitis: inflammation within the pulp chamber

Inflammation is the fundamental response of all vascular connective tissues to injury and is provoked in the dental pulp by stimuli above the threshold which results in the physiological defence reactions which have just been outlined. The inflammatory process in the pulp is considered in more detail later in this chapter (section 7.10), but at this stage it is important to emphasise that, although the process is reversible and its purpose protective, excessive and uncontrolled inflammation leads to increase in tissue damage. Indeed, it is the rule rather than the exception that severe acute pulpitis results in death of the tooth.

7.2 The Nature of Dead Tract Dentine

The so-called 'dead tract' is frequently regarded as part of the spectrum of dentinal defences, but it is a much misused term. This term, also, was coined originally by Sir Wilfred Fish, who placed dyes into the pulp chambers of extracted teeth, later cutting ground sections and observing the diffusion of dye into the surrounding dentine. He noted that, whereas normal dentine was freely penetrated, there were frequently areas (or 'tracts') of tissue beneath carious lesions and beneath areas of attrition which the dye was unable to reach. This, he concluded, was due to a physical obstruction within the tubules at the pulpal end of the affected area. If a tubule does not communicate with the pulp, it clearly cannot contain a vital odontoblast process in continuity with its cell body. The tubule is thus 'dead' and groups of such tubules form a 'dead tract'[11]

Obstructions of this sort may be produced by tubular sclerosis, by the discontinuity between some tubules at the junction of normal and reactionary dentine, particularly if the latter is dysplastic, and by eburnoid. Remnants of necrotic cells may also have this effect.

Tubules within the dead tract itself may contain gases, fluids and degenerating cell remnants, and may be even more permeable than normal tissue. Bacteria and toxic substances may thus progress rapidly through dead tract dentine, but will ultimately reach the obstruction which has caused the tract to form. This is of considerable practical importance, since, because it does not contain vital tissue and is isolated from the pulp, it is likely to be relatively insensitive and can be cut with a burr or other instrument with relatively little discomfort to the patient.

When ground sections of carious dentine are prepared, the largely empty tubules within dead tracts readily become filled with air, and the tract appears dark or even opaque when viewed in transmitted light.

Figure 7.3 **(a) Longitudinal decalcified section of a molar tooth showing extensive deposition of reactionary dentine (R) on the roof of the pulp chamber beneath occlusal caries. (b–d) Higher power views of a range of reactionary dentine from several different teeth. In (b) the reactionary dentine is evenly calcified and contains many tubules, though there is some irregularity of tubule pattern between the primary and reactionary dentine. In (c) the reactionary dentine is also tubular but unevenly mineralised, as indicated by the many interglobular areas present. In (d) the reactionary tissue has fewer tubules and is very poorly mineralised with a wide predentine layer. Vacuoles have formed between the odontoblasts and the formative front of the predentine. D, primary dentine; RD, reactionary dentine; IG, interglobular dentine; PD, predentine; Ob, odontoblast layer; P, pulp.**

7.3 The Structure of Carious Dentine Prior to Cavitation of the Enamel and Consequent Infection of the Dentine

With this knowledge of the defensive reactions of the pulp–dentine complex it is now possible to construct a picture of the histopathology of caries in dentine by adding the degenerative or destructive changes. Dental caries is, by definition, a process of destruction of tooth substance so that the detailed appearance of a lesion in dentine at any time depends on the balance reached between the defence reactions and the destructive processes.

Figure 7.4 is a diagram of a tooth in which a slow but progressive enamel lesion is developing into a slow but progressive dentine lesion. The advancing front of the enamel lesion has reached the enamel–dentine junction, but the enamel surface is still intact and no cavity has formed. Because of the extent of the lesion, however, the full thickness of the enamel in this area has an increased permeability, and acid, enzymes and other chemical stimuli from the tooth surface will reach the outer dentine and cause the pulp–dentine unit to respond. The visible features (figure 7.5), from the pulp outwards, are likely to be first the formation of some reactionary dentine, then a zone of unaffected normal dentine until the translucent zone is met; this walls off and encloses the remainder, or body of the lesion, which will obviously constitute a dead tract as defined above. Translucent and reactionary dentine are, as we have seen, defence reactions. Even at this stage the outer portion of the body of the lesion may be partially demineralised and this is, naturally, a destructive change; however, because the enamel surface is not breached, the dentine cannot yet be infected with bacteria.

Lesions on approximal tooth surfaces may be detectable at this stage by clinical bite-wing radiography[13,14], but should not automatically have a restoration inserted. If the cariogenic challenge at the tooth surface is controlled the lesion may progress no further[15,16]; indeed, it

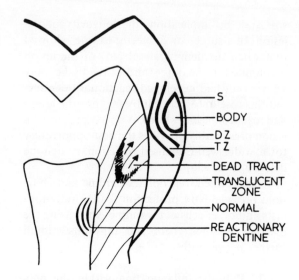

Figure 7.4 Diagram of carious lesion developing on the smooth surface of a tooth. There is not yet a cavity in the enamel but its structure has been affected resulting in the formation of a surface zone (S), body of the lesion, dark zone (DZ) and translucent zone (TZ). The reactions on the part of the dentine and pulp are indicated.

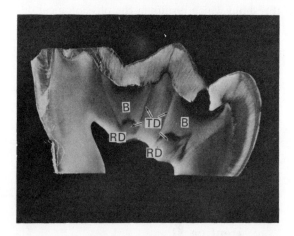

Figure 7.5 Ground section of molar crown photographed by reflected light. Two fissure lesions are present and these have provoked extensive reactions in the dentine and pulp in spite of the absence of overt cavitation of the enamel in at least one of the lesions. Features visible are reactionary dentine (RD) and well marked conical zones of sclerosed or translucent dentine (TD), enclosing the body of the dentine lesion (B). Because of the obstruction caused by tubular sclerosis the body of the lesion would constitute a dead tract. The black region towards the enamel–dentine junction is produced by demineralisation, and possibly also limited proteolysis, of dentine. (From Johnson *et al.*[1]; courtesy of *Caries Research*)

may even regress and this possibility is discussed in more detail at the end of the chapter.

7.4   The Shape of Lesions Arising on Different Tooth Surfaces

Once a carious lesion in enamel reaches the enamel–dentine junction, spread is usually relatively rapid along this interface, the anatomical discontinuity between the two tissues apparently being less resistant to penetration of the destructive agents. Fissure and smooth-surface lesions thus tend to develop different overall shapes: in the case of lesions on the smooth surfaces of teeth (figure 7.6) the enamel lesion tends to be conical with its apex touching the enamel–dentine junction. Lateral spread from this point results in a broadened base to the dentine lesion which is then itself conical; it follows the primary curvature of the dentinal tubules so that its slightly narrowed apex approaches the pulpal surface further cervically than the level at which the lesion entered the dentine.

In the case of fissure caries (figure 7.6) the enamel lesion, as it spreads guided by the prism direction, broadens as it approaches the dentine. With lateral spread at the enamel–dentine junction, the area of involved dentine is larger, initially, than in a smooth-surface lesion and because the tubules are relatively straight over the occlusal aspect of the pulp chamber, it does not taper so much toward the pulp. This explains why, when an apparently small occlusal lesion is entered, it is often found to have extensively undermined enamel and a surprisingly large area of softened dentine.

Nevertheless, dentine lesions, wherever they arise, are characteristically conical, the shape initially being determined by the distribution of the translucent zone. It is not entirely clear why the distribution of translucency should be so reproducible. However, one would expect a physiological defence reaction such as this to be placed approximately equidistant from the focus of stimulant—in this case the enamel–dentine

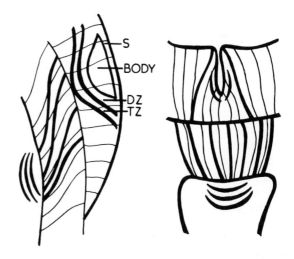

Figure 7.6   Diagram showing how, with fissure caries (right), the enamel lesion broadens as it approaches the dentine–enamel junction and thus involves a larger area than that initially involved by a lesion on a smooth surface (left).

junction beneath the centre of the enamel lesion. Close to this focus the stimulus may be too intense to permit the odontoblast processes to function, causing them to retreat closer to the pulp before they can respond by producing extra peritubular tissue. Laterally, however, a level of intensity of stimulant will be reached which permits the odontoblast processes to function in this way along their whole length—thus walling off the sides of the lesion.

It is useful to have a mental image of the characteristic morphology of dentine lesions during the preparation of a cavity for restoration of the tooth, although this is understandably more difficult if lesions commencing in one or more points in a pit or fissure have coalesced with lesions commencing on one or more of the smooth surfaces.

7.5   Progression of the Infected Dentine Lesion after Cavitation of Enamel

Once there is a cavitation of enamel and bacteria have reached dentine, progress of the lesion is likely to be more rapid. The spectrum of defence reactions described above will be seen, together with destructive or degenerative changes. These are represented progressively in figure 7.7 (A, B, C): moving from the pulp outwards, the features likely to be present (figure 7.7A) are first a mild degree of inflammation in the pulp, secondly the production of some reactionary dentine, thirdly an area of normal dentine, and then the translucent zone. Enclosed within this translucent zone we again have the body of the dentine lesion, but this is now divisible into three structural components[1, 17]: first, immediately within the translucent zone, a narrow area of demineralised dentine which does not yet contain bacteria; next a zone of penetration, so called

because the tubules have become penetrated by microorganisms; and finally a zone of destruction, or necrosis, in which microbial action has completely destroyed the substance of dentine.

This distribution of destructive processes, enclosed by the translucent zone, is brought about because the first wave of bacteria infecting dentine are primarily acidogenic (section 7.6). Acid presumably diffuses ahead of the organisms, as there is widespread agreement in the literature that a zone of demineralised tissue surrounds the advancing front of bacteria[18-21]. Toward the dentine enamel junction there is a more mixed bacterial population, in which proteolytic and hydrolytic enzymes are added to the acid effect, resulting in destruction of the organic

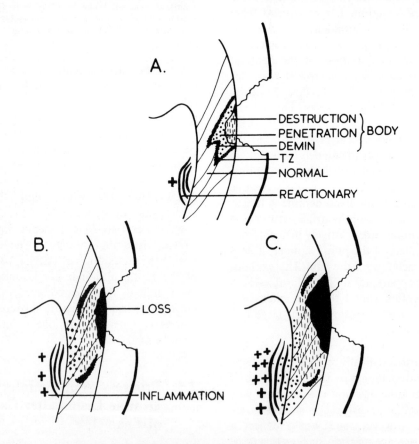

Figure 7.7   A–C. Diagram of the increasing destruction of tissue once cavitation of enamel has occurred and micro-organisms invade the dentine.

matrix of the tissue (sections 7.6 and 7.7).

Microorganisms, initially confined to tubules and their lateral branches, now invade the peritubular and intertubular dentine[1, 8, 22, 23] (figure 7.8). Small aggregations of bacteria and necrotic tissue coalesce to form what are known as liquefaction foci (figure 7.9). Destruction is sometimes more advanced along the incremental lines of growth, producing 'transverse clefts', and this explains why carious dentine can often be excavated with hand instruments in large sheets in a plane parallel to the enamel—dentine junction.

During restoration of a tooth the major objective of 'caries removal' is to excavate infected and necrotic tissue. Indeed when we speak, commonly but erroneously, of 'caries' as a substance, we are referring loosely to demineralised and infected tooth tissue, usually dentine. The zone of demineralisation is, therefore, an ideal plane

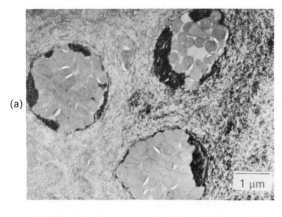

(a)

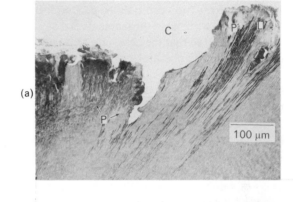

(a)

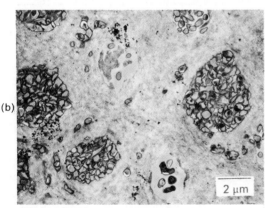

(b)

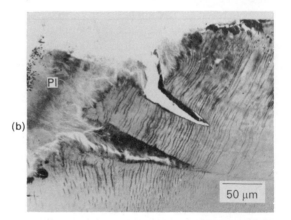

(b)

Figure 7.8 Electron micrographs of ultrathin sections of carious dentine cut transverse to tubule direction. In (a) the section is taken from close to the advancing front of bacterial penetration. Organisms are mostly confined to the original tubule lumens and there has been variable destruction of the peritubular tissue. The intertubular dentine is partially demineralised though many crystals remain. In (b), from a region of more advanced destruction, no peritubular dentine remains and organisms are beginning to invade the intertubular matrix which is completely demineralised. (From Johnson *et al.*[1]; courtesy of *Caries Research*)

Figure 7.9 Decalcified section of carious dentine forming the floor of a carious cavity (C). (a) Dentinal tubules penetrated by bacteria stain deeply (P) and several liquefaction foci have formed (L). (b) Tubules penetrated by bacteria are again visible and there is a thick bacterial plaque (Pl) on the cavity floor. Two transverse clefts have opened up and bacteria are proliferating within them. The incremental growth line associated with one of the clefts is clearly visible.

in which to attempt separation of diseased tissue from the tooth substance which is to remain, both because it is softened and therefore technically easier, and because the translucent zone, an important component of the tooth defence reaction, will be retained. A knowledge of the morphology and histopathology of dentine caries is thus an important basis for clinical procedures. Furthermore, because recognition of the translucent zone – demineralised zone interface depends on difference in hardness, as well as on prior knowledge of its likely distribution, successful excavation can only be accomplished at this level with hand instruments or slowly rotating burrs, so that the necessary sense of feel is retained by the operator.

Because the shape of the advancing front of bacterial penetration, of demineralisation and of translucent zone formation is irregular on the 'floor' of a lesion undergoing restoration it is, in practical terms, difficult to excavate infected tissue with precision. Indeed, studies have shown that, in addition to leaving obviously harmless areas of softened but sterile dentine after excavation of caries, microorganisms are often left *in situ* even when excavation has been carried to the point of removing all clinically softened and discoloured tissue. Shovelton[20] showed, in a series of 102 teeth in which cavities were prepared as would have been done clinically, that 36 per cent still contained bacteria on subsequent histological examination. In spite of this, however, restorative procedures are normally successful, so it is not regarded as essential to remove all organisms from the cavity floor so long as the walls are rendered sterile and the cavity is well sealed and mechanically sound[20,24,25]. The chances of leaving organisms behind may be greater in rapidly advancing caries in children and adolescents than in older patients in which the lesions are more likely to be slow or even arrested[26].

With further progress of the lesion, the destructive processes come to overtake the defence reactions, (figure 7.7c). The degree of inflammation in the pulp is likely to increase. There may or may not be an increase in the thickness of the reactionary dentine; in fact, the presence of significant pulpal inflammation will cause any reactionary dentine formed to be at best dysplastic or, more likely, completely to arrest further dentinogenesis. The translucent zone will ultimately be broken down by acids and enzymes diffusing from the zone of penetration, and bacteria will come closer and closer toward the pulp. The frequent observation that the characteristic conical shape of large lesions is truncated as the pulp is approached[24] has led to the suggestion that circumpulpal dentine is more resistant, in spite of its relatively low mineral and hydroxyproline content, when compared to the main mass of dentine; the effect has been attributed to its relatively high fluorine content[9,27]. In the progressing lesion, organisms will ultimately invade reactionary dentine and reach the soft tissue within the pulp chamber (figure 7.10). Concomitantly, the area of total loss of dentine toward the surface of the cavity will increase.

It has been shown[18,21,28] that inflammation in the pulp is not normally seen until the leading organisms are within 0.3–0.8 mm of the pulp itself. The first pulp reactions are therefore due to bacterial toxins rather than infection of the pulp itself[24]; indeed, the application of bacterial products to exposed dentine in experimental cavities which do not, therefore, have underlying defence reactions can be very severe[29]. If organisms are sealed beneath a satisfactory restoration they may remain viable for many months[30,31] but are apparently dormant because an area of low pH cannot be demonstrated under sound fillings[32] and the lesion does not progress. There is no need, therefore, to excavate deep lesions to hard shining dentine at the risk of exposing the pulp. The technique of 'indirect pulp capping' in which a lining material is placed over the remaining infected dentine is to be preferred and it has been shown that several of the materials commonly used for this purpose actually cause the organisms to die over a period of several months[33,35]. Zinc oxide–eugenol and calcium hydroxide formulations are especially effective in this regard, and the latter also promotes remineralisation of the

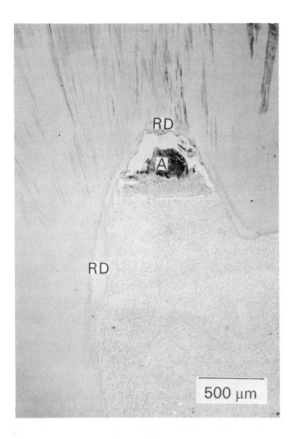

Figure 7.10 Portion of the coronal pulp beneath an advanced occlusal carious lesion. Bacteria can be seen penetrating the full thickness of the primary dentine and entering the reactionary dentine (RD). A small abscess (A) has formed at the top of the pulp cornua and the rest of the pulp contains a diffuse inflammatory infiltrate. The odontoblasts have degenerated.

softened dentine, drawing calcium and phosphate ions from the pulp fluid[25,34,36,37].

7.6 The Microbiology of Dentine Caries

Studies which have attempted to identify and classify the types of microorganisms which infect dentine once there is cavitation of the enamel and, by extrapolation, to associate their presence with causing the destruction observed, have been based on sampling, under aseptic conditions, layers of dentine from the pulp outwards. This avoids misinterpretation due to contamination with organisms from saliva or from plaque on the tooth surface.

The first organisms to be isolated are acid-producing (acidogenic) and capable of surviving under acid conditions (aciduric) and, although often comprising a number of species, the flora is less complex than that of plaque on the enamel surface. Lactobacilli are especially common and McKay[38] showed, in a small series of permanent molar teeth with rapidly progressing dentine caries beneath occlusal fissures, that there is often a primary wave of advancing organisms consisting entirely of homofermentative lactobacilli.

With successive samples further into the body of the lesion and thus closer to the zone of destruction, the flora becomes progressively more mixed and includes many more proteolytic species; it contains a mixture of aerobic, micro-aerophilic and anaerobic bacteria and varies considerably from tooth to tooth and from site to site in the same lesion. Conditions in the deep dentine lesion are likely to vary from place to place in terms of substrate availability, pH and oxygen tension, and thus to favour overgrowth of certain organisms at certain sites. In general, however, conditions are likely to be markedly anaerobic and if highly sophisticated isolation and culture techniques are employed, the anaerobic to aerobic recovery ratio may be as high as 7 to 1[39].

With more slowly progressing lesions, in which the dentine defence reactions slow the rate of invasion, the second wave of bacterial ingrowth may overtake the first, so that sampling the advancing front of the lesion produces a more complex result. Nevertheless, lactobacilli still constitute at least 20 per cent of the dentine flora and are at least as common as cariogenic streptococci including *Streptococcus mutans*[39]. Lactobacilli constitute only a small proportion of plaque bacteria on the tooth surface (approximately 4 per cent[39]; see chapter 3). Plaque ecology must therefore change considerably once it occupies space in the enamel cavity and becomes more remote from salivary influences, so that when it contacts the dentine lactobacilli are the dominant survivors.

One of the more comprehensive recent studies is that of Edwardsson[40] who found the dominating organisms in the deeper portions of infected dentine to be Gram-positive bacteria. Gram-positive rods and filaments were isolated from 93 per cent of the teeth, Gram-positive cocci from 32 per cent, Gram-negative cocci from 11 per cent and Gram-negative rods from 5 per cent. Most of the teeth studied were third permanent molars with either fissure or smooth surface lesions, so that the patients were presumably in an age-group in which caries activity was lower than that in children or adolescents. None of the genera or species was demonstrated in all teeth examined, so that these results do not favour a specific pathogenic organism or group of organisms in established lesions of this type. The relative frequency of the most common isolates in the teeth examined were:

Lactobacillus	48 %
Streptococcus	22 %
Bifidobacterium	20 %
Arachnia	17 %
Propionibacterium	17 %
Eubacterium	17 %
Anaerobic streptococci	13 %
Actinomyces	11 %

Note that lactobacilli are again found most frequently; when present they constituted more than 50 per cent of viable organisms isolated. Thus it seems likely that these organisms play a particularly important role in dentine caries. Indeed, several studies have also shown that lactobacilli may outnumber non-haemolytic streptococci in infected pulps and root ca-

nals[41,42]. It is always wise, however, to bear in mind the possibility that large numbers of a particular type of organism may be the result of particularly favourable growth conditions rather than the primary cause of disease.

7.7   Biochemical Mechanisms in the Destruction of Dentine by Caries

That the decalcification of dentine by caries is largely due to acid is suggested by the distribution of areas of low pH within lesions. These are readily detectable by staining split teeth or sections with pH reactive dyes and show how acid diffuses ahead of the bacteria, producing the zone of demineralisation surrounding the zone of penetration referred to earlier[32]. Most of the infected dentine is acidic, except for areas of advanced destruction toward the surface of the cavity, where neutral or even alkaline conditions are sometimes found.

Gas chromatographic analysis[43] reveals that most of the acid present is lactic acid and that other Krebs cycle acids cannot be detected. High activities of lactate dehydrogenase, the enzyme required for the production and catabolism of lactic acid, are found not only in infected dentine but also in the zone of demineralisation, so the enzyme as well as the acid itself must diffuse ahead of the organisms which actively produce it. Other dehydrogenases characteristic of the glycolytic pathway, of the Krebs cycle and of the pentose-phosphate shunt can also be detected diffusing away from the advancing front of bacteria, so that a number of the possible pathways for glucose utilisation and energy production are probably being employed by the organisms. In liquefaction foci and other areas of advanced destruction, strong activity of these enzymes is demonstrable; it is not possible to be certain, however, about the flux through any of these pathways, given the artificial substrates and incubation conditions so commonly used for their detection.

Nevertheless, it seems reasonable to conclude that lactate is the major acid produced and that it is this substance, as in plaque on the tooth surface, which is primarily responsible for demineralisation of the tissue. Amino acids released by proteolysis of dentine matrix, and citrate ions, may complex Ca in regions of higher pH, thus contributing to demineralisation, but their relative importance is unknown. The dissolution of the small hydroxyapatite crystals of dentine seems to take place from their external surfaces so that they become progressively smaller and irregular in outline[1, 8, 44]. Any amorphous calcium phosphate present as part of the structure of the tissue will dissolve even more readily.

The mineral ions thus liberated will diffuse along a concentration gradient away from the advancing front of demineralisation. Because the tubules between the area of active demineralisation and the pulp are likely to be sclerosed, most of the movement of calcium and phosphate ions will be outward through the zones of bacterial penetration and of tissue necrosis toward the tooth surface. *En route*, areas of tissue with a relatively high pH may be encountered and reprecipitation of these ions may occur. Such 'remineralisation crystals' have been described by several authors[1, 45, 46] within the lumen of tubules close to the advancing front of bacterial penetration (figure 7.11). They may appear as large rhombohedral structures, thought to be composed of β-tricalcium phosphate, or as thin flat plate-like structures resembling octacalcium phosphate. More extensive reprecipitation of mineral, much of it as hydroxyapatite, is deposited in both inter- and intratubular locations in arrested dentine lesions close to and on the surface exposed to oral fluids (section 7.8).

In those areas of the zone of bacterial penetration with a mixed flora, a range of hydrolytic enzymes with the potential for destruction of the organic matrix of dentine can be identified. An extensive study of these enzymes has been made by Larmas and his colleagues in Finland[43, 47–49]. Enzymes identified include esterases with activity against a wide range of substrates including esters of fatty acids, phosphate and sulphate esters and glycosidic and peptide bonds, thus

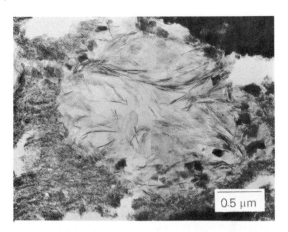

Figure 7.11 Electron micrograph of a single dentinal tubule close to the advancing front of the zone of bacterial penetration. Remineralisation crystals of rhombohedral and plate-like morphology fill the lumen. The surrounding peritubular dentine has fractured during specimen preparation. (From Johnson *et al*[1]; courtesy of *Caries Research*).

supporting a view put forward as long ago as 1926[50] that 'fatty degeneration' was an important early change in dentine caries. Other more recent histochemical studies reveal that caries first unmasks lipids in the peritubular dentine matrix[51].

A range of proteolytic enzymes have been detected, including arylaminopeptidases and endopeptidases with collagenase activity[52]. The progressive loss of collagen from the zones of destruction has been monitored by measurement of hydroxyproline content[3].

Most of these enzymes are thought to be produced by the bacteria so that, in histochemical studies, they appear confined to the tubules close to the advancing front of the lesion, but are more widely distributed in the area of more advanced destruction. Finally, as with the early lesion in enamel, parts of the tissue may acquire an increased organic content, derived from bacteria and from saliva[53].

7.8 Active and Arrested Caries

We have seen that because of the balance between attacking and defensive forces, the rate of progress of caries in dentine is highly variable. It is not surprising, therefore, that under suitable environmental conditions progress can be completely arrested and the lesion may even regress[24].

Clinically, actively progressing caries is soft and light brown or yellow in colour. There are actively growing bacteria on the surface and a wide zone of demineralisation beneath. Because of the rapid progress of the lesion, the defence reactions will not be well developed. Consequently such lesions are often painful, pain being elicited by sudden change in temperature, by osmotic shock such as the intake of concentrated sugar, by acid foodstuffs, or by mechanical pressure from impacted food or probing by the dentist[54].

If, however, the cariogenicity of the environment is controlled and, particularly if the cavity has become open and more readily kept free of accumulations of food and bacterial plaque, the tissue will become dark brown in colour and take on a harder, somewhat leathery consistency[55]. Spontaneous pain and painful responses to sweet or acid foods are generally absent in teeth with such arrested lesions. Arrest of the caries process can be confirmed microscopically by the presence of new layers of reactionary dentine showing an incremental pattern and by new translucent zone reactions. The previously destroyed tissue in the body of the lesion accumulates organic matter and mineral from oral fluids; unusual crystal forms can be detected in such regions in the electron microscope[1,45] and these may result in considerable rehardening of the tissue. The most striking remineralisation takes place on and within the surface exposed to the oral environment. This layer contains reformed crystals in a matrix derived from saliva, food and bacterial products. The crystals are predominantly apatitic[56] but are larger than those of sound dentine with a high Ca : P ratio[57] and high F content[58]. A number of non-apatitic calcium phosphates may also be found[59].

Such observations suggest the possibility of encouraging this rehardening with artificial mineralising solutions, and such compounds are currently being developed[60-62].

7.9   Caries of Exposed Root Surfaces

Our knowledge of the mechanisms of root surface caries is scanty compared to the immense amount of research conducted on enamel caries and the underlying dentine/pulp response. This is in spite of the fact that, on a global basis, it may well be the most common form of the disease, being particularly common among certain primitive peoples[63-65]. There is also a positive correlation between increased age and cemental caries, as shown in the classical Vipeholm study where more than half of all new lesions in patients around 50 years of age were of this type[66]. In Western communities, root surface caries is becoming increasingly common with the lengthening of life span and the increasing effectiveness of preventive measures directed against coronal caries[67]. It may have been neglected in the past because affected teeth frequently have advanced periodontal disease necessitating tooth extraction[68].

Root surface caries is initiated by bacterial plaque residing on the surface of cementum following gingival recession. Such plaque is likely to be different in composition from that residing further coronally, in particular by containing more anaerobic, more Gram-negative and more filamentous species[69]. Sumney and Jordan[70], in a study of surface plaque overlying cemental lesions in 15 teeth, found numerous strains of *Streptococcus mutans*, *S. sanguis* and *S. mitis*, and also large numbers of *Neisseria* and *Actinomyces* species. Syed *et al.*[71] suggest that *A. viscosus* may be of particular significance.

The initial lesion in cementum appears to involve sub-surface demineralisation with a relatively intact surface layer somewhat akin to the early enamel lesion[67]. The greater porosity of cementum and its higher organic content modify the pattern of attack, however. Several early workers commented on the fact that the remnants of Sharpey's fibres seemed to provide pathways for penetration[72,73] and the electron microscope study of Furseth and Johansen[74] has revealed microorganisms in lacunae within the structure of the tissue.

It is likely that root surface caries is initiated at several points over a wide area of the exposed cemental surface and that, because of the thinness and porosity of this tissue, dentine changes rapidly supervene. Tubular sclerosis has been described[67] and it is generally assumed that a sequence of dentine/pulp responses similar to those which occur in the crown can take place. However, because there are fewer tubules per unit area in the root than in the crown, and because most of the patients are older, the defensive capacity of the dentine may well be impeded. It is not surprising, therefore, that of a group of 99 lesions studied by Westbrook *et al.*[67], 70 per cent showed active invasion of the dentine by microorganisms and a further 18 per cent showed established pulpitis, pulp exposure or pulp necrosis. The pattern of demineralisation and proteolysis of infected dentine is not detectably different from that in coronal lesions[75].

Little is known of the nature of the bacteria in the advancing front of the dentinal lesion, although one study[70] has suggested the flora may differ from that in the crown, with large numbers of diphtheroids present, together with a possibly unique species of Gram-positive obligatory aerobic coccus resembling Arthrobacter species. However, the true nature of these interesting bacteria remains to be established by further investigations.

7.10   The Response of the Dental Pulp: Pulpitis

Inflammation is the fundamental response of vascular tissue to injury, and the dental pulp is no exception. Of the two major types of inflammatory reaction classically recognised, acute and chronic, the latter is by far the more common, but clinically less obvious, occurrence in dental pulp.

Whether an acute or chronic inflammation results from injury to any vascular tissue depends largely on the duration and intensity of the stimulus. By and large a low-grade, long-lasting stimulus will result in chronic inflammation and a sudden severe stimulus will promote an acute inflammatory response. However, the type of inflammation also depends on the *nature* of the stimulus (or injurious agent). Even the response to bacteria varies—organisms like streptococci and staphylococci, when they infect tissue, always produce an acute inflammatory response, whereas organisms like those responsible for tuberculosis or syphilis, after a fleeting acute phase, characteristically provoke chronic inflammation.

Because with a slowly progressing carious lesion in dentine the stimulae reaching the pulp are toxins and other diffusable products from bacteria and not the bacteria themselves (section 7.5), together with mild thermal and osmotic shocks from the external environment, the overall stimulus is low grade and sustained so that chronic inflammation is the usual pulp response. When the organisms actually reach the pulp—a 'carious exposure'—acute inflammation is then likely to supervene.

Inflammatory reactions have vascular and cellular components. The cellular component is most marked in chronic inflammation and such a focus in the pulp beneath a carious lesion will contain aggregations of lymphocytes and plasma cells, monocytes and macrophages (figure 7.12a). If of long standing, there may be increased numbers of fibroblasts with increased collagen production, leading to fibrosis (figure 7.12b). Such chronic inflammatory foci in the dental pulp are, however, defence reactions and probably do not endanger the vitality of the tooth.

In contrast to the above, many of the significant events in acute inflammation (figure 7.13) are related to vascular changes, in particular the dilatation of blood vessels, acceleration of blood flow and exudation of fluid, all of which normally lead to swelling of tissue. In time there is retardation of blood flow, due to concentration of blood following exudation, and vascular stasis may supervene.

The active emigration of leucocytes, particularly polymorphonuclear leucocytes, further contributes to the swelling.

In general terms the possible theoretical se-

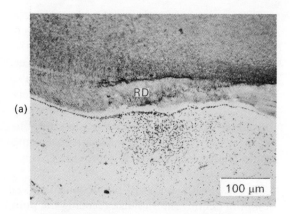

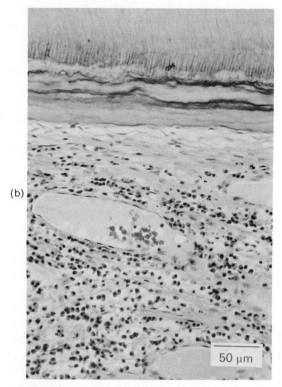

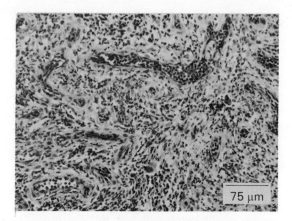

Figure 7.13   Acute pulpitis. Numerous capillaries are visible and these are engorged with blood containing many more leucocytes than usual. Polymorphonuclear leucocytes can be seen migrating through the vessel walls and many lie free in the extravascular spaces. A significant number of plasma cells is also present, suggesting that the acute episode may have arisen on a more long-standing chronic pulpitis.

Figure 7.12   Two examples of chronic pulpitis. In (a) a small localised cluster of lymphocytes and monocytes has formed beneath a band of reactionary dentine (RD). The odontoblast layer is intact and the cellularity of the rest of the pulp is normal. (b) This shows a more diffuse and possibly longer-standing pulpitis. Whilst capillaries are prominent they are not noticeably engorged with blood. The infiltrate within the tissue is dominated by plasma cells, though smaller numbers of lymphocytes and polymorphonuclear leucocytes are also visible. There is some fibrosis. The reactionary dentine is atubular and may best be termed 'eburnoid'. The odontoblasts have degenerated.

quelae of this type of acute inflammation are: resolution, repair—if tissue has been destroyed, suppuration, necrosis, extension of the lesion, and reversion to a chronic inflammation.

When applied to the unique situation of acute inflammation in the pulp chamber of a tooth, suppuration and necrosis are particularly likely outcomes. Suppuration with abscess formation is common. If the abscess is small and confined to the pulp chamber (figure 7.10), clinical pulpotomy may be successful but more extensive necrosis is, unfortunately, likely. This is thought to be because we are dealing with a delicate connective tissue in a rigidly enclosed calcific chamber receiving its blood supply from a limited number of vessels passing through narrow root foramenae. The possibility of the exudate, within the rigid confines of the tooth, raising the intrapulpal pressure above the local blood pressure has long been considered of key importance[76]. According to this view, the thin-walled and lower pressure veins draining the pulp are likely to collapse, arresting the blood flow at the apex of the tooth and leading to necrosis. Recent experimental studies however, utilising pressure transducers inserted into the pulps of monkey teeth[77] suggest that this is an oversimplification. Local pressure may be as high as 60 mmHg, and this is more than sufficient to collapse local blood vessels, but because the effects are so localised it is possible that the inflammation can be contained locally. The concept of self-strangulation of the pulp is now, therefore, regarded as an oversimplification[78].

In an infected pulp, however, the situation is made more critical because the influx of inflammatory cells will have increased the demand for oxygen. Necrosis will also result partly from the direct action of bacterial toxins and enzymes, and from by-products of the inflammatory reaction such as cytotoxic lymphocytes, lymphotoxins and hydrolytic enzymes liberated by disintegrating polymorphonuclear leucocytes.

Immunological mechanisms must play an important role in the pulp response to dental caries. Before bacteria themselves reach the pulp bacterial products, diffusing ahead of the organisms, provoke inflammation (section 7.5). Many of these toxins, enzymes, cell wall components such as lipopolysaccharides from Gram-negative bacteria and lipoteichoic acids from Gram-positive bacteria are known to be antigenic, and to provoke an antibody response in gingival tissue when they diffuse to the soft tissues through inflamed crevicular epithelium[80,81]. Similar mechanisms must operate in the pulp, although they have received surprisingly little attention.

The plasma cell aggregations seen in heavily inflamed pulp chambers in carious teeth represent deployment of the humoral arm of the immune response[82]. Immunoglobin, particularly IgG but also IgA and IgE, is synthesised locally by these cells, as well as carried in the fluid exudate from the dilated blood vessels[83]. It is not known, however, whether specific antibodies to the invading microorganisms are made to any significant extent by these local plasma cells. Likewise it is not known whether the past caries experience of an individual patient, and the possibility of an anammestic response to antigens derived from a subsequent dentine infection, influence the prognosis for the particular tooth to any significant degree.

The small foci of mononuclear round cells often seen in localised chronic pulpitis contain lymphocytes and macrophages. Nothing is known, however, of the ratio of T:B lymphocytes in these lesions, so that it is difficult to know, pending further research, whether or not specific cell-mediated immune processes are operating.

7.10.1 Symptoms of pulpitis

Over the years, many studies have attempted to correlate the clinical signs of caries in a tooth and the symptoms of which the patient complained with the level of inflammation in the pulp, determined by histological examination after extraction of the tooth[84-89,93,94]. Although the results have usually been disappointing, some generalisations are possible.

First, a chronically inflamed pulp is usually symptomless, as are most chronic inflammatory conditions in the body until they are well advanced. Periodontal disease is a very good example of slowly progressing chronic inflammatory disease of which the patient frequently is not aware. Pulmonary tuberculosis is another good example; no pain may be felt by the patient in spite of a significant degree of destruction of the lungs. Secondly, and in contrast to the above, acute inflammation is almost always painful. We have all had the experience of an acute inflammatory lesion resulting perhaps from a traumatic injury or from the presence of a 'boil' in the skin which causes considerable discomfort. Pain is produced in acute inflammation by the presence of kinins and other chemical mediators[79], and by pressure which is built up due to exudation of fluid and cells so that in a generalised acute pulpitis pain is likely to be severe, continuous and throbbing in character, and to be exacerbated by lying down due to a rise in venous pressure in the tooth. Intermittent pain from the tooth or pain in response to hot or cold stimuli may result from a mild acute inflammation, perhaps because heat transmitted to the pulp results in further hyperaemia and further increase in pressure. The third generalisation possible is that necrotic pulps are themselves painless, because there are no viable nerves to transmit pain stimuli. Once periapical tissues are involved, however, an extra set of symptoms develops such as pain on pressure—the tooth may be tender to bite upon or tender to percussion by the clinician.

Accurate assessment of the nature and extent of pulpal inflammation is essential to successful treatment of teeth with advanced caries. We have already seen that localised chronic inflammation precedes the actual arrival of microorganisms into the pulp chamber and that indirect pulp capping is often successful in obtaining resolution of such inflammation.

Acute inflammation, and even micro-abscess formation, is also sometimes localised to a pulp horn or to the coronal pulp without necessarily involving radicular pulp[90]. In these circumstances the procedure called 'pulpotomy', in which the affected pulp is excised and a bland dressing placed over the remaining pulp, is theoretically possible. In practice, it is usually the whole of the coronal pulp which is removed, the dressing being placed over the openings of the root canals. This procedure is usually applicable only to those teeth with open root apices and thus a good blood supply to the pulp, and is most often carried out on deciduous molars. As before, however, success depends on accurate diagnosis: if due weight is given to the history of pain experience, the size of the physical exposure of the pulp after excavation of infected dentine, the type and extent of bleeding from the exposed pulp and radiographic evidence of periapical involvement, the correlation between clinical and histologic findings can be high[91].

Once acute pulpitis is well established and generalised, however, necrosis of the pulp is probable, leaving full root canal therapy or tooth extraction as the only treatment possibilities.

7.10.2   Open and closed pulpitis

Apart from division into acute and chronic forms, it is usual to classify pulpitis as either open or closed. A so-called closed pulp is one with a normal, fully developed, root with a narrow apical foramen and an intact crown. Inflammation within a tooth of this type would be a '*closed pulpitis*' and most of the foregoing discussion applies to this situation. A pulp may however be 'open' if it has a wide apical foramen, either because the root is incompletely formed or because it is undergoing resorption, such as preparation for the exfoliation of deciduous teeth. The pulp also becomes 'open' when a large carious lesion or operative intervention has destroyed the overlying hard tissue of a tooth or when a fracture involves the pulp.

The prognosis for an inflamed pulp with an open apex is improved because it has a better blood supply and because less pressure can build up within the pulp space. Consequently, resolution of inflammation, reversion to a chronic inflammatory state, or the production of a localised abscess are more likely sequelae in this situation. As stated earlier, acute inflammation with a closed apex is a potentially dangerous situation in which pulpal necrosis is likely.

With the pulp chamber open to the mouth via the crown, inflammatory change is of course inevitable, because of the presence of bacteria and other irritants in oral fluids. There may be less spontaneous pain than with a closed chamber, because oedema fluid and pus can now drain and pressure cannot build up to the same extent, although sensitivity to pressure, thermal and osmotic shock will be marked. Reversion to chronic inflammation is likely and it is usual to speak of two types of chronic open pulpitis— ulcerative and hyperplastic.

An ulcer, by definition, is a break in the continuity of an epithelium i-lined surface. The term 'chronic ulcerative pulpitis' is therefore a misnomer but it is an analogous situation to a true ulcer of the skin or mucous membrane, because in both situations connective tissue, normally covered and protected by another tissue, is now exposed to the external environment. Some pain is inevitable because of the exposure of nerve endings within the pulp and because there would be a superimposed acute inflammatory process at the surface.

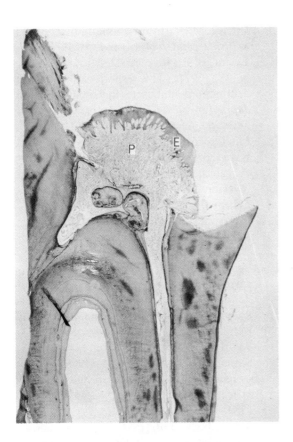

Figure 7.14 Deciduous molar tooth with massive coronal caries exposing the whole of the pulp chamber. Granulation tissue has proliferated into the cavity to form a pulp polyp (P), which has become covered by a thick stratified squamous epithelium (E).

Chronic hyperplastic pulpitis, or *pulp polyp* (figure 7.14), results when the crown is exposed in teeth which also have a very good blood supply from the apical vessels. The endothelial cell and fibroblast proliferation characteristic of granulation tissue forms a mass projecting outwards from the pulp chamber. This mass then becomes epithelialised either by growth of cells from the gingival margin if the carious cavity is in continuity with the gingiva or because epithelial cells which have been shed into the saliva have fallen on to the surface and proliferated to form an epithelial lining[92]. Because a good apical blood supply is a necessary prerequisite to the formation of a pulp polyp, these lesions are most

common in first permanent molars in young children in which the roots have not been completely formed and also in resorbing deciduous molars. Once epithelialisation is complete, the inflammation within the polyp and within the pulp itself subsides and such lesions are usually painless.

The extension of pulpal infection and inflammation to involve the periapical and more distant tissues is common, but is beyond the intended scope of this chapter; good accounts exist in many of the standard texts of oral pathology and oral surgery.

Further Reading

Baume, L. J. (1970). Diagnosis of diseases of the pulp. *Oral Surgery*, **29**, 102–16

Finn, S. B. (1968). *Biology of the Dental Pulp Organ*, University of Alabama Press

Fish, E. W. (1948). *Surgical Pathology of the Mouth*, Pitman, London

Massler, M (1967). Pulpal reactions to dental caries. *International Dental Journal*, **17**, 441–60

Seltzer, S. and Bender, I. B. (1975). *The Dental Pulp*, Lippincott, Philadelphia and Toronto

Symonds, N. B. B. (Ed) (1968). *Dentine and Pulp: Their Structure and Reactions*, University of Dundee

References

1. Johnson, N. W., Taylor, B. R. and Berman, D. S. (1969). The response of deciduous dentine to caries studied by correlated light and electron microscopy. *Caries Research*, **3**, 348–68

2. Weber, D. F. (1974). Human dentine sclerosis: a microradiographic survey. *Archives of Oral Biology*, **19**, 163–9

3. Levine, R. S. (1972). The distribution of hydroxyproline in the dentine of carious teeth. *Archives of Oral Biology*, **17**, 127–35

4. Bradford, E. W. (1960). The dentine, a

barrier to caries. *British Dental Journal*, **109**, 387–98

5. Frank, R. M. (1970). Etude autoradiographique de la dentinogènese en microscopies électronique à l'aide de la proline tritiée chez le chat. *Archives of Oral Biology*, **15**, 583–96

6. Nalbandian, J., Gonzales, F. and Sognnaes, R. F. (1960). Sclerotic age changes in root dentine of human teeth as observed by optical, electron and X-ray microscopy. *Journal of Dental Research*, **39**, 598–607

7. Miles, A. E. W. (1976). Age changes in dental tissues, in *Scientific Basis of Dentistry* (Eds Cohen, B and Kramer I. R. H.), Livingstone, Edinburgh and London, pp. 363–75

8. Frank, R. M., Wolff, F. and Gutmann, B. (1964). Microscopie électronique de la carie au mileu de la dentine humain. *Archives of Oral Biology*, **9**, 163–79

9. Levine, R. S. (1974). The microradiographic features of dentine caries. *British Dental Journal*, **137**, 301–6

10. Barber, D. and Massler, M. (1964). Permeability of active and arrested carious lesions to dyes and radioactive isotopes. *Journal of Dentistry for Children*, **31**, 26–33

11. Fish, E. W. (1948). *Surgical Pathology of the Mouth*, Pitman, London

12. Corbett, M. E. (1963). Incidence of secondary dentine present in carious teeth. *British Dental Journal*, **114**, 142–6

13. Darling, A. I. (1959). The pathology and prevention of caries. *British Dental Journal*, **107**, 287–302

14. Dwyer, D. M., Berman, D. S. and Silverstone, L. M. (1973). A study of approximal carious lesions in primary molars. *Journal of the International Association of Dentistry for Children*, **4**, 41–6

15. Backer Dirks, O. (1966). Posteruptive changes in dental enamel. *Journal of Dental Research*, **45**, 503–11

16. Berman, D. S. and Slack, G. L. (1973). Caries progression and activity in approximal tooth surfaces: a longitudinal study. *British Dental Journal*, **134**, 51–7

17. Taylor, B. R., Berman, D. S. and Johnson, N. W. (1971). The response of pulp and dentine to dental caries in primary molars. *Journal of the International Association of Dentistry for Children*, **2**, 3–9

18. MacGregor, A. B., Marsland E. A. and Batty, I. (1956). Experimental studies of dental caries I: The relation of bacterial invasion to the softening of the dentine. *British Dental Journal*, **101**, 230–5

19. Fusayama, T. (1972). Structure and removal of carious dentine. *International Dental Journal*, **22**, 401–11

20. Shovelton, D. S. (1968) A study of deep carious dentine. *International Dental Journal*, **18**, 392–405

21. Shovelton, D. S. (1972) The maintenance of pulp vitality. *British Dental Journal*, **133**, 95–107

22. Sarnat, H. and Massler, M. (1965) Microstructure of active and arrested dentinal caries. *Journal of Dental Research*, **44**, 1389–1401

23. Symonds, N. B. B. (1970). Electron microscopic study of the tubules in human carious dentine. *Archives of Oral Biology*, **15**, 239–51

24. Massler, M. (1967). Pulpal reactions to dental caries. *International Dental Journal*, **17**, 441–60

25. Paterson, R. C. (1974). Management of the deep cavity. *British Dental Journal*, **137**, 250–2

26. Whitehead, I., MacGregor, A. B. and Marsland, E. A. (1960). Experimental studies of dental caries II: The relation of bacterial invasion to softening of the dentine in permanent and deciduous teeth. *British Dental Journal*, **108**, 261–5

27. Yoon, S. H., Brudevold, F., Gardner, D. and Smith, F. (1960). Distribution of fluoride in teeth from areas with different levels of fluoride in the water supply. *Journal of Dental Research*, **39**, 845–56

28. Reeves, R. and Stanley, H. R. (1966). The

relationship of bacterial penetration and pulpal pathosis in carious teeth. *Oral Surgery*, **22**, 59–65

29. Bergenholtz, G. (1977). Effect of bacterial products on inflammatory reactions in the dental pulp. *Scandinavian Journal of Dental Research*, **85**, 122–9

30. Fisher, F. J. (1966). The viability of micro-organisms in carious dentine beneath amalgam restorations. *British Dental Journal*, **121**, 413–16

31. Fisher, F. J. (1969). The viability of micro-organisms in carious dentine beneath amalgam restorations. *British Dental Journal*, **126**, 355–6

32. MacGregor, A. B. (1962). The extent and distribution of acid in carious dentine. *Proceedings of the Royal Society of Medicine*, **55**, 1063–6

33. King, J. B., Crawford, J. J. and Lindahl, R. L. (1965). Indirect pulp capping: a bacteriologic study of deep carious dentine in human teeth. *Oral Surgery*, **20**, 633–71

34. Mjör, I. A., Finn, S. B. and Quigley, M. B. (1961). The effect of calcium hydroxide and amalgam on non carious, vital dentine. *Archives of Oral Biology*, **3**, 283–91

35. Fisher, F. J. (1972). The effect of a calcium hydroxide/water paste on micro-organisms in carious dentine. *British Dental Journal*, **133**, 19–21

36. Mjör, I. A. (1967). Histologic studies of human coronal dentine following the insertion of various materials in experimentally prepared cavities. *Archives of Oral Biology*, **12**, 441–52

37. Eidelman, E., Finn, S. B. and Koulorides, T. (1965). Remineralization of carious dentine treated with calcium hydroxide. *Journal of Dentistry for Children*, **32**, 218–25

38. McKay, G. S. (1976). The histology and microbiology of acute occlusal dentine lesions in human permanent molar teeth. *Archives of Oral Biology*, **21**, 51–8

39. Loesche, W. J. and Syed, S. A. (1973). The predominant cultivable flora of carious plaque and carious dentine. *Caries Research*, 7, 201–16

40. Edwardsson, S. (1974). Bacteriological studies on deep areas of carious dentine. *Odontologisk Revy*, **25**, suppl. 32

41. Crawford, J. J. and Shankle, R. J. (1961). Application of new methods to study the importance of root canal and oral microbiota in endodontics. *Oral Surgery*, **14**, 1109–23

42. Winkler, K. C. and Van Amerongen, J. (1959). Bacteriologic results from 4000 root canal cultures. *Oral Surgery*, **12**, 857–75

43. Larmas, M. (1972). Histochemical demonstration of various dehydrogeneses in human carious dentine. *Archives of Oral Biology*, **17**, 1143–53

44. Johnansen, E. and Parks, H. F. (1961). Electron microscopic observations on soft carious human dentine. *Journal of Dental Research*, **40**, 235–8

45. Lester, K. S. and Boyde, A. (1968). Some preliminary observations on caries ('remineralisation') crystals in enamel and dentine by surface electron microscopy. *Virchows Archives of Pathology and Anatomy*, **344**, 196–212

46. Vahl, J., Höhling, H. J. and Frank, R. M. (1964). Elektronen strahlbeugung am rhomboedrisch aussebenden Mineralbildungen in kariösem dentin. *Archives of Oral Biology*, **9**, 315–20

47. Larmas, M. (1972). A chromatographic and histochemical study of non-specific esterases in human carious dentine. *Archives of Oral Biology*, **17**, 1121–32

48. Larmas, M. (1972). Alanine and aspartate aminotransferases in sound and carious human dentine. *Archives of Oral Biology*, **17**, 1133–41

49. Karjalainen, S. and Larmas, M. (1975). Quantitative study of the arylaminopeptidase activity in normal and altered states of human dentine. *Caries Research*, **9**, 340–50

50. Willner, H. (1926). Untersuchungen über des Vorkommen von Fett in der Zahn

Pulpa. *Zeitschrift fur stomatologie*, **24**, 1084–92

51. Allred, H. (1969). The staining of the lipids in carious human dentine *Archives of Oral Biology*, **14**, 271–6

52. Mäkinen, K. K. (1970). Characteristics of the hydrolysis of 4-phenylazobenzyloxy-carbonyl-1-prolyl-1-leucylglycyl-1-prolyl-D-arginine (a collagenase substrate) by enzyme preparations derived from carious dentine. *Acta Odontologica Scandinavica*, **28**, 485–97

53. Bergman, G. and Anneroth, G. (1972). A semiquantitative microradiographic study of the distribution of organic mass in human carious dentine. *Archives of Oral Biology*, **17**, 201–9

54. Miller, W. A. and Massler, M. (1962). Permeability and staining of active and arrested lesions in dentine. *British Dental Journal*, **112**, 187–97

55. Kuwabara, R. K. and Massler, M. (1966). Pulpal reactions to active and arrested carious lesions. *Journal of Dentistry for Children*, **33**, 190–204

56. Takuma, S., Ogiwara, H. and Suzuki, H. (1975). Electron probe and electron microscope studies of carious dentinal lesions with a remineralised surface layer. *Caries Research*, **9**, 278–85

57. Levine, R. S. (1973). The differential inorganic composition of dentine within active and arrested carious lesions. *Caries Research*, **7**, 245–60

58. Levine, R. S. (1972). Distribution of fluoride in active and arrested carious lesions in dentine. *Journal of Dental Research*, **51**, 1025–9

59. Rowles, S. L. and Levine, R. S. (1973). The inorganic composition of arrested carious dentine. *Caries Research*, **7**, 360–7

60. Levine, R. S. (1972). Remineralisation of human carious dentine *in vitro*. *Archives of Oral Biology*, **17**, 1005–8

61. Levine, R. S. and Rowles, S. K. (1973). Further studies on the remineralisation of human carious dentine *in vitro*. *Archives of*

Oral Biology, **18**, 1351–6

62. Causton, B. E., Samarawickrama, D. Y. D. and Johnson, N. W. (1976). Effects of calcifying fluid on bonding of cements and composites to dentine *in vitro*. *British Dental Journal*, **140**, 339–42

63. Mehta, F. S. and Schroff, B. C. (1965). Aspects of dental diseases in Indian Aborigines. *Indian Dental Journal*, **15**, 182

64. Jordan, H. U. and Sumney, D. I. (1973). Root surface caries: review of literature and significance of the problem. *Journal of Periodontal Research*, **44**, 158–63

65. Hazen, S. P., Chilton, N. W. and Mumma, R. D. (1973). The problem of root caries with literature review and clinical description. *Journal of The American Dental Association*, **86**, 137–44

66. Gustafsson, B. E., Quensel, C. D., Lanke, L. S., Lundqvist, C., Grahnen, H., Bonow, B. E. and Krasse, B. (1954). The Vipeholm dental caries study: the effect of different levels of carbohydrate intake on caries activity in 436 individuals observed for 5 years. *Acta Odontologica Scandinavica*, **11**, 232–364

67. Westbrook, J. C., Miller, A. D., Chilton, N. W., Williams, F. L. and Mumma, R. D. (1974). Root surface caries: a clinical, histopathologic and microradiographic investigation. *Caries Research*, **8**, 249–55

68. Keyes, P. H. (1970). Reappraisal of various types of dental caries, in *Proceedings 27th Annual Meeting of American Institute of Oral Biology*, Palm Springs, pp. 101–11

69. Krasse, B. (1977). Microbiology of the gingival plaque, in *The Borderland between Caries and Periodontal Disease* (Ed. Lehner T.), Academic Press, London

70. Sumney, D. L. and Jordan, H. L. (1974). Characterisation of bacteria isolated from human root surface carious lesions. *Journal of Dental Research*, **53**, 343–51

71. Syed, S. A., Loesche, W. J., Pape, H. L. Jr.

and Grenier, E. (1975). Predominant cultivable flora isolated from human root-surface caries plaque. *Infection and Immunity*, **11**, 727–31

72. Williams, N. B. (1955). In *Kronfelds Histopathology of the Teeth and their Surrounding Structures*, 4th ed. (Ed. Boyle, P. E.), Lee and Febiger, Philadelphia chap. 5, pp. 258–72

73. Kostlan, J. (1963). L'image histologique de la carie du cement dentaire. *Bulletin du Groupment International pour la Recherche Scientifique en Stomatologie*, **6**, 339–53

74. Furseth R. and Johansen, E. (1970). A microradiographic comparison of sound and carious human dental cementum. *Archives of Oral Biology*, **13**, 197–1206

75. Furseth, R. (1971). Further observations on the fine structure of orally exposed and carious human dental cementum. *Archives of Oral Biology*, **16**, 71–85

76. Boling, L. R. and Robinson J. B. G. (1938). Vascular changes in the exposed pulp. *Journal of Dental Research*, **17**, 310 (abstract)

77. Stenvik, A., Iversen, J. and Mjor, I. A. (1972). Tissue pressures and histology of normal and inflamed tooth pulps in macaque monkeys. *Archives of Oral Biology*, **17**, 1501–11

78. Van Hassel, J. H. (1971). Physiology of the human dental pulp. *Oral Surgery*, **32**, 126–34

79. Ahlberg, K. F. (1978). Functional studies on experimentally induced inflammatory reactions in the feline tooth pulp. *Thesis*, Univ. of Stockholm

80. Cowley, G. and MacPhee, T. (1975). *Essentials of Periodontology and Periodontics*, 2nd edn Livingstone, Edinburgh

81. Schluger, S., Yuodelis, R. A. and Page, R. C. (1977). *Periodontal Disease*. Lee and Febiger, Philadelphia

82. Brandtzaeg, P. (1975). In *Oral Mucosa in Health and Disease*, (Ed. Dolby, A. E.),

Blackwell Scientific Publications, Oxford and Edinburgh

83. Pulver, W. H., Taubman, M. A. and Smith, D. J. (1977). Immune components in normal and inflamed human dental pulp. *Archives of Oral Biology*, **22**, 103–11

84. Stephan, R. M. (1937). Correlation of clinical tests with microscopic pathology of the dental pulp. *Journal of Dental Research*, **16**, 267–78

85. Herbert, W. E. (1945). A correlation of the clinical signs and symptoms and histological conditions of the pulps of 52 teeth. *British Dental Journal*, **78**, 161–74

86. Langeland, K. (1959). Histological evaluation of pulpal reactions to operative procedures. *Oral Surgery*, **12**, 1235–48, 1357–71

87. Seltzer, S., Bender, I. B. and Zionitz, M. (1963). The dynamics of pulpal inflammation: correlations between diagnostic data and actual histologic findings in the pulp. *Oral Surgery*, **16**, 846–71; 969–77

88. Eidelman, E., Touma, B. and Ulmansky, M. (1968). Pulp pathology in deciduous teeth: clinical and histological considerations. *Israel Journal of Medical Science*, **4**, 1244–8

89. Garfunkel, A. (1973). Dental pulp pathosis: clinico-pathologic correlations based on 109 cases, *Oral Surgery*, **35**, 110–17

90. Schröder, U. (1977). Agreement between clinical and histologic findings in chronic coronal pulpitis in primary teeth. *Scandinavian Journal of Dental Research*, **85**, 583–7

91. Koch, G. and Nyborg, H. (1970). Correlation between clinical and histological indications for pulpotomy of deciduous teeth. *Journal of the International Association of Dentistry for Children*, **1**, 3–10

92. Radden, H. G. (1939). Chronic hypertrophic pulpitis. *Thesis*, Univ. of Melbourne.

93. Tyldesley, W. R. and Mumford, J. M.

(1970). Dental pain and the histological condition of the pulp. *Dental Practitioner and Dental Record*, **20**, 333–6

94.   Mathews, B., Searle, B. N., Adams, D. and Linden, R. (1974). Thresholds of vital and non vital teeth to stimulation with electric pulp testers. *British Dental Journal*, **137**, 352–5

Chapter 8

Kinetics of Enamel Dissolution

J. S. Wefel

Division of Cariology, Dows Institute for Dental Research, College of Dentistry, University of Iowa, USA

8.1   Summary

The fact that enamel dissolves in acidic media has contributed to the universal problem of dental caries. The occurrence of this disease is dependent on many factors of which one is tooth enamel. Since enamel consists mainly of inorganic calcium and phosphate in the form of hydroxyapatite (HAP), studies on the dissolution of enamel have often used synthetic apatites as models. These models have proved to be quite successful in describing many aspects of enamel dissolution and will be mentioned throughout this chapter. Since the mathematics needed to describe thoroughly the dissolution rates of enamel can become rather complex, this summary is intended to describe the dissolution process without the detail found in the main body of the chapter.

In describing the kinetics of dissolution of any material it must first be realised that dissolution is controlled by the solubility of the material. This may be expressed as the thermodynamic solubility product, which for HAP would be as follows:

$$K_{HAP} = [Ca^{2+}]^{10}[PO_4^{3-}]^6[OH^-]^2$$

Therefore, the solubility product for HAP is dependent on the activities of calcium, phosphate and hydroxide in solution. When this solubility product is exceeded, HAP will precipitate and, likewise, HAP will dissolve when a solution is undersaturated. Another important factor in describing enamel dissolution is the kinetics or rate at which enamel dissolves. In reaction kinetics, the rate-controlling step is the slowest reaction step in the total process. Physical–chemical concepts should make it possible to distinguish between diffusion-controlled reactions and surface-controlled reactions.

One of the first quantitative descriptions of bulk enamel dissolution was made by Gray[1]. He found that initial enamel dissolution was a function of the total buffer concentration, pH, and buffer acid strength. This led to the following differential equation for enamel dissolution:

$$\frac{dEn}{dt} = k_1[H^+] + k_2 K^{1/2}[HB]^{3/4}[B^-]^{-1/4}$$

where k_1 and k_2 are functions of temperature and agitation, K is the equilibrium constant for the acid buffer employed, and $[H^+]$, $[HB]$ and $[B^-]$ are the concentrations of hydrogen ion, undissociated buffer and buffer anion, respectively. Gray also showed that enamel dissolution in his system was controlled by the diffusion rates of the reactants and products of the dissolution process. The success of Gray's semi-empirical equation led other workers to postulate more detailed mathematical models.

Higuchi and co-workers[2,3] developed a physical model based on Fick's law of diffusion that met with moderate success and was generally applicable. The driving force for the dissolution is again governed by the solubility product of the mineral phase in contact with the acid buffer, and the dissolution is a diffusion-controlled process in the diffusion layer adjacent to the enamel. Some of the shortcomings of this model are the uncertainties in the equilibrium constants, the solubility product for HAP, the diffusion layer thickness, and the mathematical modelling which then occurs. The model also requires that diffusion of ions be independent when, in fact, the diffusion of various ions during a steady-state process is almost surely coupled and therefore not independent.

Several of the above problems were eliminated with the development of rotating disc experiments in which well-controlled fluid dynamics allowed the calculation of the diffusion layer thickness. One such study[4] revealed that as the initial dissolution proceeds, the rate-controlling step may change from diffusion to a surface reaction involving the solution of the lattice ions. Another investigator[5] noted that additives changed the dissolution behaviour of his apatite discs. This led to the development of a two-site dissolution model for dental enamel. In this model two sites of dissolution occur and are governed by separate solubility products. Only one site is affected by additives such as EDTA, while the other is not. A consequence of such a model is that a zone of dissolution rather than surface dissolution is predicted. This may have consequences in the development of a white spot lesion.

The investigation by White and Nancollas[6], using the rotating disc, included the addition of an inert electrolyte to minimise any charge gradients, as well as consideration of coupled diffusion and concentration gradients. This work has led to a semi-empirical equation which included coupled diffusion of ions as well as a change in the thickness of the diffusion layer due to reaction within this layer. The overall dissolution rate was:

$$R_d = \frac{-SD_{HAP}}{10^3 \delta_N} [(HAP_0) - (HAP)] [a[H^+] + b]$$

This work was carried out at similar concentrations and solution conditions as employed by previous investigators and showed that dissolution of bovine enamel, like synthetic apatite, may be described by conventional thermodynamics and kinetics.

In summary, the pH, acid buffer concentration, and buffer acid strength are the main variables in enamel dissolution. The effect of other ions such as calcium and phosphate must also be considered, especially in the case of white spot formation. Most studies seem to support diffusion as the rate-controlling process in initial enamel dissolution, although several reports have mentioned a possible surface reaction becoming rate controlling as the reaction proceeds. The mathematical models are limited in describing all parameters and must be used as guides in describing more complicated systems.

8.2   Introduction

The formation and histological appearance of enamel caries has been described in chapter 6. Enamel caries is the result of the chemical dissolution of enamel and may be described in terms of physical–chemical principles. At its simplest level the caries process must include the

diffusion of the reactants (acids) to the reaction site (dental enamel), followed by reaction (dissolution) and diffusion of the reaction products away from the reaction site. The reaction between solution and solid is a heterogeneous one and is normally dependent on the rate of diffusion of the reactants to the solid surface. It is also possible, however, that the reaction at the tooth interface is the rate-controlling step.

In chemical reactions the rate-determining step is the slowest reaction in the total process. Physical–chemical concepts should enable one to develop a quantitative description of enamel dissolution. The dissolution of dental enamel by acid occurs as a result of the reaction between hydrogen (H^+) ion and the inorganic materials of dental enamel. This material is predominantly hydroxyapatite, $Ca_{10}(PO_4)_6(OH)_2$ and its dissolution may simply be described as follows:

$$Ca_{10}(PO_4)_6(OH)_2 + 8H^+ \rightarrow 10Ca^{+2} + 6HPO_4^{-2} + 2H_2O$$

$$(8.1)$$

with the form of the phosphate ion being determined by the pH of the system. This simplified concept of dissolution is affected, however, by the environment surrounding the enamel surface. Thus plaque, salivary pellicle, saliva, and surface mineral phases may influence the overall reaction rates of enamel dissolution. In this chapter several mathematical approaches to enamel dissolution, together with a current model of caries formation, will be described.

8.3   Kinetics of Bulk Enamel Dissolution

Several early attempts to correlate acid diffusion with demineralisation[7] and the use of Donnan membrane theory to explain sub-surface demineralisation[8] failed to result in an adequate mathematical expression of the carious process. One of the first quantitative descriptions of the carious process was made by Gray in 1962[1]. He prepared enamel blocks from human incisors which were placed into lactic acid buffer solutions. Initial solubility rates were determined by measuring the concentration of calcium and phosphate ions in the solution and expressing these quantities as grams of enamel dissolved/cm^2 area. He was then able to vary the pH, lactate concentration, temperature of reaction, agitation speed and foreign ion concentration.

The results showed that the enamel solubility rate was greatly affected by agitation speed and hardly affected by a 10°C temperature change. As agitation will directly affect diffusion but not surface reactions, these results clearly showed that the reaction was diffusion controlled and not surface controlled. Thus, the reaction rate depends on how fast the hydrogen ions reach the enamel surface. As weak acids are only dissociated to a limited extent, the undissociated acid buffer (HB) becomes the principle source of hydrogen ions (H$^+$) and must also diffuse to the enamel surface. The overall reaction rate can be expressed as follows:

$$\frac{dEn}{dt} = f[H^+] + f([HB], [B^-], K) \quad (8.2)$$

where dEn/dt = grams of enamel in solution/cm^2 of surface/second of exposure, and is a function (f) of the dissociated acid buffer concentration in mol/l (B$^-$); the buffer dissociation constant (K); the hydrogen ion (H$^+$); and undissociated acid buffer (HB) concentrations. Thus, the first term in equation (8.2) represents the action of dissociated hydrogen ions or a strong acid on enamel. Since the rate of diffusion of hydrogen ions depends on the concentration of hydrogen ions in the bulk solution, the enamel dissolution is a function of the hydrogen ion concentration. Likewise, enamel dissolution is also a function of the concentration of undissociated buffer, since it may diffuse to the enamel surface and dissociate (HB $\rightleftharpoons$ H$^+$ + B$^-$). Gray then applied the usual rate function (kC^n) for diffusion-controlled reactions[9] to each variable in equation (8.2). The following expression results from this substitution:

$$\frac{dEn}{dt} = k_1[H^+]^{n_1} + k_2 K^{n_2}[HB]^{n_3}[B]^{n_4} \quad (8.3)$$

where the k's are rate constants and the n's are also constants. Total buffer concentration (TB) may be used for ease of calculation by substituting the following equations:

$$[TB] = [HB] + [B^-] \quad (8.4)$$

$$K = \frac{[H^+][B^-]}{[HB]} \quad (8.5)$$

Now by substituting and rearranging, the equation obtained can be used to evaluate the exponents (n) and rate constants (k) by holding the pH or buffer concentration constant. The results of the experiments on enamel blocks yielded the exponents to be substituted into equation (8.3). This gives the following differential rate equation:

$$\frac{dEn}{dt} = k_1[H^+] + k_2 K^{1/2}[HB]^{3/4}[B^-]^{-1/4}$$
$$(8.6)$$

The constants k_1 and k_2 are functions of temperature and agitation, while K depends on the acid buffer system employed. As expected, the [B$^-$] term has a negative exponent which implies an inhibiting effect. It was also verified by Gray's experiments with varying buffers that as K decreased, the rate increased, reached a maximum, and decreased.

The effect of common ions such as calcium and phosphate and other inhibitors such as magnesium were incorporated into the model by adding a kC^n term for each ion. Interestingly, each inhibitor had the same exponent (1/2) when measured experimentally. According to Gray, this may be related to the mechanism of their inhibiting action. In the case of cations, Gray postulated that the irreversible dissolution of enamel provides calcium and phosphate (see equation (8.1)) which may react to form surface phases. With calcium, the surface phase formed would be dicalcium phosphate dihydrate (CaHPO$_4$.2H$_2$O). Likewise, other cationic inhibitors of enamel dissolution would form insoluble phosphate salts and the more insoluble the salt, the more effective is the inhibition. This behaviour was illustrated in Gray's work by the fact that enamel dissolution in acid approached equilibrium as the reaction products accumulated.

The same inhibition should also occur with anions (for example, phosphate and fluoride) that form insoluble calcium salts. In the case of fluoride, the inhibition of enamel dissolution is well known and will occur if the fluoride is added to the buffer solution or occurs naturally in the enamel.

In summary, Gray has deduced a semi-empirical equation for the rate of dissolution of dental enamel which satisfactorily describes the experimental findings. This equation shows that initial enamel dissolution is a function of the total buffer concentration, buffer acid strength and pH. When present, the effect of other ions is described by additional terms in the equation. A mechanism for the retardation of enamel dissolution by foreign ions was also postulated.

8.3.1 Mathematical models

The success of Gray's theories and experiments led Higuchi to use detailed mathematical models based on Fick's laws of diffusion. In 1965, the first in a series of papers[2] tested two mathematical models for relevance. The two models (figure 8.1) involve the use of either hydroxyapatite (model A) or dicalcium phosphate dihydrate (DCPD; model B) as the dissolving phase. In model B it is assumed that the buffer solution is in contact with DCPD, which may be more stable under the acidic conditions of demineralisation and has been identified as a reaction product of enamel dissolution[10]. In both cases the dissolution process may be described similarly. The acid buffer and hydrogen ions must diffuse from the bulk solution across a diffusion layer of constant thickness, h, to the surface. The acidic components diffusing inward will meet the phosphate species that are diffusing outward and may interact within the diffusion layer to an extent determined by the dissociation of both phosphoric acid and the buffer acid, and the concentration of all the species involved. Outward diffusion of the reaction products, calcium ion

and unreacted phosphate species, continues out of the diffusion layer into the bulk solution. The appropriate equations can now be formulated to describe mathematically the dissolution process.

Using Fick's laws of diffusion[11] and mass balances in the steady state, coupled with the simultaneous diffusion and rapid chemical reaction expressions, the following differential equations are obtained:

$$D_{Ca}\frac{d^2[Ca^{2+}]}{dx^2} = 0 \tag{8.7}$$

$$D_{HP}\frac{d^2[HPO_4^{2-}]}{dx^2} - \phi_1 - \phi_2 = 0 \tag{8.8}$$

$$D_{H_2P}\frac{d^2[H_2PO_4^-]}{dx^2} + \phi_1 + \phi_2 = 0 \tag{8.9}$$

$$D_B\frac{d^2[B^-]}{dx^2} + \phi_2 - \phi_3 = 0 \tag{8.10}$$

$$D_{HB}\frac{d^2[HB]}{dx^2} - \phi_2 + \phi_3 = 0 \tag{8.11}$$

$$D_H\frac{d^2[H^+]}{dx^2} - \phi_1 - \phi_3 = 0 \tag{8.12}$$

The D's in equations (8.7)–(8.12) are the respective diffusion coefficients for Ca^{2+}, HPO_4^{2-}, $H_2PO_4^-$, the buffer ion B^-, monobasic buffer acid molecule HB, and H^+. The bracketed terms are the concentration of the individual species. The ϕ_1, ϕ_2 and ϕ_3 terms are the respective rates of reaction per unit volume for the following reactions:

$$HPO_4^{2-} + H^+ \rightarrow H_2PO_4^- \tag{8.13}$$

$$HPO_4^{2-} + HB \rightarrow H_2PO_4^- + B^- \tag{8.14}$$

$$H^+ + B^- \rightarrow HB \tag{8.15}$$

These reaction rates are assumed to be entirely diffusion controlled so that if other reactions, such as calcium complexation, occurred in the solution phase, equations (8.7)–(8.12) would not describe the situation fully. Even though the extent of complexation would need to be extensive to affect the overall calculations, incorporation of terms for calcium complexing with

Model A

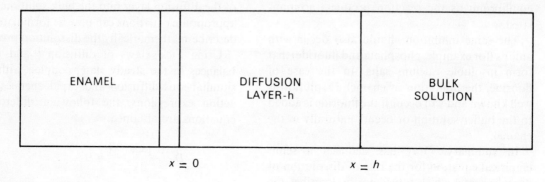

Layer of
HAP-$Ca_{10}(PO_4)_6(OH)_2$

Model B

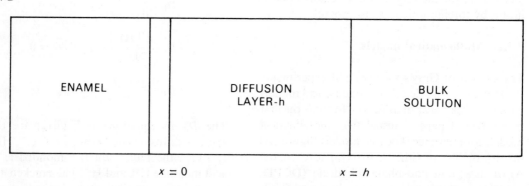

thin layer of
DCPD-$CaHPO_4.2H_2O$

Figure 8.1   Dissolution of enamel in acidic buffer solution, assuming solution adjacent to surface is in equilibrium with hydroxyapatite (model A) or dicalcium phosphate dihydrate phase (model B). (After Higuchi et al.[2])

phosphate or other agents should eventually be performed.

Within the diffusion layer the following equilibrium expressions must also hold:

$$\text{at } x \geq 0, \qquad K_B = \frac{[H^+][B^-]}{[HB]} \qquad (8.16)$$

$$K_{2P} = \frac{[H^+][HPO_4^{2-}]}{[H_2PO_4^-]} \qquad (8.17)$$

$$K_{3P} = \frac{[H^+][PO_4^{3-}]}{[HPO_4^{2-}]} \qquad (8.18)$$

$$K_w = [H^+][OH^-] \qquad (8.19)$$

$$\text{at } x = 0, K_{HAP} = [Ca^{2+}]^{10}[PO_4^{3-}]^6[OH^-]^2 \qquad (8.20)$$

These equilibrium expressions determine the relative concentrations of the species at any point in the diffusion layer.

The other boundary conditions that may be established within the diffusion layer show that the rate of HB reaching the enamel interface must equal the amount of B^- leaving:

$$-D_{HB}\frac{d[HB]}{dx} = D_B\frac{d[B^-]}{dx} \quad (8.21)$$

Also, from the net dissolution reaction of

$$Ca_{10}(PO_4)_6(OH)_2 + 8H^+ \rightleftharpoons 10Ca^{2+} \\ + 6HPO_4^{2-} + 2H_2O$$

it can be shown that

$$10\left(D_H\frac{d[H^+]}{dx} + D_{H_2P}\frac{d(H_2PO_4^-)}{dx} + D_{HB}\frac{d[HB]}{dx}\right) \\ = -8D_{Ca}\frac{d[Ca^{2+}]}{dx} \quad (8.22)$$

and

$$10\left(D_{HP}\frac{d[HPO_4^{2-}]}{dx} + D_{H_2P}\frac{d[H_2PO_4^-]}{dx}\right) \\ = 6D_{Ca}\frac{d[Ca^{2+}]}{dx} \quad (8.23)$$

The integration of equations (8.7)–(8.12) may now be carried out if it is assumed that the diffusion coefficients and equilibrium constants are independent of their position in the diffusion layer.

It is seen that the constant of the first integration of equation (8.7), C_1, is the negative rate of diffusion of Ca^{2+} through the layer. Therefore, let $G = -C_1$, where G is the diffusion rate of Ca^{2+} and is the quantity giving the rate of enamel dissolution. The value of G is the theoretical value that may be compared to actual measured values of enamel dissolution. In order to solve for G, the quantity Gh is taken as a single unknown. A second integration, substitution and rearrangement yields the two working equations for model A:

$$\frac{0.6Gh + D_{HP}[HPO_4^{2-}]_h + D_{H_2P}[H_2PO_4^-]_h}{D_{H_2P} + (D_{HP}K_{2P})/([H^+]_0)} \\ = [H_2PO_4^-]_h + \frac{D_H}{D_{H_2P}}[H^+]_h - \frac{D_H}{D_{H_2P}}[H^+]_0$$

$$+ \frac{D_{HB}}{D_{H_2P}}[HB]_h - \frac{D_{HB}}{D_{H_2P}}\left(\frac{D_{HB}[HB]_h + D_B[B^-]_h}{D_{HB} + (D_B K_B)/([H^+]_0)}\right) \\ - \frac{0.8Gh}{D_{H_2P}} \quad (8.24)$$

and

$$[H^+]_0^{14} = \frac{K_{3P}^6 K_W^2}{K_{HAP}}\left([Ca^{2+}]_h + \frac{Gh}{D_{Ca}}\right)^{10} \times \\ \left(\frac{0.6Gh + D_{HP}[HPO_4^{2-}]_h + D_{H_2P}[H_2PO_4^-]_h}{(D_{H_2P})/K_{2P} + (D_{HP})/([H^+]_0)}\right)^6 \quad (8.25)$$

When $[H^+]_0$ is eliminated from equations (8.24) and (8.25), an evaluation of Gh for any set of values for the diffusion coefficients, K's and species concentrations at $X = h$ may now be made.

In model B a further assumption is made that the thickness of the surface dicalcium phosphate dihydrate layer remains constant over the time of reaction under study. All the equations in model A will apply in model B, except for the boundary conditions of a DCPD surface versus HAP. Thus, equation (8.20) will become

at $x = 0$, $K_{DCPD} = [Ca^{2+}][HPO_4^{2-}] \quad (8.26)$

The working equations for model B will become equation (8.24) and the following expression:

$$K_{DCPD} = \left([Ca^{2+}]_h + \frac{Gh}{D_{Ca}}\right) \\ \left(\frac{0.6Gh + D_{HP}[HPO_4^{2-}]_h + D_{H_2P}[H_2PO_4^-]_h}{D_{HP} + (D_{H_2P}[H^+]_0)/K_{2P}}\right) \quad (8.27)$$

The application of the theoretical models may now be made. Higuchi used Gray's data on enamel blocks to test the relevance of both models. The main problem encountered was the choice of equilibrium constants consistent with the experimental conditions used in Gray's work. Thus, two sets of values were used in the calculations with each model together with more than one value of h, the diffusion layer thickness. Under controlled hydrodynamics, h is constant for any given stirring speed and may be determined experimentally, but in this case was varied to find the best fit.

The results of comparing the models with the experimental values of pH, buffer concentration, acid buffers and common ion effect gave generally acceptable agreement. Both models, however, showed rough quantitative agreement and suggested that the present method may be insensitive with regard to distinguishing the phases that are dissolving. Since the experimental conditions were close to those approximating an equilibrium between DCPD and HAP, Higuchi suggests that the similarity between predictions of the two models supports the likelihood of a surface phase conversion of HAP to DCPD.

A more critical evaluation revealed that model B did not show good agreement with the observed common ion effects. Model A, however, showed better quantitative agreement when acid buffers such as acetic and chloroacetic were used. One must also keep in mind that model B requires a very fast conversion of HAP to DCPD for initial dissolution rates. Therefore, model B may be applicable at a point in time which is closer to equilibrium, where DCPD has already been identified by independent means.

In general, the results show that a diffusion-controlled mechanism, involving dissolution from an hydroxyapatite surface, best explains all the data. Both pH and buffer concentration, together with common ion effects, give satisfactory agreement. At very high initial rates of dissolution, conversion of HAP to DCPD may occur, according to the theory. Uncertainties exist in the chosen thermodynamic value for K_{HAP} (Reference 12), the value for the diffusion layer thickness, and the use of the physical model versus experimental models.

The assessment of Gray's enamel block data involved several problems in view of the uncertainties in chosen equilibrium values. In 1969, however, Higuchi and co-workers[3] presented a critical examination of the hydroxyapatite model both theoretically and experimentally. Both synthetic apatite powder and powdered enamel were used in the dissolution experiments as well as rotating disc experiments. The advantage of the rotating disc method is that it allows calculation of the diffusion layer thickness, h. In the pow-

dered experiments, a weighed amount of powdered enamel or synthetic apatite (TVA or Victor's HAP) was placed in a flask with acid buffer and continuously shaken. Samples were then withdrawn at specified times, filtered and analysed for calcium and phosphate.

Flat round discs of 1/2 in. diameter were prepared from the synthetic-apatite samples and mounted to lucite blocks such that only one side was exposed to the solution. The apparatus employed affords reproducible hydrodynamics which allow for the calculations of h, the diffusion layer thickness, and the concentration of all species using the established Levich theory[13] for fluid flow at a rotating disc. Higuchi found that the use of TVA synthetic apatite did not yield smooth curves for the initial rates due to an abrupt curvature in the amount of hydroxyapatite dissolved versus time. No explanation of this finding was given, although subsequent experiments used 'predissolved' TVA apatite [TVA(PD)] samples, because smooth curves were then obtained with this material.

The results showed that all powdered-enamel data were in good agreement with the previously described model A. Thus, the model satisfactorily described the experimental values in two different buffers, at several buffer concentrations and pH values, as well as predicting the common ion effects of calcium and phosphate. With the choice of one K_{HAP} value, the model also described Gray's enamel block dissolution rates. The value found for K_{HAP} ranged from 10^{-130} to 10^{-132} and is noteworthy in that the normal range of the thermodynamic solubility product of hydroxyapatite is known to be between 10^{-110} and 10^{-120} (Reference 12). The use of a variable solubility product provides better agreement with the theory, but implies an unclear picture of the thermodynamics and driving potential of the dissolution reaction. The fact that one value of K_{HAP}, even though smaller than previously reported values, showed good agreement with the experimental parameters is encouraging, since it implies a constant thermodynamic driving force for dissolution. As stated by the authors, 'the proposed hydroxyapatite model for the dissolution rate of enamel in acidic media is a very generally applicable one'.

8.4   The Role of Fluoride

An extension of Higuchi's hydroxyapatite model of enamel dissolution was published in 1969 by Mir, Higuchi and Hefferen[14]. This work considers the role of fluoride in enamel demineralisation, because of its relevance to dental caries[15, 16]. A similar approach was used to derive the theoretical equations, and most of the equations mentioned above apply. The basic assumption in this model is that when hydroxyapatite is exposed to a low concentration of fluoride in acidic buffers, a thin layer of fluorapatite is formed around the HAP crystals. Thus, fluorapatite and not hydroxyapatite becomes the thermodynamically governing phase during dissolution. It does not matter for the model whether the FAP phase is formed by surface exchange with the hydroxyl group or surface precipitation of FAP from solution. This model is similar to model B mentioned earlier, except that FAP is assumed to have formed on the enamel crystals instead of DCPD. The same reactions are expected to occur in the diffusion layer, equations (8.13)–(8.15), and the same equilibrium expressions, equations (8.16)–(8.18), will govern. At the interface between solid and solution ($x = 0$), however, the following reaction for fluorapatite holds:

$$K_{\text{FAP}} = [\text{Ca}]^{10}[\text{PO}_4]^6[\text{F}]^2 \qquad (8.28)$$

This replaces equation (8.20) of the hydroxyapatite model. The expressions for Fick's law of diffusion in a steady state, equations (8.7)–(8.12) are also applicable, but an additional expression must be formulated to account for the fluoride in solution, namely:

$$D_{\text{F}}\frac{\text{d}^2[\text{F}^-]}{\text{d}x^2} = 0 \qquad (8.29)$$

Integration of these equations gives similar results as before along with

$$D_{\text{F}}\frac{\text{d}[\text{F}]}{\text{d}x} = 0 \qquad (8.30)$$

which states that fluoride is neither consumed nor generated during the steady-state dissolution period. The second integration yields two equations which describe the hydroxyapatite dissolution rate, G, for this FAP model:

$$[\text{H}^+]_0^6 = \frac{(K_{3\text{P}})^6(K_{2\text{P}})^6}{K_{\text{FAP}}}$$

$$\left([\text{Ca}^{2+}]_h + \frac{Gh}{D}\right)^{10}[\text{F}^-]^2$$

$$\times \left[\frac{(0.6Gh)/D + [\text{HPO}_4^{2-}]_h + [\text{H}_2\text{PO}_4^-]_h}{K_{2\text{P}} + [\text{H}^+]_0}\right]^6 \qquad (8.31)$$

$$0.8Gh = D[\text{H}_2\text{PO}_4^-]_h + D[\text{HB}]_h$$

$$- \left[\frac{0.6Gh + D[\text{H}_2\text{PO}_4^-]_h + D[\text{HPO}_4^{2-}]_h}{1 + (K_{2\text{P}})/[\text{H}^+]_0}\right]$$

$$- \frac{D[\text{HB}]_h + D[\text{B}^-]_h}{1 + (K_\text{B})/[\text{H}^+]_0} \qquad (8.32)$$

All of the concentration terms with the subscript h are known since these are the bulk solution concentrations. The only unknown terms are G (the congruent dissolution rate of hydroxyapatite), h (the diffusion layer thickness) and $(\text{H}^+)_0$ (the concentration of hydrogen ions at $x = 0$). Since G and h always occur together (Gh), they may be treated as one unknown and hence $(\text{H}^+)_0$ may be eliminated from the two equations by successive approximation methods with a computer. The mathematical expressions may now be used to compare the theoretical values with those obtained experimentally.

The experiments consisted of placing weighed amounts of either synthetic HAP or enamel powder into acetate buffers at pH 4.5 or 6.0. Aliquots are then withdrawn at specified times and analysed for calcium, phosphate and fluoride. Fluoride was added to the buffer solutions in concentrations up to 100 p.p.m. Concentrations above 100 p.p.m. caused the formation of CaF_2 which is not considered in the present model. The results showed that fluoride decreased the rate of enamel dissolution, as expected, with all hydroxyapatite preparations. In the case of the synthetic hydroxyapatite [TVA(PD)], the model gave good agreement with and without common ions present by using the same K_{HAP} value of 10^{-131}. The value found for K_{FAP} was very similar to K_{HAP} and implied that the FAP was formed by the isomorphous substitution of surface hydroxyls by fluoride ions rather than bulk precipitation. The good agreement of model and experimental results with the TVA(PD) samples showed that all the data may be described by a single unified physcial model.

The experiments with enamel powder and acidic buffer solutions containing fluoride did not give good agreement between the model and the experimental results. The theoretical model was then modified to account for the amount of fluoride originally in the enamel powder. The correction procedure improved the agreement between model and experimental data regarding pH effects, although the assumption that all the fluoride is evenly distributed within the enamel sample is highly unlikely. The same correction procedure was used in the analysis of the fluoride-treated enamel powder, and produced a good correlation with the model. The K_{HAP} value used with enamel is 10^{-116} to 10^{-120} which is higher than that for synthetic apatites. This is most probably due to the improved purity and crystallinity found in the synthetic samples when compared with enamel powder. The K_{FAP} found to give the best consistency with enamel powder was 10^{-119}. This was also similar to the K_{HAP} value found for enamel powder.

The use of a single value for K_{HAP} for a given hydroxyapatite sample (either synthetic or natural) is desirable. It is not expected that one sample should change its thermodynamic solubility product to meet the needs of a model. Thus far, the investigations of Higuchi and co-workers have given much encouragement to the use of a physical model. These studies should serve as baselines for more complex situations. The more complex models would involve the kinetics of dissolution in white spot formation, a plaque or pellicle layer at the enamel interface, and the formation of surface phases during dissolution.

The work by Higuchi and co-workers up to 1969 may now be summarised. A physical model has been developed that describes the dissolution rate behaviour of human dental enamel and synthetic hydroxyapatite in weak acid buffers. The driving force of the dissolution is governed by the solubility product of the hydroxyapatite phase, and dissolution is a diffusion-controlled process in a diffusion layer adjacent to the enamel surface. The model is able generally to account for the effects of buffer types, buffer concentration, pH, and common ions. An extension of the model showed that solution fluoride influences the reaction rates and was explained by assuming that a surface exchange of OH^- by F^- occurs rapidly during dissolution.

Thus, we have discussed two possible models for the dissolution of dental enamel. The first involved a semi-empirical approach which gave a rate expression dependent on pH, buffer concentration and buffer type. The experimental work by Gray showed the dissolution reaction to be diffusion controlled and suggested to Higuchi and co-workers that Fick's law of diffusion may be used to describe the dissolution of dental enamel. This approach has been criticised from several viewpoints. Brown[17] has stated that the diffusion of various types of ions during a steady-state process is so strongly coupled that it is questionable whether one should attempt to designate diffusion of any one component or ion as rate controlling. This concept was reiterated by Nancollas[18] at the workshop on Physiochemical Mechanisms of Dental Caries. He also suggested that the dissolution studies be performed with well-characterised fluid dynamics. This is possible when rotating disc experiments are performed where one can apply the Levich equations to study the fluid dynamics. Several publications now exist which have used the rotating disc experimental design and these will now be discussed.

8.5 Rotating Disc Dissolution Experiments

One of the first studies using a rotating disc experimental design for examining the dissolution of dental enamel was published in 1973 by Linge and Nancollas[4]. This work examines the enamel dissolution under simple chemical and well-defined hydrodynamic conditions, which practically conserve the enamel surface. Bovine enamel was mounted in a self-curing resin and machined to the required shape. The exposed enamel surface was polished with suspensions of Al_2O_3 and stored in synthetic HAP solutions to prevent dissolution. The tooth and resin were then mounted on a metal spindle with fixed rotation speeds from 300 to 3000 rev/min. The dissolution experiments were performed by placing the specimen in solutions containing various amounts of added calcium and phosphate. The rate of enamel dissolution was measured as a function of the proton uptake needed to maintain a constant pH. Two factors are important in the current design. The experiments revealed no subsurface demineralisation nor any effective surface area changes. This eliminates inherent uncertainties in assessing surface area changes. Also, the levels of calcium and phosphate from the dissolution of the enamel were less than 1 per cent of the calcium and phosphate added; therefore, the amounts added reflected the solution compositions.

The results showed no systematic variation in the rate of proton uptake compared to total Ca released $d[H^+]/d[T_{Ca}]$ under different experimental conditions. In this experiment, this value was found to be 1.42, which agreed well with the theoretical value of 1.40. Congruent dissolution was also apparent from separate experiments and confirmed HAP as the dissolving phase. Substantial changes in dissolution rate with rotation speed of the source confirmed the results of Gray, showing that mass transfer in the Nernst boundary layer contributes significantly as a rate-determining step in the reaction. In order to use mass transport calculations, an inert electrolyte must be present in the system to minimise the development of electrical field-gradients normally set up in the boundary layer by the moving ions having different intrinsic mobilities. Thus, Fick's law of diffusion is not applicable when more than two ions are transferred in the boundary layer unless charge gradients are suppressed. Experiments designed to determine the amount of inert electrolyte required, showed an initial increase in dissolution rate below a concentration of 0.02 mol/l KNO_3. This was a consequence of the elimination of the electric field gradient in the diffusion layer by the addition of the electrolyte, and not due to a variable solubility of HAP.

Dissolution-rate experiments were conducted at 6, 25 and 60° C and showed that enamel solubility decreases with increasing temperature. An Arrhenius plot with this experimental data gave an apparent solubility activation energy of -4.0 kcal/mol T_{Ca} and provides support that the nature of the calcium phosphate surface phase does not change during dissolution over this temperature range.

Theoretical calculations of the diffusion process under steady-state conditions of dissolution involved expressions of the following type[19]:

$$\int_0^\delta R_d dl = \int_0^\delta F\left(\frac{\partial \tilde{\mu}(i)}{\partial l}, \mu^0(i)\right) dl \qquad (8.33)$$

where R_d is the steady-state dissolution rate, l is the distance parameter perpendicular to the rotating disc surface, and F is a complex function of the mobility $\mu^0(i)$ and electrochemical potential $\tilde{\mu}(i)$ of each ion (i) in the diffusion layer (δ), The dependence of R_d on stirring, therefore, has the form:

$$R_d = \omega^a \phi \qquad (8.34)$$

where ϕ is a complex integral, dependent on the solution and surface concentration of each ion, and ω is the angular velocity. The parameter a has a value between 1/2 and 1 depending on the type of flow (laminar or turbulent) occuring at the disc surface[20]. Plots of the dissolution rate, R_d, versus $\omega^{1/2}$ should give a linear relationship if diffusion is the rate-controlling step. Initially these plots gave straight lines, but marked deviations from linearity occurred at higher stirring speeds as the reaction proceeded. Thus, the initial dissolution rate appeared to be diffusion controlled but as the reaction proceeds, the surface-dissolution step becomes rate controlling. Several possible semi-empirical equations were tested by Linge and Nancollas and the one found to be consistent with the data had the following form:

$$R_d = k(C_\infty - C)^N = kC_\infty^N(1 - \alpha)^N \quad (8.35)$$

where R_d is the dissolution rate, k is a specific rate constant, C_∞ is the solute solubility, C is the solution concentration at time t, and $\alpha(0 \leqslant \alpha \leqslant 1)$ describes the extent of the reaction. This type of equation is frequently found to describe the kinetics of surface reactions whenever simple solvation of the lattice ions govern crystal dissolution[21]. Quantitative analysis using this equation was to follow in a subsequent publication, but has not been published at this time.

In summary, Linge and Nancollas have studied the dissolution of enamel using a rotating disc method, which gave well-defined hydrodynamic conditions. As the undersaturation is decreased, a slow reaction at the crystal surface gains increasing control of the dissolution. This reaction was described qualitatively by a semi-empirical equation for the dissolution of enamel. The approach used by the authors has allowed a study of the mechanism of the chemical reaction at the crystal surface during dissolution. In the earlier work by Higuchi, this was not possible since the diffusion step was always assumed to completely determine the reaction rate.

Further studies by Nancollas and co-workers using the rotating disc design complemented the earlier findings[22] and confirmed that a surface reaction controlled the dissolution rate as the reaction proceeds. The effectiveness of additives on the dissolution rate of both sound and white spot enamel were investigated. The results indicated that the assumption of chemical equilibrium at the enamel surface during demineralisation may not be justified. This assumption is basic to the physical model, which assumes

diffusion control throughout the dissolution reaction.

Another study using the rotating disc was presented at the same meeting by Young[23]. This work was performed by Higuchi and co-workers on human dental block enamel and compressed pellets of HAP. Their data revealed that 'there are at least two solution partial saturation regions in which the dissolution rate patterns for apatite are significantly different'. They state that when the solution activity product for K_{HAP} is less than 10^{-128} the dissolution rate obeys the Levich predictions for rotating discs. This activity product corresponds to the initial dissolution reaction, since very little calcium and phosphate have yet dissolved. As dissolution continues, the calcium and phosphate concentrations increase and the solution activity product reaches a value of $10^{-115} > K_{HAP} > 10^{-128}$. In this region, the dissolution rates were found to be independent of rotation velocities and therefore not diffusion controlled in the boundary layer. The authors interpreted the initial dissolution site as the one previously investigated[3], and related this site to the rapid dissolution of individual crystals. In the second region ($K_{HAP} \equiv 10^{-115} \sim 10^{-128}$), dissolution occurred slowly from individual crystals and a zone of decalcification rather than surface dissolution resulted.

Subsequent work in Higuchi's laboratories with EDTA solutions showed that at pH 3–4 EDTA decreased the dissolution rates, while at pH 5–6 it did not appreciably change the rates. This phenomenon was not consistent with the physical model developed earlier. This study[5] suggested that there may be two sites of enamel dissolution. The authors then formulated a two-site dissolution model for dental enamel. The enamel crystals are assumed to have two different sites, one of which is inhibited by EDTA and the other is not. The site unaffected by EDTA, however, may not be in instantaneous equilibrium with its surroundings. The initial model gave an expression for the rate of release of material from this second site:

$$R_s = k_s^*[Cs - C(x)] \quad (8.36)$$

where Cs is the equilibrium solubility character of the site, and $C(x)$ is the concentration at a given point in the system. This expression was combined with equations for Fick's law of diffusion and the chemical equilibrium in the boundary layer. A consequence of this model is that a zone of dissolution rather than surface dissolution is predicted. This only seems to occur at partial saturation or when an additive such as EDTA is present. The use of a rotating disc system and weak acid buffers under sink (site 1) conditions showed similar deviations from the model. In 1976, a quantitative treatment of rotating disc systems was published by Wu *et al.*[24]. In this treatment the equilibria in the diffusion layer are the same as those mentioned previously in the bulk dissolution section, but the dissolution behaviour within the pellet must also be examined. For the steady state the authors expressed this behaviour as:

$$D' \frac{\mathrm{d}^2 C}{\mathrm{d}x^2} + k(Cs - C) = 0 \qquad (8.37)$$

where D' is the effective diffusivity in the pellet, Cs is the 'solubility' of the solute, C is the solution concentration in the pores of the pellet, and k is the apparent first-order surface reaction rate constant. In the other region of concern, the diffusion layer, the flux of solute was expressed by the Noyes–Nernst equation[25]:

$$J = \frac{DA}{h}(C_o - C_h) \qquad (8.38)$$

where A is the area of the pellet, h is the diffusion layer thickness, and C_o and C_h the concentrations at the pellet solution interface and the bulk solution, respectively. The dissolution rate equations were obtained by applying equation (8.38) to all species and assuming that the apparent diffusivities for all species are equal. This gave the following expressions:

$$\frac{J_{T_P}}{A} = \frac{[T_P]_s - [T_P]_h}{k' + h/D} \qquad (8.39)$$

$$\frac{J_{T_{Ca}}}{A} = \frac{[T_{Ca}]_s - [T_{Ca}]_h}{k' + h/D} \qquad (8.40)$$

$$J_{T_{Ca}} = 1.67 J_{T_P} \qquad (8.41)$$

where $[T_P]$ is the total concentration of all phosphate species, $[T_{Ca}]$ is the total concentration of all calcium species, and k' is equal to $(kD')^{1/2}$. The use of a single k for the surface reaction rate constant implies that the interfacial transfer coefficient is equal in all species. It should be mentioned that diffusion of more than one ion may well involve coupled reactions at different rates.

In the dissolution experiments, compressed hydroxyapatite pellets were employed and nearly sink conditions were maintained. The results once again showed that at low agitation speeds the rates become almost linear with $\omega^{1/2}$, which is to be expected with diffusion-controlled dissolution. At higher speeds, however, the rates significantly deviate from linearity indicating a surface-controlled reaction. The authors refer to this as a 'substantial contribution of surface resistance to the dissolution reaction rate'. This deviation from linearity is described in the model by the k' term and gives fairly good agreement then between model and experiments.

The results are explained on the basis of a predominant dissolving site under sink conditions being the one possessing a solubility that is significantly less than the true thermodynamic one. When the two-site model is used the predicted dissolution rate only differs by 4–5 per cent under these sink conditions. The model developed for the rotating disc experiments is then able to establish the ionic activity product (K_{HAP}) that governs the dissolution reaction and the apparent surface dissolution reaction rate constant. The model appears to be applicable for sink conditions but may not describe the dissolution kinetics in partially saturated solutions.

In contrast to the above model, White and Nancollas[6] have described enamel dissolution based wholly on conventional thermodynamic methods. The rotating disc design was again employed to study the dissolution of bovine enamel. The experimental procedures were similar to those used previously[4] and discussed above. The rate of reaction was followed by the rate of acid uptake. A range of rotational speeds and partially saturated calcium and phosphate solutions were used with the same disc. The pH of the solutions were varied between 4.4 and 5.6 and the Ca : P ratio was varied from 3/5 to 5/3.

In order to quantify the ion transport process in solutions containing calcium, phosphate and hydrogen ions, one must consider the differences in ionic charge and diffusion coefficients, which may lead to charge as well as concentration gradients. The addition of an inert electrolyte minimises the development of charge gradients. Without the inert electrolyte, the application of Fick's first law is inappropriate. As described previously, the dependence of the steady-state dissolution rate on the stirring rate for laminar flow is $R_d = \omega^{1/2}\phi$. All experiments performed by White and Nancollas showed that laminar flow and diffusion-controlled kinetics occurred. Previous work[4] showing a considerable dependence on a surface reaction at higher spin speeds was not confirmed by the current investigation. Since an inert electrolyte was used to suppress charge gradients, Fick's law may be used to represent the measured rate of dissolution. This could be done provided the diffusion of each species is independent. However, the diffusion processes are coupled by both the solubility product and stoichiometry. Thus an empirical equation was used to relate the rate of diffusion of HAP in mol/s/cm^2 to solution concentration:

$$R_d = V\frac{d(\text{HAP})}{dt} = \frac{-SD_{\text{HAP}}}{10^3\delta_N}[(\text{HAP}_o) - (\text{HAP})]$$

(8.42)

In equation (8.42), V is the volume of the cell solution, in litres; S is the area of enamel exposed, in cm^2; D_{HAP} is the 'overall' diffusion coefficient of HAP in cm^2/s; δ_N is the thickness of the Nernst diffusion layer; (HAP) is the molar activity of aquated HAP in the bulk solution; and (HAP$_o$) is the value of the activity at the enamel surface corresponding to saturation. The activity of (HAP) is defined as follows:

$$(\text{HAP}) = \left(\frac{[\text{Ca}^{2+}]f_2}{5}\right)^{5/9}\left(\frac{[\text{PO}_4^{3-}]f_3}{3}\right)^{3/9}\left([\text{OH}^-]f_1\right)^{1/9}$$

(8.43)

where square brackets denote concentrations of the individual species, and f_Z the activity coefficient of an ion of charge Z.

This model showed satisfactory agreement with the experimental data, except for a small non-zero intercept. This was due to an error in the choice of K_{SP} for HAP, and the use of 5.9×10^{-59} was found to give satisfactory convergence of the data. The overall diffusion coefficient found for HAP was 1.4×10^{-5} cm^2/s and is similar to that used by Higuchi. However, when the ratio of the theoretically calculated rates to experimental rates are plotted as a function of the hydrogen ion concentration, it was found that there is a dependence of Rd on the hydrogen ion activity that is not explained by the simple model of equation (8.42). A straight line with positive slope and intercept gave a correlation coefficient of 0.9996 over the experimental range. This was explained as coupled diffusion of hydrogen ions inward and dissolution products outward. The term δ_N must be considered for each ion and may well be shortened in the case of PO$_4^{3-}$ and OH$^-$ by reactions within the diffusion layer. This model involving a decrease in the diffusion distance explained the observed dissolution rate, which is more rapid than diffusion control for a single species and less mobile than a hydrogen ion. The overall dissolution rate was then expressed as follows:

$$R_d = \frac{-SD_{\text{HAP}}}{10^3\delta_N}[(\text{HAP}_o) - (\text{HAP})][a(\text{H}^+) + b]$$

(8.44)

where the constants are $a = 6.469 \times 10^6$ and $b = 32.99$. At constant hydrogen ion concentration this equation reduces to a form similar to equation (8.42).

In summary, the rotating disc method was used to study enamel dissolution and led to a simple equation based on fundamental solution chemistry and diffusion theory. Conditions of pH, ionic concentration and ionic strength similar to those in regions of carious lesions were adequately explained by the model. For the first time, an enamel dissolution model considers the coupled diffusion of ions and forms the basis of a rigorous representation of the reaction. The solutions used represented partial saturation conditions from 0 to 30 per cent and the coupled diffusion model showed good agreement over all experimental ranges. This work has also shown that the dissolution of bovine enamel, like synthetic apatite, may be described by conventional thermodynamic methods.

8.6 Kinetics of Incipient Caries Formation

The enamel dissolution described so far concerns only surface dissolution, which bears little resemblance to the development of a carious lesion. In the natural lesion the enamel is dissolved from the sub-surface and this decalcified region is covered with a relatively sound surface layer. In the oral environment the sound outer layer would be covered by salivary pellicle and probably also by plaque. The production of incipient carious lesions in vitro has involved the use of inhibitors,[26] organic polymers,[27] gelatin gels[28] and non-agitation conditions in acidic buffers.[29] In 1963, Gray and Francis[10] reported an *in vitro* system for creating lesions which decalcify subsurface enamel and produce a white spot without incurring surface damage. The system consisted of an organic, non-ionic polymer (hydroxyethyl cellulose) and acidic buffers. The rate of enamel dissolution during formation of the lesions was measured as a function of pH, buffer concentration, calcium concentration and temperature. The rate was found to be directly proportional to the total acid concentration ($[H^+]$ and $[HB]$) and was not significantly affected by temperature. This system of lesion formation was used by Gray in 1966[30] to study the kinetics of incipient caries-like lesion formation. The enamel samples were placed in various acid buffers, pH and buffer concentration for a specified time period. Samples were changed for each measurement at a different time period. The dissolution rates became an average for various enamel samples. At the end of the demineralisation time period the solution calcium and phosphate concentrations were measured. The resulting infor-

mation was used to establish a semi-empirical equation of the dissolution kinetics.

It should be mentioned that in strictly empirical curve-fitting operations, mathematical equations which describe differently shaped curves are used. By adjusting the constants and adding more terms to the equation, the data could be made to correlate perfectly with some equation, but the equation would have little or no physical meaning. In the semi-empirical approach, variables are observed experimentally and are related in an expression using physical–chemical concepts. Deviations may be expected if not all the effects have been taken into account.

In the 1966 paper, Gray found that the dissolution rate was constant over the first 96 hours of caries-like lesion formation. He therefore used the data at 96 hours and a differential approach to establish the expression for lesion formation. The basic equation takes a similar form to the one used earlier for surface dissolution:

$$R = k_0[H^+]^{n_0} + k_1 K_A{}^{n_1}[H^+]^{n_2}[HB]^{n_3} \tag{8.45}$$

where R is the rate of enamel dissolution in mg/cm^2/96 h; k_0 and k_1 are rate constants; K_A is the dissociation constant of the acidic buffer, HB; $[H^+]$ is the concentration of hydrogen ions; and $[HB]$ is the concentration of undissociated buffer. In a static system, sufficient calcium may well build up at the reaction interface and therefore inhibit the dissolution process. This was accounted for by adding a third term to the equation, which gave the following expression:

$$R = k_0[H^+]^{n_0} + k_1 K_A{}^{n_1}[H^+]^{n_2}[HB]^{n_3} \\ + k_2[H^+]^{n_1}[Ca^{2+}]^{n_2} \tag{8.46}$$

since it was found experimentally that the calcium ion effect was pH dependent. To solve this expression several basic equilibria are involved:

$$K_A = \frac{[H^+][B^-]}{[HB]} \tag{8.47}$$

$$K_c = \frac{[Ca^{2+}][B^-]}{[CaB^+]} \tag{8.48}$$

The end result when the exponents are evaluated from the experimental data is:

$$R = k_0[\text{H}^+] + k_1 K_A^{1/4}[\text{H}^+]^{1/4}[\text{HB}] -$$

$$k_2 \frac{K_A[\text{HB}]^2}{[\text{H}^+]^{3/4}} \left(\frac{K_c}{[\text{B}^-] + K_c} \right)^{3/2} \quad (8.49)$$

This equation was used to evaluate the agreement between model and experimental results. The results indicated that the important variables affecting the rate were undissociated acid concentration, hydrogen ion concentration, acid dissociation constant and dissociation constant of the acid anion complex of the calcium ion. A relatively sound outer layer resulted from the presence of a protective agent. The amount of enamel dissolved was also found to increase almost linearly with time.

The caries-like lesion model may now be described in non-mathematical terms. The protective agent, HEC, adsorbs on the surface and acts as a protective coating against acid dissolution but otherwise is assumed to be inert. The undissociated acid buffer and hydrogen ions diffuse through the spaces between enamel crystals, particularly at prism junctions where they migrate to reaction sites in the enamel. After reaction (dissolution) the products must diffuse back along the channels to the bulk solution. At this time the buffer anion may complex with the calcium ion and slow down the diffusion into the bulk solution. This fact necessitates the third term in the equation.

It is interesting to compare the initial rate equations for surface and sub-surface dissolution. The previous model for surface dissolution when rearranged gave the following:

$$R_{\text{surface}} = k[\text{H}^+] + k_1 K_A^{1/4}[\text{H}^+]^{1/4}[\text{HB}]^{1/2} \quad (8.50)$$

while the current model for caries-like lesion formation gave the following if the third term is neglected:

$$R_{\text{sub-surface}} = k_0[\text{H}^+] + k_1 K_A^{1/4}[\text{H}^+]^{1/4}[\text{HB}] \quad (8.51)$$

The only difference between the two expressions

was the exponent for the undissociated acid. This result was not totally unexpected, since surface dissolution and sub-surface dissolution should be the same at the level of enamel crystalites. The difference would lie in the extra diffusion steps in the case of sub-surface dissolution and this seems to have been absorbed in the undissociated acid term.

This expression for sub-surface dissolution, however, does not depend on any physical model of the lesion nor is decalcification a function of exposure time. In 1968, Holly and Gray[31] extended the study of the formation of incipient carious lesions based on a physical model and diffusion concepts. Experimentally, the amount of enamel dissolved and depth of penetration of the lesion into enamel was measured as a function of exposure time to acid buffers with 6 per cent HEC added. It was found that both acid consumption and depth of lesion increased with exposure time. Normally, the consumption of reactant and penetration of the decalcification front would be expected to vary with the square root of time. The data, however, showed that the time dependence was almost linear. This was explained by the restriction on diffusion by the sound outer layer. Since diffusion through a relatively intact layer would be the slowest process, it would mask the normal time dependence that originated from increasing the distance between the place of reaction and the source of the reactant.

The model was treated as a mass transport process of acidic reactant through a double membrane, the relatively sound outer layer representing one membrane of constant thickness, d, and the sub-surface decalcified region representing another membrane which increases in thickness, x, with time.

The assumptions in constructing the model were as follows: (1) An intact layer, d, separates the reactant solution from the decalcified region and is constant in thickness. (2) The diffusion pathways within the intact layer are formed quickly and have a constant cross-sectional area, A_1. (3) The sub-surface layer has a thickness of x and cross-sectional area, A_2. (4) At a certain degree of decalcification in the second layer, the reaction stops (A_2 becomes maximum) and the reaction advances into the sound enamel. (5) Reaction occurs only at the boundary between the decalcified region and normal sound enamel, therefore the reacting interface continues to advance deeper into the enamel. (6) The rate of diffusion of HB is rate controlling. Since the reaction at the interface is fast compared to the diffusion of HB, no considerable accumulation of acid will occur at the interface (C_R) and the bulk solution concentration (C_B) will be large by comparison. This will be the case as long as the reaction is diffusion controlled.

The mathematical treatment of this model involves the use of Fick's first law:

$$dQ/dt = -DA(dc/dk) \qquad (8.52)$$

where Q is the amount of reactant that has diffused into enamel of unit surface area at time, t, D is the diffusion coefficient of the reactant in the solution phase of enamel, and A is a measure of the fractional cross-sectional area. By equating the diffusion rate of acid through the outer surface and through the sub-surface region, the following expression is obtained:

$$\frac{dQ}{dt} = \frac{DA_2(C_B - C_R)}{A_2 d/(A_1) + X} \cong \frac{DA_2 C_B}{A_2 d/(A_1) + X} \qquad (8.53)$$

when $C_B \gg C_R$ as mentioned above. X is then replaced in the equation using the assumptions above and the conservation of matter to obtain:

$$\frac{dQ}{dt} = \frac{DA_2 C_B}{A_2 d/(A_1) + Q/SA_2} \qquad (8.54)$$

Solving the differential equation with the initial conditions of $Q = 0$ when $t = 0$ yields the following:

$$Q = (\alpha^2 + 2\beta t)^{1/2} - \alpha \qquad (8.55)$$

where

$$\alpha = SA_2^2 d/A_1$$

$$\beta = 2SA_2^2 Dt_B$$

This equation was then used to evaluate the data on bovine and human enamel. The agreement

between the calculated and experimental results was reasonably good, with the largest deviation being for human enamel at longer reaction times. This deviation was explained by the slight apparent increase in the value A_2 which was assumed to be constant.

Although the model gave fairly good agreement with the experimental data, several comments should be made in regard to recent observations. Diffusion of more than one ion either to the reaction site or away from it cannot be treated separately since charge and mass coupling occur, as pointed out by Nancollas. Also, salivary pellicles which may be compared to the protective coating (HEC) have been shown to be perm-selective membranes[32] and would definitely affect the ionic diffusion of reactants and products. In the model system the protective coating may have only a passive role, but the salivary pellicle has an active part in the prevention of dental caries.[33]

During white spot formation a considerable build up of calcium and phosphate concentration may occur. Experiments without any added calcium and phosphate would describe only surface dissolution. In the rotating disc study by White and Nancollas, partially saturated solutions of up to 32.5 per cent were used without appreciable deviations from the coupled diffusion model. Studies with partially saturated solutions are believed to be important to the clinical situation of white spot formation. In contrast to the predictable behaviour observed with 32.5 per cent saturated solutions, Fawzi Higuchi and Hefferen[34] have recently published results of enamel dissolution with 50 per cent saturated solutions. These studies have shown an unusual dissolution behaviour and will be described here.

A rotating disc method was again used to study the dissolution of both tooth enamel and pellets of synthetic hydroxyapatite under conditions of relatively high partial saturation (for example 50 per cent saturated with respect to HAP). The dissolution of enamel was followed by withdrawing aliquots of fluid for calcium and phosphate analysis.

The results showed congruent dissolution (stoichiometric amounts of calcium and phosphate) and an unusual cyclic stepwise pattern of dissolution. This cyclic pattern was found with various calcium to phosphate ratios, with both lactic and acetate buffers and with experiments at 30° C and 37° C. The behaviour was also found to be independent of stirring rate and thus implied a surface-controlled reaction. According to the authors, calculations showed that no other phase could be precipitating and therefore affecting the overall rate of dissolution.

This unusual pattern of dissolution was explained by assuming a synchronisation among an assembly of crystals and a large variation in chemical potential at the sites of dissolution. This was related to substantial chemical potential differences among different planes in domains of the order of dimensions of the unit cell. Thus variations in the 'driving force' for dissolution may occur that would be dependent on the stage of dissolution of these domains.

Synchronisation was believed to occur when the ambient solution ion activity product can oscillate about a critical value. The oscillations resulted from bursts of dissolution from the crystals followed by diffusional relaxation of the ambient ions into the bulk solution. Thus, when ambient solution conditions are appropriate, the faster dissolving crystals slow up, while the slower dissolving crystals catch up, and the whole assembly of crystals becomes synchronised. When the ambient solution activity again drops below a critical value, sudden dissolution of all the synchronised crystals takes place. Thus, the ambient solution activity is raised and the process repeats itself.

This mechanism is more likely to occur during *in vivo* dental caries than the model described under sink conditions. The sub-surface demineralisation present in incipient carious lesions is consistent with the zonal dissolution of the proposed mechanism. Since this is the first reported case of this unusual dissolution behaviour, further studies are necessary to confirm the results.

Support for the synchronous dissolution model was provided in a companion paper[35] that evaluated the above model. The study used suspensions of HAP crystals in a dialysis bag which was placed in a partially saturated acetate buffer. The dissolution of the HAP crystals and diffusion of ions out of the bag was followed by analysing the amount of calcium and phosphate within the bulk solution and the dialysis bag. The values obtained from the solution inside the bag corresponded to the microenvironment surrounding the enamel crystals, while the ion concentrations outside the bag would correspond to those seen in the bulk solution.

The results showed a steady increase in ion concentration outside of the bag, but revealed the cyclic pattern of dissolution inside the bag. The oscillation of ion concentration inside the bag strongly supports the synchronised dissolution hypothesis. When the ion concentration difference between the inside and outside of the bag was large, a very rapid diffusion out of the bag occurred and the oscillations were not observed. It was also observed that when this concentration difference was very small, only initial transient decay was observed. Thus, under certain conditions the oscillatory pattern of dissolution was observed and supported the synchronised dissolution model for those conditions. This unusual behaviour has not been reported by other workers and may be the result of the experimental conditions employed. Further independent studies of the proposed model should be carried out in the future.

The kinetics of caries-like lesions have been described in terms of a semi-empirical model and a physical diffusion model. The unusual behaviour of enamel under conditions of relatively high partial saturation have also been described in terms of a synchronised dissolution model. All of the models proposed explain some aspect of enamel dissolution, but have been simplified to allow the mathematical formulations. It is certainly difficult to express the *in vivo* situation of plaque, pellicle, intact surface and sub-surface demineralisation in mathematical terms. The coupled diffusion, complexation and reprecipitation of ions further complicates the expressions used for enamel dissolution. Thus, several very good descriptions of enamel dissolution have been formulated for the experimental conditions used, but caries is a dynamic, multifactorial process which is still not totally understood and requires continued investigation.

References

1. Gray, J. A. (1962). Kinetics of the dissolution of human dental enamel in acid. *Journal of Dental Research*, **41**, 633–45
2. Higuchi, W. I., Gray, J. A., Hefferren, J. J. and Patel, P. R. (1965). Mechanisms of enamel dissolution in acid buffers. *Journal of Dental Research*, **44**, 330–41
3. Higuchi, W. I., Mir, N. A., Patel, P. R., Becker, J. W. and Hefferren, J. J. (1969). Quantitation of enamel demineralization mechanisms: III. A critical examination of the hydroxyapatite model. *Journal of Dental Research*, **48**, 396–409
4. Linge, H. G. and Nancollas, G. H. (1973). A rotating disk study of the dissolution of dental enamel. *Calcified Tissue Research*, **12**, 193–208
5. Fox, J. L., Higuchi, W. I., Fawzi, M., Hwu, R. C. and Hefferren, J. J. (1974). Two-site model for human dental enamel. *Journal of Dental Research*, **53**, 939
6. White, W. and Nancollas, G. H. (1977). Quantitative study of enamel dissolution under conditions of controlled hydrodynamics. *Journal of Dental Research*, **56**, 524–30
7. Hals, E., Morch, T. and Sand, H. F. (1955). Effect of lactate buffers on dental enamel in vitro as observed in polarizing microscopy. *Acta Odontologica Scandinavica*, **13**, 85–122
8. von Bartheld, F. (1958). Decalcification in initial dental caries. *Tijdschr. Tandheelk.*, **65**, 76–89
9. Laidler, K. J. (1950). Chemical kinetics, in *The Measurement of Reaction Rates* McGraw-Hill, New York, chap. I, p. 1
10. Gray, J. A. and Francis, M. D. (1963). Physical chemistry of enamel dissolution in *Mechanisms of Hard Tissue Destruction* (Ed. Sognnaes, F.) American Association for the Advancement of Science, pp. 213–60
11. Crank, J. (1957). *The Mathematics of Diffusion*, Clarendon Press, Oxford
12. Rootaire, H. M. Dietz, V. R. and Carpenter, F. G. (1962). Solubility product phenomena in hydroxyapatite water systems. *Journal of Colloid Science*, **17**: 179–206
13. Levich, V. G. (1962). *Physiochemical Hydrodynamics*, Prentice Hall, Englewood Cliffs, NJ
14. Mir, N. A., Higuchi, W. I. and Hefferren, J. J. (1969). The mechanism of action of solution fluoride upon the demineralization rate of human enamel. *Archives of Oral Biology*, **14**, 901–20
15. Brudevold, F., Savory, A., Gardner, D. E., Spinelli, M. and Spiers, R. (1963). A study of acidulated fluoride solutions. *Archives of Oral Biology*, **8**, 179–82
16. Newbrun, E. (Ed.) (1975). *Fluorides and Dental Caries*, Charles C. Thomas, Springfield, Illinois
17. Brown, W. E. (1970). Physiochemical aspects of decay and decalcification. *Dental Tissues and Materials*. Proc. int. Symp. on Calcified Tissues, Dental and Surgical Materials and Tissue Material Interactions, pp. 69–84
18. Nancollas, G. H. (1974). Physiochemistry of demineralization and remineralization. *Journal of Dental Research*, **53**, 297–302
19. Jones, A. L., Linge, H. G. and Wilson, I. R. (1972). The dissolution of silver chromate into aqueous solutions. I. Analysis of mass transport of the lattice ions from the crystal surface during the reaction. *Journal of Crystal Growth*, **12**, 201–8
20. Riddiford, A. E. (1966). The rotating disk system. *Advances in Electro-chemical Engineering*, **4**, 47–116
21. Linge, H. G. (1970). The dissolution of silver chromate. *Ph.D. Thesis*, Melbourne Monask Univ.

22. Bishop, D. W., Eick, J. D., Nancollas, G. H. and White, W. D. (1974). Dissolution kinetics of rotating discs of sound and white spot enamel. *Journal of Dental Research*, **53**, 575 (abstract)

23. Young, F., Fawzi, M., Dedhiya, M. G., Wu, M. S. and Higuchi, W. I. (1974). Dual mechanisms for dental enamel dissolution in acid buffers. *Journal of Dental Research*, **53**, 576 (abstract)

24. Wu, M., Higuchi, W. I., Fox, J. L. and Friedman, M. (1976). Kinetics and mechanisms of hydroxyapatite crystal dissolution in a weak acid buffers using the rotating disk method. *Journal of Dental Research*, **55**, 496–505

25. Higuchi, W. I. (1967). Diffusion model useful in biopharmaceutics. *Journal of Pharmaceutical Science*, **56**, 315–24

26. White, W. D. and Nancollas, G. H. (1975). The kinetics of enamel dissolution and white spot formation. *Journal of Dental Research*, **54**, 448 (abstract)

27. Gray, J. A., Francis, M. D. and Griebstein, W. J. (1962). Chemistry of enamel dissolution, in *Chemistry and Prevention of Dental Caries* (Ed. Sognnaes, R. F.), Charles C. Thomas, Springfield, Illinois, chap. 5, pp. 164–79

28. Silverstone, L. M. (1966). The primary translucent zone of enamel caries and of artificial caries-like lesions. *Caries Research*, **1**, 261–74

29. Sperber, G. H. and Buonocore, M. G. (1963). Effect of different acids on character of demineralization of enamel surfaces. *Journal of Dental Research*, **42**, 707–23

30. Gray, J. A. (1966). Kinetics of enamel dissolution during formation of incipient caries-like lesions. *Archives of Oral Biology*, **11**, 397–421

31. Holly, F. J. and Gray, J. A. (1968). Mechanism for incipient carious lesion growth utilizing a physical model based on diffusion concepts. *Archives of Oral Biology*, **13**, 319–34

32. Zahradnik, R. T., Moreno, E. C. and Burke, E. J. (1976). Effect of salivary pellicle on enamel subsurface demineralization *in vitro*. *Journal of Dental Research*, **55**, 664–70

33. Moreno, E. C. and Zahradnek, R. T. (1974). Chemistry of enamel subsurface demineralization in vitro. *Journal of Dental Research*, **53**, 226–35

34. Fawzi, M. B., Higuchi, W. I. and Hefferren, J. J. (1977). Unusual dissolution behavior of tooth enamel and synthetic HAP crystals under high partial saturation conditions. *Journal of Dental Research*, **56**, 518–23

35. Fawzi, M. B., Sonobe, T., Higuchi, W. I. and Hefferren, J. J. (1977). Synchronized crystal dissolution behavior for tooth enamel and synthetic (NBS) hydroxyapatite. *Journal of Dental Research*, **56**, 394–406

Part II
The Scientific Basis of Caries Prevention

Part II

Chapter 9

Possibilities for Caries Control by Modification of the Diet

The total food and drink intake of an individual, including non-nutrient components, is termed the *diet*. The constituents of the diet come into contact with the external surfaces of the teeth, with the gingivae and with dental plaque. A dietary effect in dental disease is defined as a local effect of substances eaten. There may be a direct effect upon the tissues by a component of the diet, or the effect may be indirect—for example, due to production of acid by interaction of dietary carbohydrate with plaque—but in either case the effect is produced from within the mouth. *Nutrition*, on the other hand, concerns the effects of digested and assimilated foods upon the host, and nutritional effects are, therefore, systemic rather than local. A nutritional effect upon the dental tissues is, therefore, an effect upon development, regeneration or repair. It is the local interactions in the mouth due to diet which will be considered in this chapter.

9.1 Evidence for the Influence of Diet on Dental Caries

The lines of evidence indicating an effect of diet, and particularly of dietary carbohydrates, upon dental caries are many, and have been referred to elsewhere in this volume, notably sections 1.4.3 and 2.2.6. It is appropriate to summarise them here before drawing conclusions as to the possibilities for control.

9.1.1 Epidemiological evidence from human populations

A marked increase in caries seems the inescapable result of the adoption of a modern 'Western' diet. A well-defined case is that of the inhabitants of Tristan da Cuhna, an isolated group who lived for many years as subsistence farmers and fishermen. Their dental state was excellent in 1932 and 1937 when their diet comprised potatoes and other vegetables, meat and fish. The sale of imported manufactured foods and the evacuation of the population to Britain was associated with an increase in caries (figure 9.1) which has continued since their return to the island[1]. Fisher states 'Tristan is probably the best example of dental deterioration associated with the consumption of sophisticated foods enjoyed

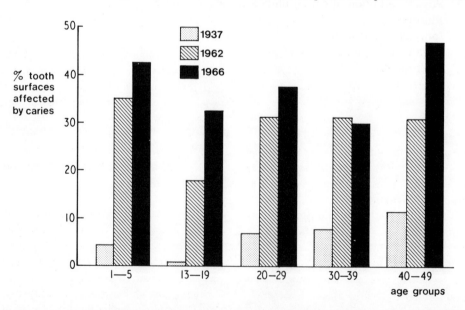

Figure 9.1 The prevalence of dental caries expressed as percentage of decayed, missing and filled teeth in various age-groups of the population of Tristan da Cunha in 1937, 1962 and 1966

by populations with an improved standard of living'.

The severe dietary restrictions in many countries during World War II were accompanied by a decrease in dental caries. The teeth that had already erupted showed the same reduced caries score as the developing teeth and the improvement was therefore due to a local dietary effect rather than a nutritional one. In studies of these phenomena, the dietary components which correlate well with caries score are sucrose and its products. In the UK the consumption of sucrose rose from 9.1 kg per capita per annum in 1835 to 54 kg in 1961. In a survey of children in Dundee in 1964, 49.6 g of sweets and candy alone were eaten per child per week, and the 13-year-olds had 10 decayed teeth per child. Although it has been possible to remark upon the coincidence of high sucrose consumption and marked caries, it has been difficult to demonstrate a relationship between degree of caries and extent of sucrose consumption within present-day urban populations. One reason for this may be that it is impossible to identify groups of individuals with a truly low-sucrose intake. The sucrose consumption of all individuals in a natural urban population may be so high that it may not be easy to show marked differences in caries experience as a function of sucrose intake.

9.1.2 Evidence from the regulation of diet in supervised human groups

The effect of sucrose upon caries was tested on a group of 436 patients of a mental hospital at Vipeholm, Sweden[2], and the frequency of consumption, together with the form in which the sucrose was administered, were found to be of paramount importance. The control group (which received the basal low-carbohydrate diet with 150 g margarine) showed little increase in caries throughout the study (figure 9.2). In the other groups (which received carbohydrate supplements in various forms in place of the margarine) there was a dramatic increase in caries when the supplements were allowed between meals. A significant group is the sucrose group in

which the supplement was 300 g sucrose per day dissolved in drinks given only at mealtimes. This group was very little different to the control group in rate of caries increase. No attempt was made in this study to test the effect of eating starchy foods between meals. The relative dental safety of taking sucrose in forms easily cleared from the mouth[3] and when consumed at mealtimes was confirmed by experiments in which large sucrose supplements were administered to children in residential homes in Britain over a 1–2-year period[4].

A population of 80 children were brought up from birth at Hopewood House, Bowral, New South Wales, according to the dietary theories of the founder. Their diet was vegetarian but did include dairy products. Refined carbohydrates were excluded, but wholemeal bread, oats, potatoes, rice, treacle and molasses were permitted. The fluoride content in the water was low (0.1 p.p.m.) and the standard of oral hygiene was poor as they had periodontal disease. However, children of 5–13 years had only 10 per cent of the caries found in the general population[5]. After leaving the home the children suffered an increase from 2 DMFT at 13 years to 11–14 DMFT at the age of 18. The teeth were, therefore, not inherently resistant to caries due to some nutritional effect during their development, and the low caries experience was therefore attributed to the absence of refined carbohydrates in the diet while the children were in the institution.

9.1.3 Evidence of the low caries incidence in hereditary fructose intolerance

The saturation of liver hexokinase by glucose, and the specificity of glucokinase for glucose, require a specific mechanism for metabolising fructose. Normally, fructose is phosphorylated by liver fructokinase to fructose-1-phosphate, which is not an intermediate of glycolysis. Liver aldolase, which splits fructose-1,6-diphosphate, also metabolises fructose-1-phosphate to glyceraldehyde and dihydroxyacetone phosphate.

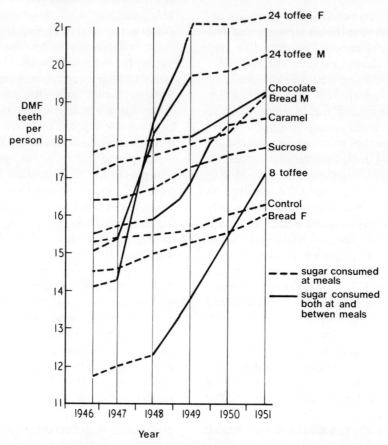

Dental caries frequency 1946-1951

Figure 9.2   **Dental caries expressed as number of decayed, missing and filled teeth per person in participants in the Vipeholm study[2]. The steepness of the curve is always less if consumption of the sugar is restricted to mealtimes. The form of administration of sucrose is also significant**

Glyceraldehyde can be phosphorylated by tri-okinase to glyceraldehyde-3-phosphate, so that fructose normally gives the same triose phosphates as glucose but by a different metabolic route.

A rare genetic defect (an inborn error of metabolism) called hereditary fructose intolerance (HFI) is due to the inability of liver aldolase to split fructose-1-phosphate, although fructose-1:6-diphosphate produced from glucose is metabolised normally. Individuals with this defect cannot tolerate fructose or sucrose. The major source of fructose in the human diet is sucrose or sucrose products. Ingestion of fructose causes

sweating, nausea and vomiting, tremors and convulsions, and may lead to coma and death. If early childhood is survived, those affected learn to avoid all foods containing sucrose and fructose, but they do consume other fermentable carbohydrates such as lactose (in milk) and starch (in bread, rice and potatoes).

The symptoms of HFI are those of hypoglycaemia and resemble those of diabetes mellitus. Fructose ingestion results in abnormally high fructose-1-phosphate concentrations in the liver and depletion of tissue ATP and plasma inorganic phosphate. The low blood glucose concentration that causes the symptoms of HFI may be caused by inadequacy of ATP for the cyclic AMP production necessary to stimulate glycogen phosphorylase, the enzyme responsible for producing glucose-1-phosphate from liver glycogen. However, the hypoglycaemia is probably explained by the inhibitory effect of high fructose-1-phosphate concentrations on liver phosphorylase, and on the deficiency of the inorganic phosphate necessary for this enzyme to function[6].

Individuals affected by HFI have remarkably little caries[7] and are often caries-free (for example, 8 out of 19 patients[8] compared with 1 in 4000 in the general population). Siblings without this autosomal recessive defect who were brought up with HFI patients had a degree of dental caries comparable to that of the general population. The low degree of caries found in individuals with HFI is restricted to occlusal fissures and is not found on the smooth surfaces of the teeth.

9.1.4 Evidence that sucrose assists implantation and maintenance in the mouth of cariogenic bacteria

The formation of a voluminous extracellular polysaccharide from sucrose is a consistent feature of cariogenic streptococci (sections 3 and 5.6.1). In numerous studies it has been shown that attempts to introduce these bacteria into the mouths of hamsters, rats, monkeys and man was more successful when sucrose was used than when other carbohydrates were included in the diet. The frequent chewing of sugar has also been shown to assist the retention of easily identifiable caries-inducing streptococci in human mouths. Restriction of dietary sucrose reduces an already established population of *Streptococcus mutans* in man and monkey, but in other studies *S.mutans* was shown to be persistent in monkeys in the absence of dietary carbohydrate. The relative success in implanting *S. mutans* in the mouths of rats has been shown to depend on the carbohydrate in the diet[9]. In one experiment, both the proportion of *S.mutans* and the incidence of caries were greatest with sucrose, less with glucose and least with starch, but in another

experiment sucrose and starch were equally effective at promoting implantation, although little caries occurred on the starch diet[9].

Sucrose has also been shown to be essential for the establishment of *S.mutans* in the dental plaque of man[10]. Furthermore, dental plaque formed in the absence of sucrose is not cariogenic. Thus, mentally retarded children who were fed routinely by stomach tube had very little dental caries. Plaque from these children showed very little fall in pH when exposed to sucrose, and hence contained few lactic acid bacteria[11].

9.2 The Relative Cariogenicity of Carbohydrates

Many studies of the effect of diet on caries have been carried out in rats and other rodents. For example, in the experiments of Stephan[12] the basal diet of skimmed milk powder and dried liver was non-cariogenic (table 9.1). In the scoring system used, a value of 10 or more for a foodstuff supplement is considered significantly cariogenic. It is notable that fruits such as apples, which contain over 10 per cent of fermentable carbohydrates and are moderately cariogenic when fed *ad libitum* to rats (table 9.1), are considered not to be cariogenic in man.

Most research of this type has concerned the relative potency of different carbohydrates, and foodstuffs containing them, as causes of caries. When carbohydrate of different types was incorporated into a skimmed milk–liver powder diet at a level of 66 per cent, sucrose (mean caries score 23 after 8 weeks) was much more cariogenic than either glucose or raw wheat starch (mean caries scores 7–8 and 2–3, respectively)[13]. Fructose had a similar cariogenicity score to glucose, and as these two sugars are the components of the sucrose molecule, it is evident that sucrose is much more cariogenic than its constituents[14]. In the many different studies of relative cariogenicity, sucrose has almost invariably been found to be the most cariogenic. Presumably part of the special effect of sucrose is due to its ability to be converted into bacterial

Table 9.1   Effects of human foods fed *ad libitum* to rats on a basal diet—rats were fed 581 s diet for two one-hour periods per day, test food available continuously (From Stephan[12])

Additional food	Mean caries score
Nil—control group	0
Corn chips, peanuts, popcorn	0
Lettuce, cabbage	0
Orange*, lemon*	0
Potato chips (crisps)	1.6
Carrots	2.1
Graham crackers (cracker biscuits)	8.7
White bread and raspberry jam	10.2
Apples*	19.4
Bananas	21.0
Grapes*	24.1
Candy mints	24.7
Cola*	29.6
Raisins	30.9
10 % sucrose solution	32.2
Dates	32.7
Milk chocolate	34.1
Sucrose	62.1

* Dental erosion caused.

extracellular polysaccharides (for example, dextran), which form part of the matrix of dental plaque (section 5.6.1). Raw wheat starch caused very little caries, and the same was true if the starch was cooked to swell the grains, and the product then dried, and powdered to resemble raw starch in physical texture prior to incorporation in the diet[15].

When starch solutions are applied to plaque no Stephan curve is observed. This may be for two reasons: starch, being a polysaccharide, diffuses slowly into plaque compared to mono- or disaccharides, and secondly, it is a polymer that must be hydrolysed by extracellular amylase before it can be assimilated and metabolised by plaque bacteria. The degree of refinement of bread seems to have little bearing upon its cariogenicity. White bread contains less than 2 per cent sucrose and about 60 per cent starch, and caused little caries in a susceptible strain of rats, as did brown bread. There is no evidence

from these experiments that substituting wholemeal for white bread would have any beneficial effect upon human caries rate[16]. Sweet biscuits (cookies) have a high sucrose content, but it is interesting to note that cooked biscuits, powdered and added to the rat diet, were much more cariogenic than the same biscuit mixture added to the diet in the same amount, but uncooked[17]. It was suggested that the cooking process produced a consistency which favoured retention in the fissures of molars. This idea is supported by the finding that very few of the carious lesions formed on the biscuit diet were on the smooth surfaces of the teeth.

It should be noted that all foods containing the lower-molecular-weight forms of the common saccharides are more cariogenic than those comprising the corresponding polymers. The corn syrup or liquid glucose (table 9.2) used extensively in British bakery products has a high content of glucose and maltose. Lately, the development of industrial enzymology has allowed corn syrup to be converted into a sweeter product by isomerisation of glucose to fructose, and this product has found extensive application in prepared foods in North America.

The syrups remaining after the crystallisation of sucrose, molasses (70 per cent sucrose), treacle (more sucrose and less impurities than molasses) and golden syrup (partly inverted syrup containing sucrose, glucose and fructose) are all highly cariogenic, as is honey (largely sucrose with some fructose and glucose). There is no convincing evidence that the less pure forms of these sugars serve any less well as substrates for oral bacteria, or that the dirt and impurities they contain in any way reduce the impact of the acids produced from them.

9.3   Possible Modifications of the Human Diet to Reduce Dental Caries

Since it is quite clear that sucrose and its products are key factors in the aetiology of caries, means of modifying its potentially damaging effects

Table 9.2 The relative sweetness and cost of carbohydrates and other sweeteners

Sweetener	Relative sweetness (sucrose = 10)		Cost in £ per kg[a]	Cost per unit of sweetness
	a	b		
Lactose	2.7	1.6	1.87	6.9
Sorbitol (glucitol)	4.8	5.4	1.75	3.6
Glycerol	4.8	10.8	2.60	5.4
Glucose	5–6	7.4	0.66	1.1–1.2
Maltose	6	—	9.24	15.4
Sucrose	10	10	0.83	0.83
Xylitol	— 10[c]	—	13.00[f]	13.0[g]
Invert sugar	8–9	13	—	—
Fructose	10–15	17.3	3.75	2.5–3.75
Sodium cyclamate	300–800	300–800		
Aspartame	—	1000–2000		
Saccharin	2000–7000	2000–7000		

a. Data from *The Carbohydrates Chemistry–Biochemistry*, vol. 1A (Eds Pigman, W. and Horton, D.), Academic Press, London and New York, 1972.
b. Data from Newbrun[18] (the relative sweetness of substances depends on physical factors in the solution used and on the taster, hence the differences between data and the ranges cited for some compounds).
c. the relative sweetness of xylitol was not quoted in either *a* or *b*, but it has been claimed to be equal to that of sucrose in 10 per cent solution.
d. Costs of 1 kg of grades suitable for bacteriological tests, or for consumption, from one supplier. Commercial quantities would undoubtedly be much cheaper, and the shop price of sucrose is half that in this table.
e. Cost with reference to relative sweetness in column *a*.
f. £25 per kg in Finland (1970). Pilot plant production (2000–5000) tons/year for the Turku study reduced the cost to £3 per kg (1975). Further cost reduction may be expected on full-scale production (Scheinin, personal communication).
g. 3.0 on the basis of the 1975 Finnish price.

have been considered extensively. There seem to be three approaches that recommend themselves:

(1)   The limitation of consumption of sucrose items, preferably in a non-sticky form, to mealtimes. This is a matter of education of the public, either en masse or by individual dentists advising their own patients.
(2)   The replacement of sucrose by other sweetening agents in foods and beverages. This is more difficult and involves economic and in-

dustrial considerations, palatability and consistency, as well as health and safety factors. Although sucrose is not an essential component of the diet, and could certainly be replaced by other carbohydrates without harm, it seems unlikely that many individuals will voluntarily reduce their consumption of sucrose (in all forms) to a degree that will reduce caries significantly. Caution should be used in giving nutritional advice. In Western countries, about 50 per cent of calories are provided by carbohydrates, and this is both nutritionally satisfactory, and also inexpensive! What is desirable for dental health is not the substitution of costly protein, or fat, for carbohydrate, but the replacement of more cariogenic carbohydrates by less cariogenic carbohydrates. In view of this the use of 'non-caloric'[18] sweeteners (for example saccharin) can only be of limited value unless in conjunction with carbohydrates that are not cariogenic.

(3)   The third possibility for dietary modification is that certain additives which are known to have an inhibitory effect on the initiation and development of caries, might be included in the diet, either by adding them to a wide range of foods, or by educating the public to choose specific items that contain them.

9.3.1   The limitation of sucrose consumption to mealtimes

The evidence that sucrose consumption at frequent intervals is associated with high caries is overwhelming. Caries could be reduced in the population solely by restricting the eating of sweet snacks between meals (figure 9.3 and section 5.3.1).

9.3.2   Possible replacement of sucrose by other sweeteners in foods

The majority of people enjoy sweet foods, and sucrose has come to represent one-third of the total carbohydrate intake (or one-sixth of the total calorie consumption) in Western nations. The reasons for this high consumption of sucrose are several. It is the traditional sweetener, and is an important ingredient in many well-loved recipes, to which it frequently imparts a desirable

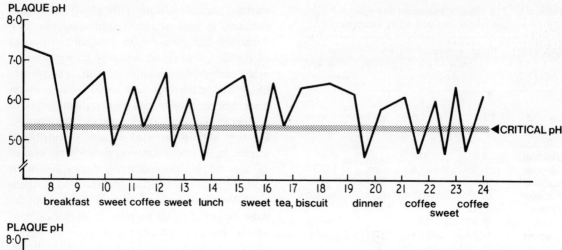

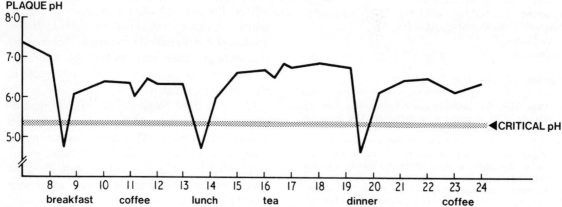

Figure 9.3   The plaque pH of individuals taking frequent snacks, above, and main meals only, below (After Jenkins[60]).

consistency. Sucrose is sweeter than any simple carbohydrate except invert sugar (a mixture of glucose and fructose obtained by hydrolysing sucrose) or its component, fructose (table 9.2), and is cheaper per 'unit of sweetness' than any other carbohydrate, although this may well be solely because of the scale on which sucrose is produced. However, it is worth remembering that huge industries are founded on the growth of sugar beet and cane, and on the purification of sucrose, so that attempts to replace sucrose on a large scale might be successfully opposed by these interests (as in the case of cyclamate[18], and the establishment of a fructose syrup industry in Europe).

It is unlikely that an item of food containing a sucrose substitute will gain acceptance if it is worse in flavour, or texture, than the sucrose

equivalent, or if it is more expensive. The situation with caries is not like that of diabetes mellitus. Diabetics who wish to eat sweets or chocolate are obliged by their disability to buy items prepared especially for them that are more expensive, and less palatable, than those available to non-diabetics. No such restriction of choice applies to the rest of the population. There is also a lack of urgency in tackling the problem. Many people are not willing to change their dietary habits in order to avoid dental caries that may occur in the months or years ahead.

In spite of these problems, trials of sucrose substitutes have been caried out, largely in Scandinavia and Switzerland. Sorbitol (glucitol) is the sweetener used in many diabetic preparations. It is prepared by catalytic hydrogenation of glucose:

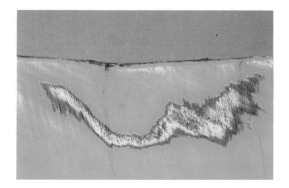 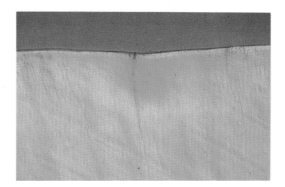

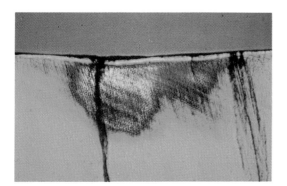 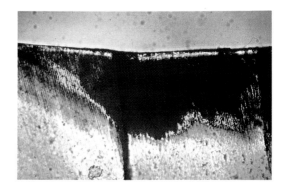

Plate 6.1 (Top left) Longitudinal ground section through an artificial caries-like lesion created in an acidified gel after 20 weeks exposure. The section is examined in quinoline with the polarizing microscope and shows a well marked, positively birefringent, dark zone at the advancing front of the lesion (X100). (Top right) Same section but now examined in Thoulet's medium, refractive index 1·62, with the polarizing microscope. The dark zone can no longer be seen since the aqueous medium has penetrated the micropore system of the zone. The lesion appears as a region of reduced negative birefringence relative to sound enamel (X100). (Bottom left) Same section seen with polarised light after imbibition with water. The body of the lesion shows as a region of positive birefringence, sharply demarcated from the surface zone which shows a high degree of negative birefringence, since it is relatively unaffected by the attack. It requires a region having a pore volume of 5 per cent to change from negative to positive birefringence, under these conditions. (Bottom right) Same section now examined dry in air with the polarising microscope. The body of the lesion appears almost black due to the excessive positive form birefringence produced within this porous region. However, the surface zone still exhibits a negative birefringence in part, showing that the pore volume in this zone is approximately 1 per cent.

D-glucose → (2H) → D-sorbitol) (D-glucitol)

Sorbitol may be oxidised to glucose and fructose in the liver of man and animals by polyol dehydrogenases that are rather non-specific, but which have sometimes been called specially sorbitol dehydrogenases:

Thus, sorbitol does not require insulin to enter cells, but produces glucose and fructose within them. The normal energy yield of hexose metabolism is available from sorbitol, together with an additional amount from the oxidation of $NADH_2$. Although it is only about half as sweet

D-sorbitol

D-fructose

D-glucose

as sucrose, and less sweet than glucose, sorbitol has apparent advantages as a 'dentally safe' sweetener. A mouth rinse with a 50 per cent solution of sorbitol produced little or no drop in pH, and neither did candies made with sorbitol[19]. This is in spite of the fact that there are bacteria in plaque (*Streptococcus mutans*) that can ferment sorbitol, and that in a pure closed culture these bacteria may produce sufficient acid to cause a decalcifying pH. It seems likely that sorbitol is fermented so slowly by whole plaque that the acid produced may diffuse away and be neutralised by salivary buffers, without generating a pH low enough to cause decalcification. This is not the case with a closed culture of fixed volume. Sweets which do not cause the plaque pH to fall below 5.7 may be described as 'safe for teeth' in Switzerland, and this designation is permitted for sorbitol candies. There are, however, problems with sorbitol. It is absorbed more slowly than glucose, and as absorption is not by active transport it is incomplete. This causes diarrhoea in some individuals, presumably by the osmotic effect of unabsorbed sorbitol retaining water in the intestine. Indeed, sorbitol has been used as a laxative. It has been suggested that the daily intake of sorbitol should be restricted to 150 mg/kg body weight (FAO–WHO Commission Report on Food Additives) which is equivalent to about two heaped teaspoonsful per day for an adult.

A product called 'Lycasin' has been produced by the partial hydrolysis of starch to glucose, maltose and larger saccharides of glucose, and then catalytical hydrogenation to sorbitol, maltitol and a mixture of reduced saccharides. Such preparations have 4.9–9.4 per cent free sorbitol and 14.5–23.8 per cent total sorbitol[20]. Lycasin caused less caries than sucrose in animals, and less plaque was formed during its use in animals, and in man. The sorbitol and maltitol (derived from maltose by reduction) largely appeared in the faeces unchanged, but the glucose components of Lycasin were absorbed and metabolised in man. Candy made with Lycasin has been tested on 3–6-year-old children[20], but there were problems in this study due to the consumption of sucrose-lemonade and sucrose-candies by the children who were supposed to be eating only Lycasin products. Many children did not like the Lycasin candy, and occasionally flatulence was reported. Nevertheless, the authors claim up to 25 per cent reduction in caries in the Lycasin group, although it is not known to what extent this may be due to a general reduction of candy consumption.

Human dental plaque forms acid from Lycasin faster than from sorbitol and maltitol but slower than from soluble starch. This indicates that amylase hydrolysis releasing maltose from the higher saccharides of Lycasin is responsible for this acid production[21]. The amylase involved was the human salivary enzyme entrained in the plaque.

Xylitol has a similar degree of sweetness to sucrose (table 9.2) and occurs naturally in a number of foods, particularly bananas and mushrooms. It may be made from xylose by exactly the same process of reduction used to make sorbitol from glucose, and Lycasin from partly hydrolysed starch:

D-xylose   D-xylitol

$$
\begin{array}{ccc}
\underset{\text{D-xylitol}}{\begin{array}{c} CH_2OH \\ | \\ H\!-\!C\!-\!OH \\ | \\ HO\!-\!C\!-\!H \\ | \\ H\!-\!C\!-\!OH \\ | \\ CH_2OH \end{array}}
& \xrightarrow[\;\; NADH_2\;\;]{NAD}
\underset{\text{D-xylulose}}{\begin{array}{c} CH_2OH \\ | \\ C\!=\!O \\ | \\ HO\!-\!C\!-\!H \\ | \\ H\!-\!C\!-\!OH \\ | \\ CH_2OH \end{array}}
& \xrightarrow[\;\; ADP\;\;]{ATP}
\underset{\text{D-xylulose-5-phosphate}}{\begin{array}{c} CH_2OH \\ | \\ C\!=\!O \\ | \\ HO\!-\!C\!-\!H \\ | \\ H\!-\!C\!-\!OH \\ | \\ CH_2OPO_3H_2 \end{array}}
\end{array}
$$

glycogen ←

→ hexose phosphates ← pentose phosphates ← D-xylulose-5-phosphate

glycolysis and tricarboxylic acid cycle

nucleotides

Xylitol is a normal metabolic intermediate in man[22], and one route by which it may be metabolised is by dehydrogenation (by the same enzyme that oxidises sorbitol) to xylulose, which is then phosphorylated and enters the pentose phosphate pathway:
Xylitol may thus be metabolised to produce energy and carbon dioxide or produce glycogen stores in muscle and liver, or to synthesise nucleotides.

Xylitol has been proposed as a dietary additive for diabetics by the WHO/FAO Joint Foods Program (1969), and is classified as a sugar-replacing substance. Its use has recently been investigated in a wide range of foods by a Finnish group. The only factor that appears to limit the dosage of xylitol is the phenomenon of osmotic diarrhoea, or soft faeces. As with sorbitol, individual susceptibility to this inconvenience varies, and tolerance of xylitol is markedly increased by frequent dosage. The percentage of xylitol absorbed in man depends on the dose (90 per cent of 5 g oral dose to 60 per cent of a 30 g test dose)[23].

During a 4.5-year study of xylitol consumption, osmotic diarrhoea only developed under abnormal conditions such as a 30–50 g dose of xylitol in the morning on an empty stomach[24].

The effect of xylitol upon plaque pH is similar to that of sorbitol. Thus, when xylitol solutions are applied to dental plaque little or no fall in pH occurs[25]. Whereas it is known that sorbitol and mannitol are metabolised by plaque bacteria, xylitol appears not to be converted to acids by plaque. Xylitol has been shown to be less cariogenic than sucrose or sorbitol in rats[26], and less cariogenic than sucrose or fructose in man[27]. The low cariogenicity is associated with a marked reduction in the quantity of dental plaque in individuals consuming a xylitol diet[28]. Some studies have shown that xylitol may inhibit certain streptococci, although this is not a universal finding. Prolonged exposure of plaque bacteria to xylitol seems to result in an adaptation, but this may well be an acquired tolerance to xylitol rather than an acquired ability to metabolise it[29].

Microorganisms that can metabolise xylitol do occur, but apparently not in plaque. From the beginning of the Finnish study it was realised that xylitol-metabolising mutants might arise in plaque. However, a selective pressure to establish such hypothetical variants might not be present, due to the regular availability of small quantities of other sugars such as glucose. Dental plaque from subjects who had consumed xylitol-sweetened foods constantly for 4.5 years produced little or no pH fall with xylitol, although acid was formed from both glucose and sorbitol.

The use of carbohydrate sucrose-substitutes as effective means of controlling caries depends heavily on the palatability of the products. In this respect the xylitol foods have proved acceptable during the Finnish study. In particular, the xylitol chewing gum, chocolate, wafers and ice-cream were considered by many people to be superior to the corresponding glucose products. Xylitol dissolves more rapidly than sucrose, and causes a slight drop in temperature in the mouth as it does so. Most people seem to find this 'cool

taste' agreeable (Scheinin, personal communication).

Another factor that is essential to the substitution of other sweeteners for sucrose is the active cooperation of the food industry. The extent to which this has been achieved in Finland is illustrated in figure 9.4[27], which shows some of the wide range of foodstuffs prepared with xylitol in place of sucrose. Any side-effects of possible sucrose substitutes also affects the likelihood of their widespread adoption. During long-term trials Scheinin found a notable absence of diarrhoea and other side-effects[30], the solid products were tolerated well by volunteers, but the intake of large amounts of xylitol-containing soft drinks resulted in osmotic diarrhoea of short duration in a minority of cases[27]. Only one of 52 participants in the xylitol group withdrew from

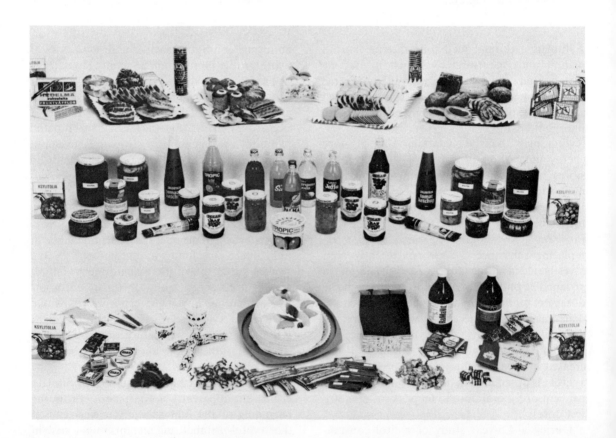

Figure 9.4   Range of foodstuffs prepared with xylitol instead of sucrose (from Scheinin *et al.*[27])

the study, and this was because of diarrhoea. Xylitol therefore seems to satisfy the requirements for a sucrose substitute.

The possibilities for the utilisation of non-carbohydrate sweeteners have been reviewed by Newburn[18]. There appears to be a wide range of such compounds available, but their flavour properties often differ perceptibly from sucrose. However, it is also possible that the use of non-sucrose sweetners may be limited by government regulations, as has already happened with cyclamates.

9.3.3 Possible addition of caries-inhibiting agents to foods

Fluoride

A wide range of naturally occurring dietary components inhibit, or have been claimed to inhibit, dental caries. Fluoride is so important among them that a whole chapter is devoted to it in this book (chapter 10). This section refers solely to food as a vehicle for fluoride. As is more fully discussed in section 10.2, fluoride is widely distributed in many dietary components (table 9.3) and is particularly abundant in calcified tissues and in tea[31]. Seafoods, of which the calcified components may be eaten, may contribute significant quantities of fluoride to our diet.

Table 9.3   Fluoride in dietary components (from Hodge and Smith[31])

	Fluoride (p.p.m.)
Meats	0.14–2
Most fish flesh	approx. 1
Sardines (whole)	8–40
Shrimp (Japan)	50
Shrimp meal (USA)	0.2–0.4
Cereals and products	0.18–2.8
Vegetables	0.02–0.9
Fruits	0.03–0.84
Tea infusion	0.1–2.0
Wine	0–6.3
Milk	0.04–0.55

The normal dietary intake of fluoride is 0.5–1.5 mg/day worldwide.

The use of food items as a vehicle for added fluoride has received some consideration in view of the opposition to water fluoridation. There is no doubt that water is the best carrier for fluoride, but unfortunately some people feel that an element of personal choice is removed if fluoride is added to tap water. The addition of fluoride to foods presents a problem in that individual consumption of many food items varies considerably. Fluoridated salt (90 mgF/kg NaCl) has been used in Switzerland. The caries reduction over a 5-year test period was approximately half that observed in children of the same ages drinking fluoridated water (1.0 p.p.m.) in Grand Rapids, Michigan. Milk has been tested as a vehicle for fluoride in small studies with apparent beneficial effects. Half a pint of milk containing 1 mg fluoride was given daily for $4\frac{1}{2}$ years. Ericsson[32] has concluded from independent experiments that fluoride in milk is available, but that more clinical data relating to the efficacy of fluoridation of milk is needed. A Dutch study of consumption of bread and flour by 20 000 people has indicated a surprising constancy which suggests that fluoridation of bread may be an effective measure. It has also been estimated that if 3.5 mg fluoride were added to each kg of cereal, 98 per cent of the Danish population would receive 0.6–1.5 mg fluoride per 3000 cal consumed.

The effectiveness of many food additives in reducing caries has been tested in experimental animals and it should be borne in mind that because of the many differences in eating habits, tooth and oral cavity morphology, etc., there are problems in applying the results of animal experiments to the human situation.

As the tooth mineral comprises calcium and phosphate these components were obvious choices for dietary supplements because increased concentrations of calcium and phosphate ions in the oral environment might be expected to suppress the dissolution of tooth mineral in acid by means of mass action. However, neither dietary calcium, nor vitamin D, which promotes calcium absorption, seems to affect caries, although deficiencies of these nutrients produce their own developmental defects.

Inorganic phosphates

When a mixed diet was ashed, the ash was cariostatic in hamsters and only the phosphate of the components of this mixture had cariostatic

$$O=\underset{\underset{OH}{|}}{\overset{\overset{OH}{|}}{P}}-O^- \qquad O-\underset{}{\overset{\overset{O}{\|}}{P}}-O^-$$

orthophosphate   metaphosphate

$$O=\underset{\underset{OH}{|}}{\overset{\overset{O^-}{|}}{P}}-O-\underset{\underset{OH}{|}}{\overset{\overset{O^-}{|}}{P}}=O$$

pyrophosphate

activity. Of the various phosphates tested, pyro- and orthophosphates were the least effective in preventing caries in rodents, and trimetaphosphate was most effective[33]. Acid and sodium salts were more effective than potassium, calcium or magnesium salts. When 2 per cent $CaHPO_4$ was added to sucrose, flour, cakes and bread in the diet of children over a 2–3-year period a 3–9 per cent reduction of decayed, missing and filled surfaces of the teeth was reported[34]. A problem in the assessment of these experiments is the fluoride content of the phosphates used. From a practical point of view, incorporation of inorganic phosphates into a range of food items is possible for experimental animals, and for small

groups of people over short periods of time, but it presents great problems for a wider public over prolonged periods. Phosphate-enriched chewing gum has been tested and apparently produced a reduction of caries in one study but not in two others[34]. The effects of inorganic phosphates on caries have been reviewed[35–38], and mechanisms for the anti-caries effect have been postulated.

One potential mechanism that has been investigated is that high concentrations of inorganic phosphate decrease the acid production by oral streptococci including *Streptococcus mutans*[39]. This may be partly due to the inorganic phosphate preventing the activation of lactate dehydrogenase by its normal allosteric activator, fructose diphosphate[40].

Organic phosphates

Many experiments have shown that purified cereals in the diet of rodents produce more caries than unrefined cereals. This parallels the epidemiological evidence from human populations eating 'primitive' and 'civilised' diets. Such results have initiated searches for cariostatic components of unrefined vegetable foodstuffs. The inclusion in the diet of rodents of the husks of oats, rice, peanuts, pecan nuts, barley, cottonseed and other seeds has commonly produced a reduction in caries of 20–40 per cent, and the effect has been as high as 75 per cent[41]. Finely ground seed hulls were used in most cases so that an abrasive action on the dental plaque seems unlikely to account for the magnitude of the effect. Such reductions in dental caries could not be achieved by adding the ash of the seed hulls to the diet nor by adding calcium hydrogen phosphate, so that the effect seems to be due to an organic component. Components in unrefined foods were shown to reduce the solubility of calcium phosphate and tooth powder[42]. Active fractions were readily extractable with water from brown flour, which contains 340 mg/100 g of organic phosphates, including 240 mg/100 g of phytic acid (myoinositol hexaphosphate).

phytic acid (phytate)

myoinositol

The solubility of calcium phosphate in acid buffers was perceptibly reduced by 0.01 mM phytate, and this effect was maximal at 3 mM phytate. In such experiments free phytate in solution decreased. Furthermore, teeth pre-treated with phytate and washed still showed reduced solubility in acids. It therefore seems likely that phytate binds to the mineral surface. Phytate may have ester phosphate groups removed hydrolytically catalysed by the enzyme phytase, and such degradation probably occurs during the early stages of cooking. However, cooked brown bread does appear to reduce enamel solubility[43], and myoinositol compounds with less than the maximum of six ester phosphates have been shown to be capable of reducing solubility, although to a lesser extent.

Aqueous extracts of the fibrous coats of various seeds and nuts were found to be capable of reducing enamel solubility. Aqueous extracts of pecan nuts only were inhibitory to bacteria, but alcoholic extracts of both wheat bran and oat husks inhibited a streptococcus and mixed salivary bacteria. The cariostatic or anticariogenic effects of these fibrous components of foodstuffs were considered to be more likely to be due to the water-soluble substances that might readily be extracted during chewing, than by the alcohol-soluble antibacterial agents[44]. One of the water-soluble agents is undoubtedly phytate (together with its partly degraded products), but other active components may play a part, including other organic phosphates.

One such phosphate that has been tested is β-glycerophosphate[45]. Monkeys given a diet containing 1 per cent calcium β-glycerophosphate showed a considerable reduction in caries compared to the control group, as well as a reduction in the quantity of plaque on the teeth. Another organic phosphate that has been tested is calcium sucrose phosphate ('Anticay'), which has been produced by phosphorylation of sucrose with phosphorus oxychloride in the presence of calcium hydroxide. The major component is the calcium salt of sucrose phosphorylated on the carbon 2 of the glucose ring, although other monophosphates occur, together with small quantities of sucrose diphosphates. In a 3-year clinical trial in which about 4.3 g 'Anticay' were given to 1500 children aged 5–17 years in Australia, the substance was added to carbohydrate foods at 1 per cent of the carbohydrate content. An overall reduction of 20 per cent in caries was claimed, with a greater protection being afforded to the proximal surfaces of posterior teeth where the caries reduction was as high as 35 per cent[46-49]. This study has been criticised in part because the sucrose phosphate contained significant amounts of fluoride, at least in the earlier batches.

CH₂OH
|
CHO PO₃H₂
|
CH₂OH

β-glycerophosphoric
acid

Sucrose-2-phosphoric acid

Dextranases

The effect of hydrolysing enzymes upon dental plaque presumably includes the reduction of adherence and coherence of those bacteria that need extracellular polysaccharides to establish and maintain themselves in plaque. Caries has been prevented in hamsters by dextranases (α1:6 glucanases) from *Penicillium* and *Streptomyces* species[50,51] and the enzyme has also reduced the caries in monkeys[52] when added to the diet. However, dextranase was apparently not effective in reducing plaque or caries in rats with indigenous cariogenic flora[53], although it was able to reduce caries in relatively gnotobiotic rats infected with *Streptococcus mutans*[54]. Caries in rats infected with three serotypes of this cariogenic species of streptococcus was reduced by dextranase from *Spicaria violacea*[55]. An enzyme specific for the hydrolysis of α1:3 bonds in the branched glucans sometimes called mutan has been purified from *Trichoderma harzianum*[56]. This enzyme, called mutanase (α1:3 glucanase) is reported to be more effective than dextranase in reducing the dental caries of rats[57]. In human subjects dextranase from *Spicaria violacea*[58] reduced the dry weight of dental plaque, while

mutanase from *Aspergillus nidulans*[59] reduced the proportion of *Streptococcus mutans* in the plaque without affecting the plaque accumulation. These enzymes, in tablets or mouthwashes, may therefore find a role in oral hygiene.

In conclusion it may be said that fluoridation of some staple foodstuffs is likely to be an effective measure, although less desirable dentally than the fluoridation of public water supplies. The effectiveness of intermittent consumption of flouride is probably because flouride is retained by the enamel and plaque. Of the organic phosphates, phytate also appears to bind enamel and may therefore have a persistent effect if added to certain items of the diet. The use of other phosphates in the human diet seems, at present, not to provide a practicable and effective approach to significantly reducing dental caries.

References

1. Fisher, F. J. (1972). The pattern of dental caries in Tristan da Cuhna. *The Dental Practitioner*, **22,** 267–70
2. Gustafsson, B. E., Quesnel, C. E., Lanke, L. S., Lundqvist, C., Grahnen, H., Bonow, B. E. and Krasse, B. (1954). The Vipeholm

dental caries study. The effect of different levels of carbohydrate intake on caries activity in 436 individuals observed for five years. *Acta Odontologica Scandinavica*, **11**, 232–64

3. Lundqvist, C. (1952). Oral sugar clearance. *Odontologisk Revy*, **3**, Suppl. 1

4. King, J. D., Mellanby, M., Stones, H. H. and Green, H. N. (1955). The Effect of Sugar Supplements on Dental Caries in Children, Medical Research Council Special Report Series No. 288, London

5. Harris, R. (1963). Biology of the children of Hopewood House, Bowral, Australia. 4 Observations of dental caries experience extending over five years (1957–1961). *Journal of Dental Research*, **42**, 1387–98

6. Hue, L. (1974). The metabolism and toxic effects of fructose, in *Sugars in Nutrition* (Eds Sipple, H. L. and McNutt, K. W.), Academic Press, New York, chap. 22, pp. 357–71

7. Linden, L. and Nisell, J. (1964). Hereditary intolerance to fructose. *Svensk Lakartidn.*, **61**, 3185

8. Marthaler, T. M. and Froesch, E. R. (1967). Hereditary fructose intolerance. Dental status of eight patients. *British Dental Journal*, **123**, 597–9

9. Huxley, H. G. (1974). The effect of dietary carbohydrate upon the colonisation of plaque by *Streptococcus mutans* in rats. *Archives of Oral Biology*, **19**, 941–6

10. Krasse, B., Edwardsson, S., Svenssen, I. and Trell, L. (1967). Implantation of caries-inducing streptococci in the human oral cavity. *Archives of Oral Biology*, **12**: 231–6

11. Littleton, R. W., Carter, C. H. and Kelly, R. T. (1967). Studies of oral health in persons nourished by stomach tube. I. Changes in the pH of plaque material after the addition of sucrose. *Journal of the American Dental Association*, **74**, 119–23

12. Stephan, R. M. (1966). Effects of different types of human foods on dental health in experimental animals. *Journal of Dental Research*, **45**, 1551–61

13. Grenby, T. H. (1963). The effects of some carbohydrates on experimental dental caries in the rat. *Archives of Oral Biology*, **8**, 27–30

14. Grenby, T. H. and Hutchinson, J. B. (1969). The effects of diets containing sucrose, glucose or fructose on experimental caries in two strains of rats. *Archives of Oral Biology*, **14**, 373–80

15. Grenby, T. H. (1965). The influence of cooked and raw wheat starch on dental caries in the rat. *Archives of Oral Biology*, **10**, 433–38

16. Grenby, T. H. (1966). White and wholemeal bread and flour in the diet of caries-susceptible rats. *British Dental Journal*, **121**, 26–9

17. Grenby, T. H. and Paterson, F. M. (1972). Effect of sweet biscuits on the incidence of dental caries in rats. *British Journal of Nutrition*, **27**, 195–9

18. Newbrun, E. (1973). Sugars, sugar substitutes and noncaloric sweetening agents. *International Dental Journal*, **23**, 328–45

19. Frostell, G. (1964). Substitution of fermentable sugars in sweets, in *Nutrition and Caries Prevention* (Ed. Blix, G.), Symposia of the Swedish Nutrition Foundation III, Almqvist and Wiksell, Stockholm, pp. 60–6

20. Frostell, G., Blomlof, L., Blomqvist, T., Dahl, G. M., Edward, S., Fjellstrom, A., Henrikson, C. O., Larje, O., Nord, C. E. and Nordenvall, K. J. (1974). Substitution of sucrose by Lycasin in candy; The Roslagen study. *Acta Odontologica Scandinavica*, **32**, 235–54

21. Birkhed, D. and Skude, G. (1978). Relation of amylase to starch and Lycasin metabolism in human dental plaque *in vitro*. *Scandinavian Journal of Dental Research*, **86**, 248–58

22. Touster, O. (1974). The metabolism of polyols, in *Sugars in Nutrition* (Eds Sipple, H. L. and McNutt, K. W.), Academic Press, New York, chap. 15, pp. 229–39

23. Brin, M. and Miller, O. N. (1974). The

safety of oral xylitol, in *Sugars in Nutrition* (Eds Sipple, H. L. and McNutt, K. W.), Academic Press, New York, chap. 33, pp. 591–606

24. Mäkinen, K. K. and Virtanen, K. K. (1978). Effect of a 4.5-year use of xylitol and sorbitol on plaque. *Journal of Dental Research*, **57**, 441–6

25. Mühlemann, H. R. and de Boever, J. (1970). Radiotelemetry of the pH of interdental areas exposed to various carbohydrates, in *Dental Plaque* (Ed. McHugh, W. M.), Livingstone, Edinburgh

26. Mühlemann, H. R., Regolati, B. and Marthaler, B. M. (1970). The effect on rat fissure caries of xylitol and sorbitol. *Helvetica Odontologica Acta*, **14**, 48–50

27. Scheinin, A., Makinen, K. K. and Ylitalo, K. (1974). Turku sugar studies I. An intermediate report on the effect of sucrose, fructose and xylitol diets on the caries incidence in man. Acta Odontologica Scandinavica, **32**: 383–412

28. Makinen, K. K. and Scheinin, A. (1974). Turku sugar studies II. Preliminary biochemical and general findings. *Acta Odontologica Scandinavica*, **32**, 413–21

29. Makinen, K. K. (1974). Sugars and the formation of dental plaque, in *Sugars in Nutrition* (Eds Sipple, H. L. and McNutt, K. W.), Academic Press, New York, chap. 37, pp. 645–87

30. Scheinin, A. (1974). The control of dental disease by prevention. *International Dental Journal*, **24**, 448–56

31. Hodge, H. C. and Smith, F. A. (1970). Minerals: fluorine and caries, in *Dietary Chemicals Versus Dental Caries* (Ed. Gould, R. F.), American Chemical Society, Washington, DC, chap. 7, pp. 93–115

32. Ericsson, Y. (1965). Effect of fluorides in foods, in *Nutrition and Caries Prevention* (Ed. Blix, G.), Symposia of the Swedish Nutrition Foundation III, Almqvist and Wiksells, Uppsala, pp. 112–22

33. Harris, R. S., Nizel, A. E. and Walsh, N. B. (1967). The effect of phosphate structure on dental caries development in rats. *Journal of Dental Research*, **46**, 290–4

34. Harris, R. S. (1970). Minerals: calcium and phosphorus, in *Dietary Chemicals Versus Dental Caries* (Ed. Gould, R. F.), American Chemical Society, Washington, DC, chap. 8, pp. 116–22

35. Nizel, A. E. and Harris, R. S. (1964). The effects of phosphates on experimental dental caries: a literature review. *Journal of Dental Research*, **43**, 1123–36

36. Ericsson, Y. (1965). Phosphates in relation to caries. *International Dental Journal*, **15**, 311–7

37. Harris, R. S. (1970). Fortification of foods and feed-products with anti-caries agents. *Journal of Dental Research*, **49**, 1340–4

38. Gilmore, N. D. (1969). The effect on dental caries activity of supplementary diets with phosphate. A review. *Journal of Public Health Dentistry*, **29**, 188–207

39. Handelman, S. L. and Kreinces, G. H. (1973). Effects of phosphate and pH on *Streptococcus mutans* acid production and growth. *Journal of Dental Research*, **52**, 651–7

40. Brown, A. T. and Ruh, R. (1977). Negative interaction of orthophosphate with glycolytic metabolism by *Streptococcus mutans* as a possible mechanism for dental caries reduction. *Archives of Oral Biology*, **22**, 521–4

41. Madsen, K. O. and Edmonds, E. J. (1962). Effect of rice hulls and other seed hulls on dental caries production in the cotton rat. *Journal of Dental Research*, **41**, 405–12

42. Jenkins, G. N., Forster, M. G., Speirs, R. L. and Kleinberg, I. (1959). The influence of the refinement of carbohydrates on their cariogenicity. *In vitro* experiments on white and brown flour. *British Dental Journal*, **106**, 195–208

43. Jenkins, G. N. (1966). The refinement of feeds in relation to dental caries, in *Advances in Oral Biology*, vol. 2, Academic Press, New York, pp. 67–100

44. Jenkins, G. N. and Smales, F. C. (1966). The potential importance in caries prevention of solubility reducing and antibacterial factors in unrefined plant products. *Archives of Oral Biology*, **11**, 599–608

45. Bowen, W. H. (1972). The cariostatic effect of calcium glycerophosphate in monkeys, *Caries Research*, **6**, 43–51

46. Harris, R., Schamschula, R. G., Gregory, G., Roots, M. and Beveridge, J. (1967). Observations on the cariostatic effect of calcium sucrose phosphate in a group of children aged 5–17 years. *Australian Dental Journal*, **12**, 105–13

47. Harris, R., Schamschula, R. G., Beveridge, J. and Gregory, G. (1968). The cariostatic effect of calcium sucrose phosphate in a group of children aged 5–17, Part II. *Australian Dental Journal*, **13**, 32–9

48. Harris, R., Roots, M., Gregory, G. and Beveridge, J. (1968). Calcium sucrose phosphate as a concentration agent in children aged 5–17 years, Part III. *Australian Dental Journal*, **13**, 345–52

49. Harris, R., Schamschula, R. G., Beveridge, J. and Gregory, G. (1969). Calcium sucrose phosphate as a cariostatic agent in children aged 5–17 years, Part IV. *Australian Dental Journal*, **14**, 42–9

50. Block, P. L., Dooley, C. L. and Howe, E. E. (1969). The retardation of spontaneous periodontal disease and the prevention of caries in hamsters with dextranase. *Journal of Periodontology*, **40**, 105–10

51. Fitzgerald, R. J., Fitzgerald, D. B. and Stoudt, T. H. (1973). Comparison of anticaries effects of different polyglucanase in limited-flora hamsters infected with *Streptococcus mutans*, in *Germ-Free Research*, (Ed. Heneghan, J. B.), Academic Press, New York, pp. 197–203

52. Bowen, W. H. (1971). The effect of dextranase on caries activity in monkeys (*Macacus irus*). *British Dental Journal*, **131**, 445–9

53. Guggenheim, B., König, K. G., Mühlemann, H. R. and Regolati, B. (1969). Effect of dextranase on caries in rats harboring an indigenous cariogenic bacterial flora. *Archives of Oral Biology*, **14**, 555–8

54. König, K. G. and Guggenheim, B. (1968). *In vivo* effects of dextranase on plaque and caries. *Helvetica Odontologica Acta*, **12**, 48–55

55. Hamada, S., Oshima, T., Masuda, N., Mizuno, J. and Shizno, S. (1976). Inhibition of rat dental caries by dextranase from a strain of *Spicaria violacea*. *Japanese Journal of Microbiology*, **20**, 321–30

56. Guggenheim, B. and Haller, R. (1972). Purification and properties of an α(1:3) glucanohydrolase from *Trichoderma harzianum*. *Journal of Dental Research*, **51**, 394–402

57. Guggenheim, B., Regolati, B. and Mühlemann, H. R. (1972). Caries and plaque inhibition by mutanase in rats. *Caries Research*, **6**, 289–97

58. Murayama, Y., Wada, H., Hayashi, H., Uchida, T., Yokomizo, I. and Hamada, S. (1973). Effects of dextranase from *Spicaria violacea* (IFO 6120) on the polysaccharides produced by oral streptococci and on human dental plaque. *Journal of Dental Research*, **52**, 658–67

59. Kelstrup, J., Funder–Nielsen, T. D. and Moller, E. N. (1973). Enzymatic reduction of the colonisation of *Streptococcus mutans* in human dental plaque. *Acta Odontologica Scandinavica*, **31**, 249–53

60. Jenkins, G. N. (1974). The biochemistry of plaque and caries with special reference to fluoride. Zyma, Nyon, Switzerland.

Chapter 10

Fluorides: Systemic Balance and Cariostatic Mechanisms

R. L. Speirs

Department of Physiology, London Hospital Medical College

10.1 Introduction

The widespread use of fluorides in combating dental caries requires the medical and dental professions to be conversant with the systemic actions of fluoride, its toxicity and the probable mechanisms by which it exerts its anti-caries effects. The purpose of this chapter is to consider these subjects. The scope of the discussion will be restricted, however, only to those aspects which are regarded as essential in helping the health scientist to discuss rationally and knowledgeably the pros and cons of fluoridation, to recognise the value and limitations of certain forms of fluoride prophylaxis and to understand how fluoride acts in affording some protection against caries. The reader is referred to several recent reviews for a more comprehensive coverage of these subjects.

10.2 Sources of Fluoride

10.2.1 Natural sources of fluoride

The widespread occurrence of fluorides in rocks, mineral deposits, soils and sea-water would be expected to result in this element being readily available to us in our diets and drinking water, but this is not so. Although most water supplies contain trace amounts of fluoride, less than 0.1 p.p.m. F (one part F in 10 million parts water or 0.1 mg F/l some do contain appreciable quantities, particularly in some deep well waters. The optimum level, from a dental health point of view, is 0.7 to 1.2 p.p.m. F (figure 10.1). The caries-reducing effect becomes progressively less below this level, while above, not only is there little further benefit to be derived, but there is the increased possibility of mottling in the permanent teeth, particularly at concentrations in excess of 2 p.p.m. F. Fluoride in drinking water exists as the ion F^-, the parent compound being completely dissociated. Because of the ease with which fluoride forms either insoluble salts or undissociated complexes[1], the influence of other ions in water upon the availability and effectiveness of fluoride must be considered.

Even in hard water the concentrations of calcium, magnesium and fluoride will not normally reach the solubility products of the fluoride salts. Only when all the concentrations are exceptionally high and above the recommended levels will any precipitation occur. The reduction in caries caused by fluoride is thought to be independent of the total hardness of water. One related issue which has been of some concern in water-fluoridated areas is the effect on fluoride levels of prolonged boiling of water. It would appear that considerable concentration of the fluoride can occur—reaching 13.5 p.p.m. F in some fluoridated water supplies, but that after this degree of evaporation has occurred the water is brackish and is not palatable. The same treatment of another fluoridated, hard-water resulted in smaller increases in the fluoride level, presumably on account of complexing or precipitation of fluoride[2]. Chemical treatment of water supplies with coagulants such as alum, ferric chloride or sodium silicate might also be expected to cause complexing of fluoride, but of these only aluminium has been shown to reduce the ionic fluoride to the extent of about 30 per cent. It is also of interest that the boiling of fluoridated water in aluminium utensils can result in a 50 per cent reduction in the ionic fluoride levels[1]. The effect upon human dental caries of interactions between fluoride and other trace elements in drinking water and diets has not received much study. Experiments in rodents have produced very conflicting results.

Among beverages and foods, only tea and soft-boned fish, such as canned sardines and salmon, can be considered as significant sources of fluoride in the UK. As normally prepared, tea contains about 1–2.5 p.p.m. F, depending upon the blend and infusion strength. The large variations observed between adults in their fluoride intakes are largely attributable to their tea-drinking habits. A cup of tea (with non-fluoridated water) contributes about 0.3 mg F. It is unfortunate that there is little known about the consumption of tea and the age at onset of tea-drinking in children. Such information for any given child ought to be sought by the dentist

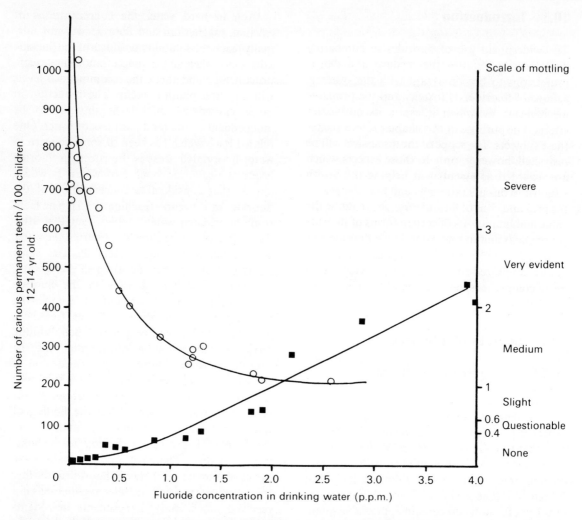

Figure 10.1   Relationship between dental caries incidences, degree of mottling and fluoride concentration in drinking water (from Wespi[43])

when fluoride supplements are prescribed. By inference from other studies in which fluoride was added to milk at a concentration of 1 p.p.m. F, the addition of milk to tea probably reduces slightly the availability of fluoride.

Milk itself contributes insignificant amounts of fluoride. Recent analytical figures suggest that human milk contains about 0.05 p.p.m. F and cows milk about 0.1 p.p.m. F[3]. Raising the fluoride intake of the mother by the ingestion of fluoridated water has no significant effect on the milk fluoride level[3, 4]. Although less than 20 per cent of the total fluoride in milk is in a free, ionic form, this does not imply that 80 per cent is non-absorbable in the conditions which exist in the gastro-intestinal tract. It is of importance to note that, in a water-fluoridated area, bottle-fed babies given milk reconstituted from powder, receive about 30 times more fluoride per day than breast-fed babies[5]. It has been calculated that the daily fluoride intake must exceed 0.1 mg F/kg body wt to produce mottling of the permanent teeth.

It has been calculated that the total intake of fluoride in persons residing in a water-fluoridated area is principally determined by the fluoride in the drinking water. Adults who drink the average 1.5 l of water per day (if such a figure means anything) will receive 1.5 mg F from this source when the fluoride level in water is 1 p.p.m. Figures reported for the water intake of children are inconsistent. Rather more conservative mean values are shown in table 10.1 than in the few earlier studies which have been carried out.

Table 10.1 Mean daily water intake of children and infants (after McPhail and Zachel[41])

Age in years:	under 1	1–2	3–4	5–6	7–8	9–10
Tap water						
ml/kg	18.3	9.8	11.2	10.9	10.7	10.7
ml/child	141	120	184	228	271	348
Total water						
ml/kg	55.2	26.3	23.4	19.8	18.6	18.0
ml/child	426	322	381	413	473	589

Figures for total fluoride intake in persons in non-fluoridated areas have been calculated from urinary fluoride levels, but these probably overestimate the intake (see page 235). They show large within-subject and between-subject variations, so that mean values must be interpreted with caution. In 1–6-year-old children in the USA, the daily intake was reported as less than 0.2 mg F, but higher mean levels of about 0.4 mg were obtained in 3–6-year-old children in Edinburgh[6]. Mean daily values of 1.6 mg F for adults in non-fluoridated districts in the UK have been reported. In recent years there has been an increase in the fluoride intake as a consequence of the widespread use of fluoride-containing dentifrice. The daily ingestion of up to 1.5 mg fluoride (near 0.49 mg) in young teenagers has been attributed to the swallowing of dentrifice after tooth-brushing[7].

Another 'natural' source of fluoride nowadays is atmospheric fluoride, which takes the form of dust particles or gases which emanate from fertiliser plants, brick works, aluminium refineries, steelworks and miscellaneous industries. Traces of these are ingested or inhaled and subsequently absorbed.

10.2.2 Artificial sources of fluoride

Fluoridation of water is effected at the water works by the controlled addition of sodium fluoride, sodium silicofluoride, or hydrofluosilicic acid. These compounds are completely dissociated when the final recommended dilutions are achieved.

Because of the rejection of water fluoridation by certain communities as a public health measure, alternative methods or vehicles for fluoride administration to children have had to be sought and tried. Most of these suffer the common disadvantage in that they each require cooperation from parent or patient.

Fluoride tablets, each containing 1 mg F as sodium fluoride or less commonly calcium or magnesium fluoride, are in use under a variety of trade names.

Fluoridized table salt, containing about 90 mg F/kg or 200 mg sodium fluoride/kg, has been available in Switzerland for many years. This source can contribute about 0.5 mg fluoride per day in adults. Very recently it has been recommended that the dosage of sodium fluoride be increased.

Fluoridized milk has been used in the USA and in Switzerland. In addition, there are fluoride preparations available for local use in the mouth—mouthwashes, topical agents and dentifrices.

10.3 Systemic Fluoride Balance

10.3.1 Absorption

Fluoride from inorganic sources is absorbed as F^- in the small intestine and possibly as HF in the stomach. It is considered to take place by diffusion across the mucosal cells rather than by active transport. Absorption is generally rapid and almost 100 per cent complete if the fluoride is in solution. The amount of fluoride absorbed can, however, sometimes be less than the quantity ingested because of the low solubility of the parent compound—for example, bone meal—or because of complex formation, precipitation or adsorption in the gut. Thus, aluminium can reduce fluoride absorption by 20 per cent in the stomach and up to 60 per cent in the small intestine. Of practical importance is the finding that fluoride from fluoride tablets (1 mg F) is absorbed to the same extent whether taken with or between meals. The addition of fluoride to milk at concentrations between 1 and 2 p.p.m. F retards the rate of absorption rather more than it reduces the amount absorbed.

10.3.2   Distribution

Over the past 15 years there has been a downward trend in the values reported in the literature for the fluoride concentrations in plasma and other body fluids. This mainly reflects the improvements in the analytical methods and raises doubts about the validity of many of the earlier results and conclusions. The total concentration of fluoride in the plasma of persons in non-fluoridated areas is now quoted as about 0.010 p.p.m. F[8]. It is no longer thought that plasma fluoride is mostly in a bound form[9].

After the oral ingestion of a few milligrams of sodium fluoride in tablet form, there is a transient

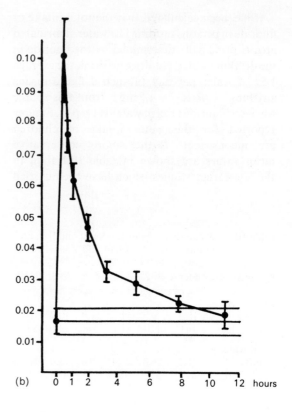

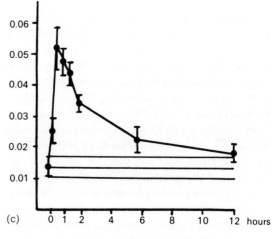

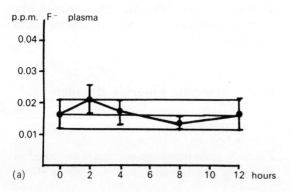

Figure 10.2 Plasma fluoride concentrations over 12 h under controlled dietary conditions; mean values ±standard deviation for 6 subjects: (a) no fluoride supplement given (normal values), (b) 1 × 2 mg F given once as NaF in tablet form, (c) 1 × 1 mg F administered once in tablet form (from Henschler, Buttner and Patz[10])

rise in the plasma fluoride level which reaches a peak within a few minutes to about 2 h and then (figure 10.2) returns slowly to the baseline within about 8 h[10, 11]. There is considerable variability in the timing of these events. On drinking fluoridated water the peaks are much smaller (figure 10.3). A curve of the decline in plasma fluoride following injection of fluoride suggests

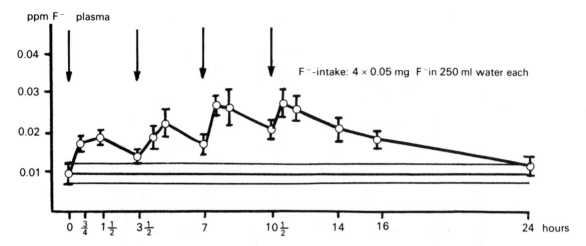

Figure 10.3 Plasma fluoride concentrations following repeated ingestion of fluoride in drinking water—each point is a mean value for 6 subjects ± standard deviation of the mean (from Henschler, Buttner and Patz[10])

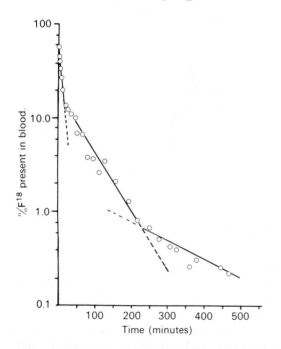

Figure 10.4 ^{18}F levels in blood following injection of the isotope into ruminants; Essentially the same shaped curve is discernible in figure 10.2(b) for orally ingested fluoride (from Perkinson[44])

three components: an initial rapid equilibration with tissue fluid, a slower, but still pronounced, fall which is attributed to skeletal deposition and finally a much slower process with a half-time ($t^{\frac{1}{2}}$) of about 3 h, which probably represents renal clearance (figure 10.4).

From this and much more evidence it can be said that fluoride homeostasis is accomplished efficiently by two principal mechanisms—deposition in the skeleton and excretion in urine. Other routes by which fluoride may be lost in small, variable amounts are through saliva and gastro-intestinal secretions (but this is mostly re-absorbed), faeces, sweat, milk and the developing fetus (figure 10.5). Soft tissues do not accumulate fluoride, apart from those in which ectopic calcification may occur.

10.3.3 Excretion by the kidney

The highest urinary fluoride concentrations occur within 2 h after the ingestion of a single small dose of sodium fluoride, about 35 per cent of the

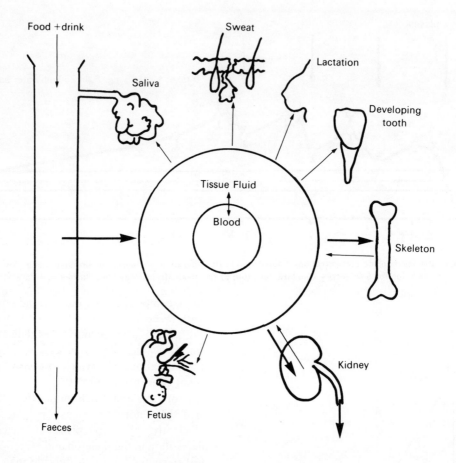

Figure 10.5   Diagrammatic representation of fluoride homeostasis

absorbed fluoride passing into the urine within 3 h and almost all of the excreted fluoride within 12 h (figure 1.6). Again the literature shows considerable variation, particularly with regard to the time taken for final elimination of the fluoride. The actual percentage of absorbed fluoride which is excreted varies according to the past history of fluoride exposure and age, both of which mainly affect the effectiveness of the skeletal component of the homeostatic mechanism; but other factors are also involved, notably the concentration of the fluoride ingested and fluid intake.

In young, unexposed children of 1–6 years in age, given small quantities of sodium fluoride, 20–30 per cent is excreted, but this rises to 50–60 per cent in adults. However, in adults ingesting fluoride in drinking water for several years, a

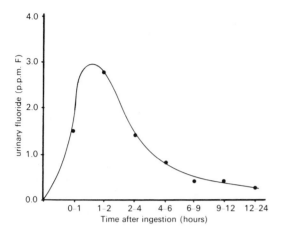

Figure 10.6 **Increment of fluoride concentration in urine as a function of time after ingestion of 2 mg F as NaF in tablet form (after Stookey[45])**

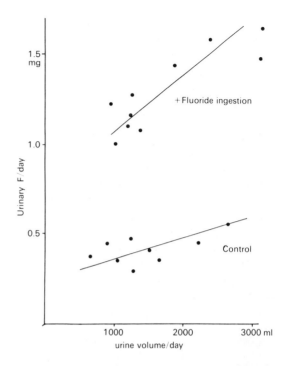

Figure 10.7 **Urinary fluoride output in 24 h in a 20-year-old subject on a variable fluid intake and relatively controlled diet—during the experimental period 2 × 0.5 mg F as NaF tablets were ingested daily. From these graphs it can be calculated that about 70 per cent of this administered fluoride was excreted in urine at normal flow-rates and about 100 per cent at the highest rates. (from Speirs, R. L., unpublished)**

situation approaching a steady state is reached in which urinary fluoride output approximates input. This again would seem to reflect decreased efficiency of skeletal fluoride deposition rather than a change in nephron activity. The adult skeleton seems to come into a near equilibrium state with a particular level of plasma or, more correctly, extracellular fluoride (near, because there is still a fluoride increment with age), but ingestion of a fluoride supplement, for example 2 mg sodium fluoride, causes a more marked elevation of the plasma level, promotes deposition of fluoride in the bones and causes a decreased percentage excretion in the urine. It is only in advanced kidney disease that urinary excretion of fluoride becomes impaired, leading to increased fluoride incorporation in bone accompanied possibly in the elderly by elevated plasma fluoride levels. The tubular reabsorption of fluoride is reduced by high urinary flowrates and thus by increased intake of fluid (figure 10.7).

10.3.4 Incorporation in the skeleton

Much of the importance of fluoride in medicine and dentistry centres on the high degree of affinity between it and hydroxyapatite. Enamel and dentine of primary and permanent teeth reflect in their fluoride contents the levels of fluoride in extracellular fluids during tooth development. After mineralisation has been completed further acquisition of fluoride occurs at the accessible surfaces, particularly at the pulpal–dentine interface, in secondary dentine, and to a smaller extent on the enamel surface[12]. In the latter case, the fluoride which accumulates after eruption originates from the oral fluids and plaque, and from tissue fluids pre-eruptively.

Fluoride is substituted for hydroxyl groups within and on the surface of the hydroxyapatite lattice and some may also be adsorbed. In consequence of the greater availability of crystal surfaces in bone than in enamel and dentine, the continued remodelling and the prolonged period during which bone accretion occurs, fluoride incorporation in bone continues throughout life, is not uniform within any one bone and varies in amount in different parts of the skeleton. Periosteal and endosteal surfaces and cancellous bone of the metaphyses tend to have the highest concentrations. Bone fluoride increases linearly with increases in water fluoride levels up to about 4 p.p.m. F, above which the increment may become less. A positive correlation has been found between concentrations of fluoride in the skeleton and in plasma[13, 14]. For example, the increase in skeletal fluoride with age is associated with a slight increase in the plasma fluoride concentration[14]. All the evidence suggests that there is an increase in bone fluoride with age, but there is disagreement as to whether the increment is less in the elderly[12]. In those studies which support this pattern, the 'steady state' or plateau concentration is related to the fluoride concentration of the drinking water (figure 10.8).

There is certainly convincing evidence in animals that the rate of fluoride incorporation in bones becomes much reduced with increasing age. Also, it has been shown experimentally that the uptake of fluoride by the skeleton of young mice is determined by the total quantity of fluoridated water ingested per day rather than the concentration of fluoride in the drinking water, whereas in older animals, as saturation of the skeleton is approached, the uptake depends more on concentration than on total intake[15]. This would suggest that the actively growing bones are virtually 'filtering off' the fluoride in the tissue fluid, whereas in the older bones further deposition of fluoride depends on a particular concentration gradient between tissue fluid and the bone crystals.

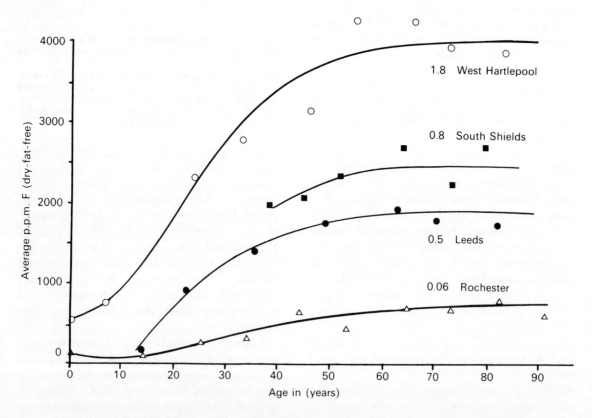

Figure 10.8 Relationship between age and the fluoride concentration in bone (from Hodge and Smith[46])

When a marked reduction in fluoride intake is instituted this is accompanied by a slight negative fluoride balance due to removal of some of the fluoride stored in the skeleton. This can continue for many months, being rapid at first then proceeding very slowly. Fluoride which is mobilised in these cases or in conditions of excess bone resorption is only partly lost in the urine, however, as some is translocated to other parts of the skeleton.

10.3.5 Placental transfer

It is now thought that fluoride passes readily across the human placenta despite evidence to the contrary in rodents[16]. Fluoride concentrations in maternal and fetal blood are similar. Fluoride in the fetal skeleton is related to the fluoride intake of the mother, but the correlation is not linear[16] (table 10.2). This lack of correspondence is presumably due to several factors besides placental transfer; one of these is the increased skeletal turnover in the mother during pregnancy which might result in increased 'trapping' of fluoride. Influences such as maternal diet, age and the number of previous pregnancies would all modify this process. From the limited evidence available it seems improbable that extra fluoride acquired by fetal teeth as a result of fluoride supplementation during pregnancy has any significant effect in protecting the teeth against caries.

Table 10.2   Fluoride content of ashed fetal femur and teeth in the full-term fetus from low and high fluoride areas (from Gedalia[16])

Fluoride in drinking water (p.p.m.)	Mean F (p.p.m.)	
	femur	teeth
0.1	43.8	40.8
0.55	92.5	69.7
1.0	85.2	53.8

10.3.6 Secretion in saliva

Because of possible topical effects of salivary fluoride on tooth surfaces and on plaque microorganisms there has been considerable interest in the secretion of fluoride in saliva of persons consuming fluoridated water or ingesting sodium fluoride tablets. Recent analytical findings quote values for fluoride concentrations which are similar to those in plasma, that is, about 0.01 p.p.m.; rising to a peak following fluoride ingestion[10]. In parotid and whole saliva there is a higher fluoride concentration in unstimulated than in stimulated samples[17, 18]. Fluoride levels in saliva are likely to be lower than in many of the oral fluids which bathe the teeth intermittently; for example fluoridated water and tea, but may be sufficiently high during times of reduced stimulation to exert an important topical effect on the tooth surface.

10.4   Effects of Fluoride on Metabolism

The magnitude of any effects of fluoride on metabolism must depend on the concentration of fluoride in the water supply, the total daily intake, and the duration of exposure to fluoride, and in any discussion on this subject it is essential to consider all these factors. We must also be cautious in extrapolating the results of studies of fluoride on isolated enzyme systems and on tissue and cell cultures to the situation in vivo in the whole organism. It is the actual fluoride concentrations naturally occurring in plasma or saliva which have to be remembered so that the significance of experimental results can be appraised. The ingestion of naturally fluoridated water by millions of people throughout the world, at concentrations even above those recommended by public health authorities, has afforded an unparalleled opportunity to study the long-term effects of fluoride on health, and extensive laboratory investigations have supported these studies. The effects of fluoride can be considered according to the level of consumption. Prolonged exposure to drinking water with 1–4 p.p.m. F or 4–8 p.p.m. F can be compared with total daily intakes of over 20 mg F for relatively short terms (months) and long terms (many years). This classification is convenient but is obviously an oversimplification.

Laboratory studies have shown that fluoride increases the size and improves the crystallinity of hydroxyapatite crystals in bones and reduces the inclusion of carbonate and citrate while increasing the magnesium, fluoride and ash contents. These changes were reported in long-term residents in a 4 p.p.m. F area and are a consequence of either the alteration of the crystal lattice or of the metabolism of the bone-forming cells. That fluoride can influence cellular metabolism at these and lower levels of intake is an inescapable conclusion, since mottling of enamel is due primarily to an effect on the ameloblasts with the result that matrix formation and mineralisation become disturbed. Severe mottling is characterised by hypoplasia of the enamel and increased porosity which permits penetration by oral fluids and staining.

A few reports suggest that bone metabolism and possibly also some aspects of liver cell function may be altered transiently in individuals who have just begun to take fluoridated water or tablets. The alterations in the urinary excretion of free hydroxyproline and in serum alkaline phosphatase levels in these studies were only of marginal statistical significance. The frequently reported sensitivity to fluoride of muscle enolase, liver lipase and various other enzymes in vitro[19] does not seem to have any relevance to physiological conditions in vivo.

The findings in tissue cultures that bone resorption can be reduced and collagen synthesis activated by fluoride added to the medium, and that prolonged high intakes of fluoride in vivo increase bone mass, have raised the possibility that the ingestion of fluoridated water might alter the structure as well as the chemical composition of bone. In a recent carefully controlled study[20] it has been shown, using photon-beam absorptiometry, that there is a tendency for increased bone mineral density in persons living in an area fluoridated for 18 years at 1.1 p.p.m. F compared with those in a non-fluoridated town (0.1 p.p.m. F). The mean difference for males and females in all age-groups studied was about 2 per cent and as such would have been undetected by older, less sensitive, methods. The clinical significance of these small changes is uncertain.

From the literature it seems that high concentrations of fluoride can be accommodated in the skeleton without any histological alterations and without any symptoms being presented. Prolonged consumption of about 8 p.p.m. F in drinking water however, leads to higher skeletal fluoride levels, increased cortical thickness and coarsened trabeculae, while even higher intakes over prolonged periods cause irregular bone accretion on the periosteal surfaces, particularly in the ribs, vertebrae and pelvis, and calcification of tendons and ligaments. Areas of increased osteoid and large resorption cavities suggest a compensatory overactivity of the parathyroid glands, but in some of these cases of skeletal fluorosis the principal histological appearance is one resembling osteosclerosis. The observation that fluoride can lead to increased bone mass has promoted its use in the treatment of senile and post-menopausal osteoporosis. The claims made for this form of therapy, in which sodium fluoride is administered in amounts ranging from 25 even up to 100 mg fluoride daily for several months, have been equivocal and do not offer much promise as a long-term measure. A more successful approach has been to combine fluoride therapy with supplementation of the diet with calcium and vitamin D. This regime has improved the osteoporotic state in less than one year.

It is difficult to define the level at which the fluoride intake becomes toxic. There are some who would suggest that mottling is a first sign of toxicity, while at the other end of the scale the finding that some patients have tolerated an intake of over 50 mg fluoride daily for months without any obvious sign of ill-health might be interpreted as an absence of toxic effects even at these levels.

As far as lethal doses are concerned, it is generally considered that a single dose of about 2.5 g would be fatal for adults. On a proportional body weight basis this would be equivalent to 35 mg F/kg in a child. Sub-lethal doses would be associated with non-specific effects such as vomiting, abdominal pain, diarrhoea and convulsions.

10.5 Cariostatic Mechanisms of Fluoride

10.5.1 Introduction

Without doubt, fluoride exerts its protective effect against dental caries in several ways. Many attempts to attribute its action entirely to one mechanism have failed. This chapter will consider the role of fluoride from sources such as water, food, beverages and preparations such as tablets, salt and milk. Topically applied fluorides, mouth-washes, chewing-gum and dentifrices will be excluded, but these agents may well share some of the anti-caries mechanisms ascribed to ingested fluorides.

Fluoride concentrations in enamel and more importantly the surface enamel are related to the fluoride levels in the drinking water at the time of tooth development (figures 10.9 and 10.10) and since the latter are related to caries experience (figure 10.1) it was logical, in trying to explain the anti-caries effect, that attention should become centred on the possible influence on enamel properties of fluoride incorporation (figure 10.11). One group of workers has gone so far as to state that 'all available evidence suggests that the caries-inhibitory effect of this element is associated with the relatively high levels present in the surface layer'. This approach was, of course, encouraged by the finding that fluoride in enamel is incorporated mainly, pre-eruptively, that it is concentrated in the outer 100 μm and that the optimal effects of fluoride on caries seem to correlate with exposure to fluoride during the late pre-eruptive phase of development and the first few years after eruption.

That there is a degree of protection post-eruptively is generally accepted from both clinical evidence and studies on experimental caries in animals. This varies on different tooth surfaces;

thus fluoride administered after eruption affords the greatest protection to buccal and lingual surfaces, presumably because of their accessibility, followed by approximal surfaces. Pits and fissures receive little benefit. Pre-eruptive exposure to fluoride gives approximal surfaces more protection than buccal, while pits and fissures receive their transient protection during this time[21]. As caries itself is a multifactorial process, it is not surprising that one cannot ascribe to a particular fluoride concentration in enamel a particular degree of caries resistance. For example, the caries susceptibility of different teeth and different surfaces of a tooth cannot be correlated with their fluoride concentrations. Analysis of the fluoride content of the enamel of teeth from fluoridated and a non-fluoridated

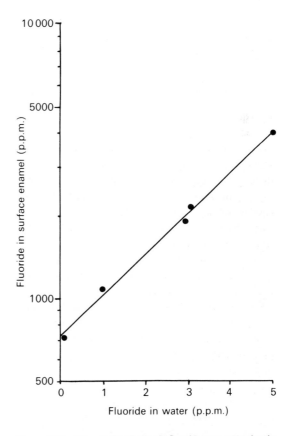

Figure 10.9 Correlation between fluoride concentration in surface enamel and that in drinking water (from Hodge and Smith[46])

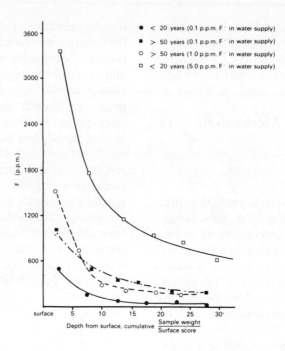

Figure 10.10   Fluoride concentration in enamel, sampled at different depths from the surface of teeth of persons differing in their exposure to fluoride in the drinking water supply (from Isaac, Brudevold, Smith and Gardner[49])

areas shows a difference in mean fluoride values. However, with respect to fluoride, there is a large overlap in frequency distribution for the two populations. Thus, it is not possible to predict whether or not a tooth will be resistant to caries simply by analysis of the enamel-fluoride content. Therefore, an actual threshold level of surface fluoride that will definitely prevent dental caries is not only unknown, but possibly also an incorrect concept to assume.

We have, therefore, to consider several theories, some dependent on the fluoride within the enamel affecting the caries process and others on fluoride acting locally on the tooth surface and plaque.

10.5.2   Effects on Enamel Solubility

It is well established that enamel, dentine and synthetic hydroxyapatite, treated with dilute fluoride solutions in vitro are rendered less soluble when subsequently tested in dilute acid. This finding was compatible with the view held by crystallographers that fluorapatite is a more stable and 'perfect' crystal than hydroxyapatite. Some fluorapatite is formed in enamel when fluoride is present systemically during the time of tooth development. After development, fluoride may be acquired by enamel pre-eruptively due to a process of ion exchange between some of the OH^- ions of hydroxyapatite and the F^- ions present in the tissue fluid bathing the tooth. The enamel may therefore be regarded as a mixture of inorganic phases and may best be described as fluorohydroxyapatite.

Several studies have been carried out to compare the behaviour in acids of natural enamel with differing fluoride concentrations, which by inference implies differing degrees of resistance to caries[22-24]. The overall conclusion from this work is a definite trend towards lower acid

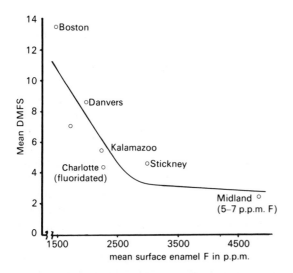

Figure 10.11 Relationship between surface fluoride concentration in enamel and dental caries experience in 12–16 yr old life time residents in fluoridated and non-fluoridated areas. It is of interest to compare this curve with that in figure 10.12. (from De Paola *et al.*[48])

dissolution rates of intact enamel surfaces or powdered enamel samples as their fluoride contents increase, particularly when teeth with widely varying histories of fluoride exposure have been compared (figures 10.12 and 10.13). However, there are many anomalies in this relationship; enamel samples with similar fluoride concentrations can show marked solubility differences (figure 10.13). Factors such as variations in surface microstructure and carbonate content, in addition to fluoride, probably influence these measurements. The significance of these small, inconsistent differences in solubility in influencing caries is difficult to assess, so also is the relevance of these *in vitro* methods to the situation in vivo[22]. As an illustration of this last point it has been found that fluorapatite and hydroxyapatite, although differing in their acid solubilities, behave similarly in acidified saliva[23].

It seems then, that if fluoride exerts an influence on enamel solubility, it does so by more subtle means than those measured by the 'sledge-

hammer' methods usually employed. One such mechanism was proposed on the basis of experimental results showing that the rates of acid dissolution of enamel from high and low fluoride areas were similar at first, but after several minutes began to show differences[25]. It was proposed that the fluoride and calcium ions released initially became redeposited as an insoluble calcium fluoride barrier. There is, however, no direct evidence for the presence of this phase in surface enamel, and extensive calculations based on equilibrium measurements of Ca^{2+}, PO_4^{3-} and F^-, in acids of different pH

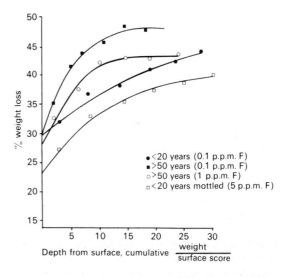

Figure 10.12 Weight loss in acid buffer (solubility rate) of powdered enamel samples obtained at different depths from the surface of teeth of persons differing in their exposure to fluoride in the drinking water supply (from Isaac, Brudevold, Smith and Gardner[47])

after exposure to enamel with known initial fluoride concentrations, suggest that this particular compound is not formed[23]. Instead the fluoride released during the early demineralisation stages will, if the pH is low enough, be avidly deposited as fluorapatite or at a higher pH will encourage the deposition of an insoluble calcium deficient

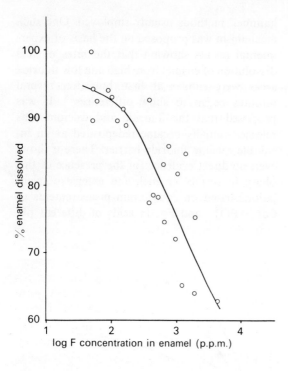

Figure 10.13 Relationship between acid solubility of powdered surface enamel samples and their fluoride concentrations (after Brudevold and McCann[22])

apatite with a more acid surface structure. The formation of either of these insoluble compounds is in sharp contrast to that of the relatively soluble octacalcium phosphate or dicalcium phosphate dihydrate which are considered to form after demineralisation of enamel with a low fluoride content.

Both of the more acid calcium phosphate phases (octacalcium phosphate OCP and dicalcium phosphate DCPD) have been suggested as precursors in the formation of hydroxyapatite. The presence of fluoride in a solution at a concentration of only 0.1 p.p.m. converts the OCP to the apatite form, while DCPD reacts directly with fluoride to form fluorapatite.

Although such hypotheses, and they are little more at the moment, seem to answer many

questions and are compatible with many experimental findings, they are very difficult to test directly.

The foregoing considerations lead inevitably to the wider issue of the role of fluoride in remineralisation. It is now generally accepted that caries is an alternating process of dissolution and remineralisation and that the overall result is a gradual decrease in carbonate, magnesium and sodium and an increase in fluoride, some other trace elements and the formation of an increasingly insoluble residue in the enamel. Relative to the intact sound surface enamel, the early carious lesion or white spot takes up fluoride preferentially. The resulting differences in fluoride content between these adjacent parts are associated with differences in acid dissolution rates, these being more marked in teeth from fluoridated than non-fluoridated areas[24].

Differences in acid dissolution rates have recently been explained by Brown[26]. Increases in the concentration of fluoride within the lesion are thought to affect the equilibrium pH as well as the activity of the basic and acidic components. In the case of $Ca(OH)_2$ and H_3PO_4, the activity of $Ca(OH)_2$ would be lowered and would therefore reduce the driving force for diffusion of calcium out of the lesion and of protons into the lesion. Conversely, a higher H_3PO_4 activity will be found with increasing fluoride and this will promote diffusion of H_3PO_4 out of the lesion, thereby lowering the acidity of the lesion.

Several lines of evidence support the concept that fluoride actually encourages remineralisation. It has been shown, for example, that not only do traces of fluoride favour the precipitation and seeding of calcium phosphate from saturated solutions, but also dictate that it is the more basic apatite form which crystallises out, even at relatively low pH values[23].

Essentially the same mechanism has been proposed as a result of rehardening studies of acid-softened enamel in vitro. The addition of 1 p.p.m. F to a saturated calcifying solution or about 20 p.p.m. F to saliva greatly accelerated the rehardening process[27]. Comparable results have been reported in newly erupted rat molars and in unerupted human teeth. In the rat, some fissures show post-eruptive maturation or mineralisation of developmental hypomineralised areas. This process was accelerated by fluoride given in the drinking water. In human teeth an increase in birefringence was observed in surface enamel on exposure to a calcifying fluid in the presence of 1 p.p.m. F[28].

Another related facet of this possible role for fluoride was provided by the demonstration that concentrations of fluoride in an acid buffer as low as 1 p.p.m. can reduce the rates of dissolution of powdered enamel or hydroxyapatite[29]. If such concentrations of fluoride can be present within an acid plaque they might, in some way, inhibit enamel decalcification. Any former doubts about the availability of such fluoride levels have been dispelled by the finding that fluoride becomes concentrated in plaque. Although most of the fluoride is in a bound form some of this is released by acidification[18,30]. Calculations suggest that about 0.5 p.p.m. F, in a free form, might be present in the aqueous phase of plaque from residents in fluoride areas but as acid is produced higher concentrations of fluoride will be present.

Thus, the readiness with which fluoride will combines with calcium and phosphate at an acid pH to form a relatively insoluble phase seems to be a recurring concept in this discussion. Fluoride is endeavouring to maintain the status quo of the mineral.

10.5.3 Effects on bacterial metabolism

Biochemical studies on muscle homogenates and pure enzyme systems had shown that fluoride could inhibit enolase and some other enzymes involved in glycolysis and cellular oxidation. Dental research workers were not slow to realise the possible implications of these findings, and the suggestion that fluoride might reduce caries by inhibiting bacterial acid production or growth was soon put to the test. The first studies on incubated pure cultures of salivary bacteria and later on saliva and salivary sediment confirmed that fluoride could inhibit acid pro-

duction, but that concentrations of 2 p.p.m. F and above were necessary to give small but significant effects. Sensitivity to fluoride was increased by an acid pH, so that at pH 5.0 as little as 6–10 p.p.m. F was shown to stop acid production completely for several hours. However, the application of these experimental results to conditions in the mouth and to caries was questionable. First, much lower concentrations of fluoride than those required in these experiments were known to be present in saliva and oral fluids and, secondly, bacteria and not plaque were being studied in grossly unphysiological circumstances. The latter criticism was subsequently answered when it was shown that fluoride in vitro could suppress acid production of plaque, although the concentrations required were higher than in the earlier studies[31]. It was argued that even in the unlikely event that these concentrations of fluoride could be available *in vivo*, from the dissolution of the surface enamel reservoir, the significance of the small differences in acid production— for example, pH 5.0 in the control incubation and 5.2 in the presence of fluoride—was difficult to assess in terms of caries prevention.

Interest in this antibacterial theory consequently waned but was revived by the important finding from two independent laboratories that fluoride is concentrated within plaque[30]. It originates mostly from oral fluids rather than from the enamel, although a tidal exchange between the inner plaque and parts of the enamel surface cannot be precluded. In the gingival crevice where plaque accumulates most readily, the tendency is for fluoride to increase in surface enamel, so there is little possibility of a predominantly one-way flow of fluoride from the enamel into the plaque. Values of 5–10 p.p.m. are representative for wet plaque samples from children from low fluoride areas[18] but very large variations are found between subjects. There is more fluoride in plaque exposed to fluoride containing drinking water.

Most of the plaque fluoride is bound at neutral pH with only about 2–5 per cent being in the free form[18]. The nature of the binding is complex and is the cause of some controversy. Some fluoride is very tightly bound and is only released by hot concentrated acids whereas another fraction is loosely bound and is liberated at pH 4–5. Whatever the nature of the loosely bound form, the significant feature, from a practical point of view, is that this represents a fluoride reservoir in that it can dissociate when acid is produced by plaque organisms to make available much more ionic fluoride. It has now been established that several strains of oral bacteria are able to concentrate fluoride in their cells so that the mean fluoride concentrations quoted for plaque are probably much higher than those in the aqueous phase of plaque. Within bacterial cells fluoride is metabolically active.

Fluoride probably has several different modes of action on bacterial metabolism. It has been shown, for example, that concentrations above 2 p.p.m. F in solution progressively decrease transport or uptake of glucose and glucose analogues into cells of oral streptococci and microorganisms in salivary sediment and that exogenous glucose metabolism is much more sensitive to fluoride than endogenous degradation of glycogen[32–34]. These effects on the cell membrane can be associated with others showing that the synthesis of intracellular iodophilic polysaccharide is inhibited by fluoride in salivary bacteria and in pure cultures of *Streptococcus mitis*[32]. Both of these actions of fluoride are pH sensitive, being enhanced by an acid pH. By reducing the storage of polysaccharide, fluoride might indirectly interfere with the acid production which occurs when plaque has been depleted of its exogenous sugar supply.

Attempts to obtain further evidence in support of the antibacterial theory have turned in recent years more to the composition and behaviour of plaque rather than to laboratory model systems. One such study revealed that samples of plaque from residents in a fluoridated area were less able to form acid when rinsed with sucrose than samples from a low fluoride area[42]. This result implies either inhibition by plaque fluoride of bacterial metabolism or an altered plaque ecology as a result of fluoride ingestion. The latter

suggestion has recently been given experimental support. In one study the percentages of *S. mutans* and iodophilic microorganisms were found to be slightly less in the plaque of children in fluoride areas[35], while in another study the percentage extracellular polysaccharide formed in such plaques was significantly reduced relative to that in plaques from low fluoride areas[36]. It is thought that this reduced synthesis is not due to interference by fluoride of the glycosyl transferase enzyme systems, but rather to a reduction in the bacterial cell population principally concerned with extracellular polysaccharide formation[37]. These findings, if substantiated by further work, could have important implications, since the retention and development of plaque and its cariogenic potential would be altered.

There is therefore considerable evidence to justify the proposal that fluoride exerts part of its protective action by affecting bacteria.

10.5.4   Effects mediated by surface adsorption

As is so often the case when several mechanisms or theories have been proposed to explain a particular observation, the time comes when yet another suggestion is put forward which appears to offer a compromise. It seemed that such a time had come when it was demonstrated that the ability of powdered hydroxyapatite to adsorb salivary proteins was reduced when partial substitution of its hydroxyl groups by fluoride had taken place[38]. Thus, the fluoride incorporated in the enamel might alter the surface charge or free energy and in this way alter the deposition of pellicle and its subsequent bacterial colonisation. The concentration of fluoride required was about 3000 p.p.m., which is quite within the range found in the extreme outermost region of enamel in teeth from a high fluoride area or after topical fluoride treatment. Unfortunately, this result with powdered material with its enormous surface area and reactivity might have little relevance to the situation on a tooth surface, and even if it did, we do not know for certain, although it is likely, that adhesion or adsorption of a surface pellicle of salivary origin is a prerequisite for further colonisation of the surface by a bacterial plaque. Certainly, there is little evidence for reduced plaque deposition in fluoride areas.

10.5.5   Effects mediated by tooth morphology

In several clinical surveys, mention has been made of apparent differences in the overall appearance of teeth in high and low fluoride areas. Where measurements of the teeth have been made these differences turn out to be quite small and by no means consistent. There is probably a greater degree of agreement about a fluoride-induced reduction in cusp height and fissure depth and an increase in fissure width than there is about alteration in the diameters of posterior teeth. Morphological changes have been observed experimentally in rat teeth also, but are associated not only with fluoride ingestion but also with the ingestion of several other trace elements. In some of the epidemiological studies in which fluoride has been implicated as the sole cause of these morphological changes other trace elements might well be contributing.

However, better control was afforded in two investigations. In one of these, comparisons were made between the teeth of children in two matched, neighbouring communities, one of which was supplied with fluoridated water[39], while in the second study, small fluoride supplements were given to a group of infants for the first three years of life[40]. An increase in the prevalance of atypically shallow pits and fissures was observed in the fluoride groups in both of these studies. Thus, we have yet another mechanism by which fluoride might exert some of its protective effect.

10.5.6   Conclusion

As stated at the outset, there is no simple explanation for the caries-reducing effect of fluoride. It is probably fair comment that the changes induced by it are beyond the detection limits of many of the laboratory methods employed for its study. After all, caries progresses at a relatively slow rate and fluoride only reduces, it does not prevent caries, thus its action must obviously be subtle. Whenever one discusses caries resistance and factors affecting it, one is considering both the attacking forces, namely the plaque and fermentable substrate on the one hand and the defensive forces, the structure of the enamel, tooth morphology and salivary composition on the other. In the early lesion and perhaps even before that stage is reached, one again envisages offensive demineralisation and defensive remineralisation. It has been shown in this chapter that fluoride has been allotted a role in almost every one of these competing processes.

Further Reading

Cariostatic Mechanisms of Fluorides (1977). Proceedings of a Workshop organised by the American Dental Association Health Foundation and the National Institute of Dental Research, Naples, *Caries Res.*, **11**, suppl. 1

Chemistry and Prevention of Dental Caries (1962). Charles Thomas, Springfield, Illinois

Ciba Foundation Symposium (1965). *Caries Resistant Teeth* (Eds Wolstenholme, G. E. W. and O'Connor, M.), Churchill, London

Fluorides and Human Health (1970). World Health Organization, Geneva

Jenkins, G. N. (1967). The mechanism of action of fluoride in reducing caries incidence. *International Dental Journal*, **17**, 552–63

Myers, H. M. (1978). *Fluorides and Dental Fluorosis*. Monographs in Oral Science. Karger, Basel

References

1.   Brudevold, F., Moreno, E. and Bakhos, Y. (1972). Fluoride complexes in drinking water. *Archives of Oral Biology*, **17**, 1155–63

2.   Jenkins, G. N. and Edgar, W. M. (1973).

Some observations on fluoride metabolism in Britain. *Journal of Dental Research*, **52**, 984–5 (abstract)

3. Backer Dirks, O., Jongeling, J., Flissebaalje, Th.D. and Gedalia, I. (1973). Total and free ionic fluoride in human and cow milk determined by gas – liquid chromatography and fluoride electrodes. *J. Dental Research*, **52**, 588 (abstract)

4. Ericsson, Y. (1969). Fluoride excretion in human saliva and milk. *Caries Research*, **3**, 159–66

5. Ericsson, Y. and Ribelius, U. (1971). Wide variations of fluoride supply to infants and their effect. *Caries Research*, **5**, 78–88

6. Hargreaves, J. A., Ingram, G. S. and Wagg, B. J. (1970). Excretion studies on the ingestion of a monofluorophosphate toothpaste by children. *Caries Research*, **4**, 256–68

7. Bloodworth, G., Ramsey, A. C., Tamacas, J. C. and Hardwick, J. L. (1979). Daily fluoride intakes in young teenagers from tea, water and fluoride dentifrices. *Journal of Dental Research*, **58**, 1128 (abstract)

8. Ekstrand, J. (1977). A micromethod for determination of fluoride in blood plasma and saliva. *Calcified Tissue Research*, **23**, 225–28

9. Ekstrand, J., Ericsson, Y. and Rosell, S. (1977). Absence of protein-bound fluoride from human blood plasma. *Archives of Oral Biology*, **22**, 229–32

10. Henschler, D., Büttner, W. and Patz, J. (1975). Absorption, distribution in body fluids and bioavailability of fluoride, in: *Calcium Metabolism, Bone and Metabolic Bone Disease*. Springer-Verlag, Heidelberg, pp. 111–21

11. Armstrong, W. D. and Singer, L. (1970). Distribution in body-fluids and soft tissues in: *Fluorides and Human Health*, WHO, Geneva, pp. 94–104

12. Weidmann, S. M. and Weatherell, J. A. (1970). Distribution in hard tissues. In: *Fluorides and Human Health*, WHO, Geneva, pp. 104–28

13. Ericsson, Y., Gydell, K. and Hammarskiöld, Th. (1973) Blood plasma fluoride: An indicator of skeletal fluoride content. *International Research Communications system* **1**, 33

14. Parkins, F. M., Tinanoff, N., Moritinho, M., Aristey, M. B. and Waziri, M. H. (1974). Relationships of human plasma fluoride and bone fluoride to age. *Calcified Tisue Research*, **16**, 335–38

15. Růžička, J. A. and Mrklas, L. (1968). Effect of the water intake on the fluoride incorporation into the skeleton of adult mice. *Caries Research*, **2**, 253–61

16. Gedalia, I. (1970). Distribution in placenta and foetus. In: *Fluorides and Human Health*, WHO, Geneva, pp. 128–34

17. Shannon, I. L., Suddick, R. P. and Edmonds, E. J. (1973). Effect of rate of gland function on parotid saliva fluoride concentration in the human. *Caries Research*, **7**, 1–10

18. Jenkins, G. N. and Edgar, W. M. (1977). Distribution and Forms of F in saliva and plaque. *Caries Research*, **11**, 226–37 (suppl. 1)

19. Venkateswarlu, P. (1970). Physiological effects of small doses of fluoride: Effects on body fluids and soft tissues. In *Fluorides and human health*, WHO, Geneva, pp. 163–85

20. Sluys Veer, J. van Der., Melman, A. P. M., Pot, T., Houwink, B. and Backer Dirks, O. (1975). Fluoridation of drinking water and bone mineral content, analyzed by monochromatic (^{125}I) radiation absorptiometry. In: *Calcium metabolism, bone and metabolic bone disease*, Springer-Verlag, Heidelberg, pp. 138–42

21. Backer Dirks, O. (1967). The relation between the fluoridation of water and dental caries experience. *International Dental Journal*, **17**, 582–605

22. Brudevold, F. and McCann, H. G. (1968). Enamel solubility tests and their significance in regard to dental caries. *Annals of the New York Academy of Science*, **153**, 20–51

23. McCann, H. G. and Brudevold, F. (1962). *Environmental variables in oral disease*, (Eds Kreshover, S. J. and McClure, F. J.), American Association for the Advancement of Science, Washington DC, pp. 103–28

24. Jenkins, G. N. (1960). *Lectures on the Scientific Basis of Medicine*, vol. 8, University of London, Athlone Press, London, pp. 442–59

25. Gray, J. A., Francis, M. D. and Griebstein, W. J. (1962). *Chemistry and Prevention of Dental Caries*, Charles Thomas, Springfield, Illinois, pp. 164–79

26. Brown, W. E., Gregory, T. M. and Chow, L. C. (1977). Effects of fluoride on enamel solubility and cariostasis. *Caries Research*, **11**, 118–24, (suppl. 1)

27. Koulourides, T., Cueto, H. and Pigman, W. (1961). Rehardening of softened enamel surfaces of human teeth by solutions of calcium phosphate. *Nature*, **189**, 226–7

28. Silverstone, L. M. and Johnson, N. W. (1971). The effect on sound human enamel of exposure to calcifying fluids in vitro. *Caries Research*, **5**, 323–42

29. Manly, R. S. and Harrington, D. P. (1959). Solution rate of tooth enamel in an acetate buffer. *Journal of Dental Research*, **38**, 910–19

30. Dawes, C., Jenkins, G. N., Hardwick J. L. and Leach, S. A. (1965). The relation between the fluoride concentrations in the dental plaque and in drinking water. *British Dental Journal*, **119**, 164–7

31. Jenkins, G. N., Edgar, W. M. and Ferguson, D. B. (1969). The distribution and metabolic effects of human plaque fluorine. *Archives of Oral Biology*, **14**, 105–19

32. Weiss, S., King, W. J., Kestenbaum, R. C. and Donohue, J. J. (1965). Influence of various factors on polysaccharide synthesis in *S. mitis. Annals of the New York Academy of Science*, **131**, 839–50

33. Sandham, H. J. and Kleinberg, I. (1969). The effect of fluoride on the inter-relation between glucose utilization, pH and carbohydrate storage in a salivary sediment system. *Archives of Oral Biology*, **14**, 619–28

34. Schachtele, C. F. and Mayo, J. A. (1973). Phosphoenolpyruvate dependent glucose transport in oral Streptococci. *Journal of Dental Research*, **52**, 1209–15

35. Houte, J. van, Backer Dirks, O., Stoppelaar J. D. de and Jansen, H. M. (1969). Iodophilic polysaccharide-producing bacteria and dental caries in children consuming fluoridated and non-fluoridated drinking water. *Caries Research*, **3**, 178–89

36. Broukal, Z. and Zajivek, O. (1974). Amount and distribution of extracellular polysaccharides in dental microbial plaque. *Caries Research*, **8**, 97–104

37. Stoppelaar, J. D. de, Houte, J. van and Backer Dirks O. (1969). The relationship between extracellular polysaccharide producing streptococci and smooth surface caries in 13-year-old children. *Caries Research*, **3**, 190–9

38. Ericson, Th. and Ericsson, Y. (1967). Effect of partial fluorine substitution on the phosphate exchange and protein adsorption of hydroxylapatite. *Helvetica Odont. Acta*, **11**, 10–14

39. Lovius, B. B. J. and Goose, D. H. (1969). The effect of fluoridated water on tooth morphology. *British Dental Journal*, **127**, 322–4

40. Aasenden, R. and Peebles, T. C. (1974). Effect of fluoride supplementation from birth on human deciduous and permanent teeth. *Archives of Oral Biology*, **19**, 321–6

41. McPhail, C. W. B. and Zachel, W. (1965). Fluid intake and climatic temperature: relation to fluoridation. *Journal of the Canadian Dental Association*, **31**, 7–16

42. Jenkins, G. N. (1974). *Forum Medici*, No. 18, Zyma, Nyon, Switzerland, p. 33

43. Wespi, H. J. (1964). *Advances in Fluorine Research and Dental Caries Prevention*, Pergamon, Oxford, p. 41

44. Perkinson, J. D., Whitney, I. B., Monroe, R. A., Hotz, W. E. and Comar, C. L. (1955). Metabolism of fluorine 18 in domestic animals. *American Journal of Physiology*, **182**, 383–89

45. Stookey, G. K. (1970). *Fluorides and Human Health*, WHO, Geneva, p. 45

46. Hodge, H. C. and Smith, F. A. (1970). Dietary chemicals vs. dental caries. *Advances in Chemistry*, The American Chemical Society, Washington DC

47. Isaac, S., Brudevold, F., Smith, F. A. and Gardner, D. E. (1958). Solubility rate & natural fluoride content of surface and subsurface enamel *Journal of Dental Research*, **37**, 254–63

48. DePaola, P. F., Brudevold, F., Aasenden, R., R., Moreno, E. C., Englander, H., Bakhos, Y., Bookstein, F. and Warran, J. (1975). A pilot study of the relationship between caries experience and surface enamel fluoride in man. *Archives of Oral Biology*, **20**, 859–64

49. Isaac, S., Brudevold, F., Smith, F. A. and Gardner, D. E. (1958). The relation of fluoride in the drinking water to the distribution of fluoride in enamel. *Journal of Dental Research*, **37**, 318–25

Chapter 11

Prevention of Caries by Control of Dental Plaque

11.1 Introduction

It is clear from the evidence reviewed in previous chapters that dental caries is initiated by microorganisms which colonise the tooth surface in the form of dental plaque. Thus, one obvious way of attempting to prevent caries is by directing prophylactic measures against these microorganisms. Theoretically, perhaps the most straightforward approach would be to eliminate all plaque deposits from the teeth, and several methods have been tried in order to achieve this objective. If complete plaque removal can be achieved and the teeth maintained in plaque-free condition, caries should not occur. From a practical viewpoint, if this approach is adopted, it does not particularly matter whether caries is regarded as a specific infectious disease or a non-specific condition which occurs as one of the sequelae of the metabolism of mixed populations of bacteria in certain sites[1].

An alternative view is that caries is a disease caused only by plaques containing certain specific pathogens, of which the prime candidate is *Streptococcus mutans*. If this hypothesis is valid, it should be possible to control caries by eliminating such pathogens selectively, or by neutralising their harmful products, while leaving the remainder of the plaque microflora relatively intact.

A number of research workers in recent years have taken the view that caries may be a specific infection caused by *S. mutans* and have tried to develop preventive methods, particularly immunological techniques, directed against this species. This approach follows logically from the many studies on experimental caries in animals. However, until further evidence from epidemiological studies on humans becomes available, it is wise to keep an open mind on the microbial specificity of caries. Should it be established that several different combinations of microbial species can be sufficiently acidogenic to produce caries in man, elimination of a single species such as *S. mutans* could not be expected to prevent caries altogether.

Caries preventive methods directed against dental plaque may have one or more of the following objectives:

(1) Prevention of plaque formation by inhibiting all bacterial colonisation of the tooth surface.
(2) Prevention of colonisation by specific pathogenic bacteria.
(3) Removal or disruption of plaque deposits that have already accumulated.
(4) Neutralisation of harmful products of plaque bacteria.
(5) Inhibition of potentially damaging metabolic pathways of plaque bacteria.

Some of these objectives are relevant only if the specific aetiology of caries is accepted. However, non-specific removal or inhibition of the whole plaque will, of course, include any specific pathogens. The methods by which these objectives might be achieved can be divided broadly into three types—mechanical, chemical and immunological.

In the sections which follow some of the evidence for and against these approaches will be reviewed briefly.

11.2 Plaque Control and Caries Prevention by Mechanical Methods

As both dental caries and periodontal disease are caused directly or indirectly by microorganisms in dental plaque, neither disease should occur in a mouth which is maintained totally free of all plaque deposits. Unfortunately, thorough removal of plaque from all surfaces of the teeth is a difficult and time-consuming activity, particularly if the most caries-susceptible sites such as occlusal fissures and approximal surfaces are to be cleaned effectively. Relatively few people, especially children, are sufficiently motivated and have developed the appropriate manual skills to maintain their teeth completely free of dental plaque.

In the Western world, the most widely available and commonly used aid for oral hygiene is the toothbrush. Many variations in size, design and texture of brushes are on the market, so that the prospective purchaser may be confronted with a bewildering selection. From time to time several different toothbrushing techniques have been advocated by dentists[2, 3]; some clinicians today recommend a 'roll' technique, while others prefer a 'scrub' or 'modified Bass' technique. Similarly, a variety of types of toothpaste are commercially available, many of which contain some form of fluoride.

The most important point about toothbrushing, regardless of the type of brush, toothpaste or brushing technique employed, is that it should actually remove plaque effectively from all accessible surfaces without traumatising the soft tissues or abrading the hard tissues. Probably the easiest way to demonstrate the efficacy of plaque removal is by the use of disclosing agents which stain residual deposits and render them clearly visible. Such disclosing agents, available in either liquid or tablet form, are now used routinely in dental surgeries and can also be used by patients at home. Without doubt, disclosing of plaque deposits is an extremely valuable aid in oral hygiene programmes.

As has been pointed out by Gillings[4], the ideal dental plaque disclosant should have the following properties:

(a) be non-toxic;

(b) have an acceptable taste;

(c) be invisible on, or easily removed from, clothing, linen, and surgery and bathroom fixtures;

(d) be invisible in daylight or, if visible, be easily removed from teeth, lips and tongue by rinsing;

(e) offer a colour contrast with the teeth and soft tissues;

(f) provide an indication of the nature of the deposit being stained with respect to age, microorganisms present and metabolic activity;

(g) be economical to use.

A variety of chemical agents have been suggested as disclosing agents, but none fulfils all the requirements listed above. Among the agents commonly used are Bismark brown, basic fuchsin, erythrosin, fast or brilliant green and fluorescein[5]. The latter substance has the advantage of being invisible in normal light, but fluoresces yellow-green under ultraviolet illumination. Iodine has also been used in the past for disclosing plaque, and a mixture of methylene blue and 2,3,5-triphenyl tetrazoleum chloride has been shown to differentiate between areas of plaque with high oxygen content (which stain blue) and more reduced anaerobic areas (red)[6]. A two-tone colour effect can also be produced by combining different dyes such as erythrosin and fast green in a single disclosing solution[7]. Several investigators have shown that disclosing agents may stain plaque in different ways; for example, erythrosin and iodine appear to stain all deposits, whereas fast green and fluorescein tend to stain only older established plaque[4]. An alternative name for erythrosin is tetra-iodo fluorescein, and its structure is very similar to that of fluorescein.

The final choice of disclosing agents is rather subjective. Fluorescein has the advantage of not causing visible staining of the teeth and soft tissues, but requires a special ultraviolet light source. Erythrosin stains all plaque deposits, but also stains the tongue, lips and other tissues. The two-tone disclosing agents have the advantage of differentiating between older deposits and newly formed plaque. Opinions vary as to the aesthetic advantages and ease of visualisation of the different coloured dyes, but any of the currently available disclosing agents can be used effectively as a valuable aid to mechanical plaque control.

No toothbrushing technique, however meticulous, is likely to remove all plaque from approximal areas. In order to clean these sites, which are particularly susceptible to caries, it is necessary to use some additional cleaning aid. The two methods commonly used are dental floss and interdental sticks. It is important that patients are properly instructed in the use of these cleaning aids, since incorrect technique may fail to remove plaque and can inflict damage on the gingival tissues. In one study, no difference was found in the interdental plaque reduction achieved by toothbrushing followed by the use of floss, either waxed or unwaxed[8]. However, daily interdental flossing carried out by research workers produced a significant reduction in approximal caries in 5–6-year-old children over a 20-month period, although there was little residual effect after the flossing regime had been discontinued[9].

Dental prophylaxis carried out professionally by dentists or ancillary personnel has several functions, including the introduction of young or nervous patients to operative procedures. It also serves to provide the patient with a good clean starting condition from which to practise home oral hygiene procedures. The caries-preventive effect of occasional polishing with a rubber cup and prophylactic paste is probably slight, although this can be used as a means of applying fluoride to the teeth. However, more frequent and regular professional prophylaxis, as discussed later, may have an extremely useful role in the prevention of both caries and gingivitis.

The ideal frequency of toothbrushing is largely a matter of opinion at present. Many dentists recommend cleaning the teeth ofter every meal, although it is arguable that brushing before meals might be more beneficial. Pre-prandial brushing should remove potential acid-producing bacteria from the tooth surface before exposure to fermentable carbohydrate and thus decrease the opportunity for carious attack. It is possible that really meticulous plaque removal, including approximal plaque, need only be carried out once a day, or even less frequently. It has been shown that thorough cleaning every 48 hours can prevent the development of gingivitis[10], but since the plaque-removing ability of many people is limited it is probably undesirable to recommend brushing less frequently than once or twice per day.

Until comparatively recently, evidence for the beneficial effects of plaque removal has been related mainly to gingivitis and periodontitis. Numerous epidemiological studies, in various populations and age-groups, have shown a direct relationship between oral hygiene status, or amount of plaque present, and the prevalence

and severity of periodontal disease[11–13]. Experimental studies on animals and in man have demonstrated that gingivitis can be prevented by regular and efficient oral hygiene procedures. The value of these procedures for maintenance of healthy periodontal tissues is well established and supported by clinical experience.

Although there has been widespread belief in the idea that toothbrushing is also valuable for preventing dental caries, evidence for this from controlled studies has, until recently, been lacking. Some investigators have attempted to show a relationship between toothbrushing and oral health by means of surveys, often retrospective in design. In many cases such surveys have failed to demonstrate an obvious connection between observed or stated frequency of toothbrushing and prevalence of caries. However, in most of these investigations the efficacy of plaque removal was not tested.

In one recent study in the USA, the caries experience of 290 12–15-year-old children was correlated with their reported frequency of toothbrushing[14]. This survey showed that subjects who claimed to brush their teeth at least twice a day had lower caries scores (DMFT) than those who brushed once a day or less. However, the possibility that this difference might have been due to increased exposure to fluoride in the frequent-brushing group could not be excluded, since 90 per cent of the subjects were using a fluoride-containing dentifrice. A small reduction in caries incidence related to oral hygiene status and toothbrushing frequency was also observed during a 3-year study on schoolchildren in Britain[15].

Surveys which depend upon the patient's own assessment of toothbrushing habits are difficult to interpret, since the data provided may not always be accurate. In any case, as pointed out previously, the efficacy of oral hygiene procedures is probably of greater importance than reported frequency of application.

Recently, research workers in Sweden have demonstrated that meticulous plaque control can be used successfully to prevent both gingivitis and caries. Studies carried out in the town of Karlstad by Lindhe, Axelsson and their colleagues initially involved 192 children aged 7–14 years. Subjects in the test group were given a fortnightly professional prophylaxis by a dental nurse, including topical application of 5 per cent sodium monofluorophosphate, and repeated instruction in oral hygiene. Dental health education, including motivation of subjects and their parents towards the importance of home care, constituted an important part of the programme. Special attention was given to the cleaning of fissures and interproximal spaces during the professional prophylaxis sessions, disclosing solutions were regularly used, and subjects were instructed in the use of dental floss. Group seminars for parents were held after 12 and 24 months. Children in the control group received neither the professional cleaning nor the intensive oral hygiene instructions. However, they did carry out monthly brushing under supervision at school, using a 0.25 per cent NaF solution.

After two years of this study, children in the test group had virtually no plaque deposits or gingivitis and had experienced an extremely low average increment of 0.1 new carious lesions per year. In contrast, the control group had higher plaque scores, showed signs of gingivitis and developed an average of 3.1 new carious lesions per year. The study was continued for a third year, during which the interval between the professional prophylaxes was increased from 2 to 4 or 8 weeks. The remarkable differences in plaque, gingivitis and caries score between test and control subjects were maintained. A summary of the caries results from this study is shown in table 11.1.

It is clear that the intensive and efficient regime undertaken by the subjects in the test groups almost entirely eliminated caries during the study period. There is a possibility that some of the caries-preventive effect could have been due to the repeated application of topical fluoride rather than the plaque removal *per se*. However, in a parallel study by the same authors[17], this proposition was tested on a further group of 82

Table 11.1   Effect of oral hygiene on caries—new carious surfaces in Swedish schoolchildren* (from Lindhe, Axelsson and Tollskog[16])

Group (age at start in 1971)	1 (7–8)		2 (10–11)		3 (13–14)	
	Test	Control	Test	Control	Test	Control
Number of subjects	40	40	37	27	16	17
1971/72	5	125	0	90	1	66
1972/73	6	57	5	83	2	115
1973/74	2	68	15	98	6	88
1971–74	13	250	20	271	9	269

* Figures show total number of carious lesions plus recurrent caries during trial.
† Test subjects = frequent professional prophylaxis and oral hygiene instruction.
‡ Control subjects = monthly supervised brushing with 0.2 per cent NaF solution.

children. In this experiment, the control group followed the regime described above for the test group (that is, fortnightly prophylaxis using 5 per cent sodium monofluorophosphate paste), whereas the test group had a similar programme, except that no fluoride was included. After 12 months there was no significant difference between the caries experience of the two groups. Thus, it seems that the plaque control rather than the topical fluoride is the important factor in these investigations.

In a subsequent large-scale field trial, using essentially the same methods but with seven newly recruited dental nurses carrying out the oral hygiene instruction and prophylaxis procedures, rather less impressive reductions in plaque, gingivitis and caries scores were obtained (59 per cent, 73 per cent and 51 per cent; respectively)[18]. However, the results are still encouraging and further studies on other populations are now required in order to evaluate this approach as a potentially viable public health measure.

A similar study has been carried out on 7-year-old children in Denmark in an attempt to establish the beneficial effect of professional prophylaxis by itself, without the added emphasis on home-care methods[19]. In this trial a statistically significant reduction in plaque accumulation between test and control groups was observed after 12 months. The experimental group, which had received fortnightly mechanical tooth cleansing (without fluoride) showed a 70 per cent reduction in caries incidence in permanent teeth compared to controls which were present at both the baseline and 12-month examinations. It appeared from this study that the fortnightly professional cleaning was effective in improving oral hygiene. These results confirmed the observations previously described that thorough and regular plaque removal can markedly reduce the incidence of dental caries.

From these studies it would appear that simple methods already exist which could be effective in preventing the major dental diseases. Efficient plaque control, together with diet regulation, use of fluorides and other measures referred to in accompanying chapters, should be capable of eliminating most, if not all, caries and gingivitis. The problems really lie with implementation of the existing knowledge.

In order to be successful in preventing caries by mechanical plaque-control methods, the following points appear to be particularly important:

(1)   All plaque deposits must be removed thoroughly.

(2)   Attention must be given to approximal surfaces; dental floss, wood points and interspace brushes can be used for this purpose.

(3)   Efficacy of plaque removal methods should be checked by means of disclosing agents.

(4)   Frequency of plaque removal may be of less importance than efficacy. For example, one thorough clean per day is preferable to three inefficient attempts at brushing.

(5)   Periodic professional prophylaxis is a useful adjunct to home tooth-cleaning procedures.

Two major factors are of importance when implementation of these measures is being considered—motivation and cost effectiveness.

Motivation of children and their families was an essential part of the Swedish studies described above, and to have any hope of success a high degree of cooperation must be achieved so that recommended oral hygiene measures are actually carried out. Good responses can be achieved on an individual basis when one operator is dealing with relatively small numbers of subjects. However, it is far more difficult to persuade large numbers of people to adopt scrupulous plaque control on a community scale. Motivation of large groups of people to change their patterns of behaviour is one of the major problems of health education in general, and dental health education is no exception[20, 21]. Much work is required in order to find out how best to encourage people to practise existing preventive procedures which are known to be beneficial[22, 23].

Individual health education and regular professional prophylaxis sessions take time, are extremely labour-intensive and, therefore, expensive. Thus, the type of preventive regime tested in the Lindhe and Axelsson studies may not be sufficiently cost effective to allow adoption on a community basis. In the Swedish studies it was found that the test subjects required 3 hours of professional time per year in order to carry out the prophylaxis and oral hygiene instruction. The equivalent amount of time which would have been needed to treat the disease prevented by this regimen was estimated to be 2.3 hours per year[70]. However, much of the preventive programme could be carried out by less highly qualified staff than the dental surgeon, so that 'preventive time' is less expensive than 'treatment time'. The feasibility and potential cost effectiveness of adopting an extensive plaque control programme on a community basis remains to be tested.

11.3   Chemical Agents for Plaque Control

A variety of chemical approaches to the control of dental plaque and caries have been considered over the years[1, 24]. Antimicrobial agents such as antibiotics and antiseptics, administered either systemically or locally, may interfere with the development of new plaque deposits and also influence the activities of pre-existing plaque bacteria. Depending upon the spectrum of antimicrobial activity of the chemical agent selected, such effects might be directed against a wide range of oral bacteria or, alternatively, restricted to a limited section of the microflora.

Interference with the formation of plaque matrix, or disruption of existing matrix, has been attempted by means of various enzyme preparations including, notably, dextranases. Fluoride, in addition to its effects on enamel, may also achieve some cariostatic action by interfering with plaque microorganisms. Thus, several quite different methods of controlling plaque by chemical means can already be considered and it is likely that many new agents and mechanisms will be suggested from time to time.

In an attempt to modify the oral microflora by means of antimicrobial agents, several potential dangers must be taken into account, particularly if the treatment is to be continued for prolonged periods of time. These include colonisation of the mouth, and possibly other parts of the body, by undesirable microorganisms (for example, *Candida albicans* following tetracycline therapy), selection of a resistant population of bacteria in the mouth and toxic side-effects of the chemotherapeutic agent.

The ideal anti-caries agent, according to Fitzgerald[40], should have the following properties:

(1)   Should not be used for treatment of other diseases.

(2)   Should be stable in storage, unaffected by components of the vehicle and active over the pH range and other ambient conditions encountered in dental plaque.

(3)   Should absorb to teeth or plaque without loss of activity.

(4)   Should have a narrow antibacterial spectrum.

(5)   Should be rapidly bactericidal against both resting and multiplying organisms and should have a low potential for inducing the emergence of resistance in the microflora.

(6)   Should be non-toxic, non-allergenic, non-absorbable and have acceptable organoleptic properties.

(7)   Should be biodegradable or destroyed in the gastrointestinal tract if ingested.

(8)   Should be inexpensive and easy to produce.

At present there does not appear to be anything available which is both an effective cariostatic agent and also satisfies all the criteria listed above. The properties of some of the numerous chemical agents which have been tested are summarised in the following sections.

11.3.1   Antibiotics

Experiments on animals have shown that addition of penicillin to the diet and drinking water can effectively prevent dental caries[25]. Similar results have also been obtained with several antibiotics, particularly those active against Gram-positive bacteria[26]. The success of these early animal studies led to clinical trials in humans in which penicillin was incorporated in toothpaste or tooth powder. Several such investigations were undertaken, but with mixed results[1]. In some cases, where toothbrushing was unsupervised, no reduction in caries was obtained, whereas in one study, with supervised brushing, a 55 per cent reduction in DMFS was observed after one year compared to control subjects[27].

The actual time of exposure of the oral microflora to penicillin in the human toothpaste experiments was short compared to the animal studies, where the antibiotic was available all the time. Because of this restricted exposure time, it is therefore not surprising that only limited success was obtained in these human studies. There is also a strong likelihood that resistant strains of bacteria could be selected by the repeated use of a penicillin dentifrice. Since penicillin is such an important antibiotic for treatment of a variety of serious infections, the use of this agent for prophylaxis against caries was wisely discontinued after the initial trials.

As mentioned in chapter 3, the fact that antibiotics such as penicillin can reduce the incidence of caries has also been demonstrated in subjects who have received long-term prophylaxis for prevention of recurrence of rheumatic fever. However, a more recent study on patients receiving such prophylaxis, while confirming the caries reduction noted in early surveys, did not show any noticeable effect on the prevalence of *Streptococcus mutans* in plaque[28]. Perhaps the main conclusion that can be drawn from various studies on penicillin and caries in humans is that caries can be reduced by means of an antimicrobial agent, even though penicillin is not the most appropriate drug for this purpose.

Several other antibiotics have been tested in humans for their ability to reduce plaque formation or to inhibit specific microorganisms within plaque[1, 24]. Usually these agents have been applied topically as gels or mouthrinses. Ideally, the drugs should not be those regarded as 'front-line' drugs for treatment of acute infections. Among the antibiotics which have been examined are vancomycin, kanamycin and spiramycin. Vancomycin has been shown to reduce the amount of plaque and gingivitis in mentally defective subjects, but was ineffective as a plaque inhibiting agent in healthy individuals with no pre-existing gingival inflammation. Topical application of kanamycin has also been tested in mentally retarded subjects. In one study, a 57 per cent reduction in plaque was observed 24 days after cessation of a 5-day course of treatment[29]. Bacteriological examination of the plaques showed that topical kanamycin treatment selectively reduced the streptococcal population, especially *S. sanguis* and *S. mitior*, which together were reduced from 30 per cent to 3 per cent of the total flora.

The use of antibiotics for control of plaque has proved to be a valuable research tool, but it is dubious whether this is the correct approach to caries prevention on a public health scale. As mentioned already, there are several theoretical objections to the widespread, long-term use of antibiotics for this purpose, including: selection of antibiotic resistant strains of bacteria; suppression of normal flora and overgrowth by less desirable species; and allergic or other adverse reactions to the drug.

However, in selected cases, such as mentally or physically handicapped patients, or immediately after surgery, there may be a case for the application of antimicrobial agents for plaque control. The agents used should ideally be those which are not used for the treatment of serious systemic infections.

11.3.2 Chlorhexidine and other antiseptics

Chlorhexidine is a disinfectant which has been in general use for many years and is known to be active against a wide range of Gram-positive and Gram-negative bacteria, as well as some yeasts. This agent is one of the bis-biguanides and is usually used in the form of chlorhexidine gluconate (trade name Hibitane). It has been shown that chlorhexidine is rapidly adsorbed to test organisms such as *Escherichia coli* and *Staphylococcus aureus* in vitro, and that it changes the permeability of the cells by interfering with the normal function of the cell membrane. Although chlorhexidine has a wide spectrum of antibacterial activity, some Gram-negative organisms, such as *Pseudomonas* species, can be extremely resistant.

Considerable interest was aroused when it was demonstrated that chlorhexidine gluconate can inhibit dental plaque formation[30, 31]. Several studies have shown that substitution of mechanical tooth cleaning by mouthrinsing or topical application of chlorhexidine can prevent plaque accumulation and the development of gingivitis. A group of research workers in Denmark have developed a system for studying experimental gingivitis and caries in student volunteers, and this system was used to investigate the potential ability of chlorhexidine to prevent caries[32]. Eight students who stopped all oral hygiene procedures and were given 9 mouth rinses per day with a 50 per cent sucrose solution, developed heavy accumulations of plaque and showed the earliest signs of caries after 22 days. Another group of students underwent the same regime, but also rinsed their mouths twice a day with 0.2 per cent chlorhexidine gluconate. These subjects had considerably less plaque and showed no signs of caries after the experimental period. The authors concluded that the prevention of plaque formation by means of the chlorhexidine mouthrinse inhibits the development of caries (and gingivitis), even in the face of the challenge of frequent sucrose rinses.

Prior to the experimental studies on the effects of chlorhexidine on plaque formation it had been shown that this agent could inhibit plaque formation and caries in animals. In recent years, investigations have been carried out in order to determine the spectrum of activity of chlorhexidine against oral microorganisms and the possible development of resistant strains of bacteria following long-term use of this agent, the mode of action of plaque inhibition, factors which may affect anti-plaque activity and methods of delivery or administration of the drug. In addition, several clinical trials have been reported. Some aspects of the numerous investigations on chlorhexidine are summarised below.

Susceptibility of oral flora

Microorganisms exhibiting some degree of resistance to chlorhexidine have been isolated from the mouths of subjects who have received local applications of this drug for some time. For example, in one study the use of chlorhexidine mouthwash for 6 months resulted in an increase in the level of chlorhexidine-resistant streptococci which could be isolated[33]. The number of *Streptococcus mutans* isolated was reduced by the chlorhexidine regime, while the proportion of *S. sanguis* was correspondingly raised. Other studies have shown that *S. mutans* levels in plaque also appear to be reduced following the use of chlorhexidine gel, and once again this is accompanied by an apparent increase in *S. sanguis*[34, 35].

The susceptibility of various microorganisms

to chlorhexidine has been studied in detail by Emilson[36]. Low minimal inhibitory concentrations (MICs) were found with staphylococci, *S. mutans*, *S. salivarius* and *E. coli*, while strains of *Proteus*, *Pseudomonas* and *Klebsiella* were less susceptible. *S. sanguis* varied in susceptibility, both low and high MICs being noted among different strains. *Propionibacterium* and *Selenomonas* were the most susceptible anaerobes examined, and the least susceptible were found to be Gram-negative cocci which resembled *Veillonella*.

Mode of action

Several workers have investigated the possible mode of action whereby chlorhexidine inhibits plaque formation, and these mechanisms have been reviewed in detail by Rölla and Melsen[37]. The plaque-inhibiting activity is apparently a unique property of the bis-biguanides, which is not due solely to any initial bactericidal effect since other agents with higher killing activities against oral bacteria do not produce the same marked clinical effects. It is likely that plaque inhibition by bis-biguanides is related to their retention in the mouth; for example, about 30 per cent of the chlorhexidine introduced in a mouthwash is retained in the mouth. Studies carried out at different pH levels indicate the acidic groups, presumably on the macromolecules of mucous secretions, are the main receptor sites. Electrostatic binding between the basic bis-biguanide molecule and acid protein groups (for example, SO_{3-}, COO^- and PO_{3-}) may be the mechanism involved. Displacement of the chlorhexidine from phosphate or carboxyl groups by divalent cations, such as calcium, could explain part of the long-term antibacterial effects in vivo. In the conclusions of their review, Rolla and Melsen suggested four possible mechanisms for the anti-plaque effects of chlorhexidine:

(1)   The number of bacteria present in saliva which are available for adsorption to the teeth is reduced.

(2)   Blocking of acidic groups on salivary

glycoproteins reduces their adsorption to tooth surfaces and thus inhibits plaque and pellicle formation.

(3) Adsorption of salivary bacterial cells to the teeth may be reduced if their surfaces are covered with bound chlorhexidine.

(4) By precipitating the acidic bacterial agglutinating factors known to be present in saliva and by displacement of calcium ions, the cohesiveness of plaque bacteria may be altered.

Some investigators have demonstrated a caries-inhibitory effect of topically applied chlorhexidine in rats[38, 39], but so far there has been no convincing demonstration of caries reduction in humans in long-term clinical trials. Short-term human studies have been reported, as discussed earlier, but the caries data here are based on early smooth lesions only. Other clinical experiments on medical and dental students have produced little or no conclusive evidence for the caries-reducing effect of chlorhexidine.

The possibility of combining chlorhexidine with some other known cariostatic agent, such as fluoride, is currently being explored and there is some evidence that such a combination can have a significant long-term caries-reducing effect in humans[71]. As already noted, short-term use of a fluoride-containing chlorhexidine gel can cause alterations in the plaque microflora including a marked reduction in *S. mutans* levels[35]. The long-term beneficial effect of chlorhexidine as a cariostatic agent remains to be demonstrated.

There are some distinct disadvantages of chlorhexidine. One of these is its unpleasant taste, which needs to be masked by addition of other flavouring compounds. The other main problem is the formation of an unsightly brown stain on the teeth, particularly around silicate restorations. Fortunately, this can be removed by polishing and it is claimed that patients can control the formation of the stain by regular use of a normal abrasive paste in addition to chlorhexide-containing gel or solution.

The methods of application of chlorhexidine which have been tried include topical application of chlorhexidine solution, mouthrinsing and brushing with chlorhexidine gel. There is little evidence available at present to indicate which particular formulation and method of application, if any, is most valuable for caries prevention.

The main advantage of chlorhexidine as a plaque-inhibiting agent, compared to other antibacterial substances, is the adsorption and slow release which takes place in the mouth. Other chemical agents which do not become so strongly adsorbed to oral surfaces probably remain in contact with plaque for too short a time during mouthrinsing or toothbrushing to exert any significant effect on the tooth surface flora.

The literature on the dental aspects of chlorhexidine is extensive, and further information can be obtained from several recent reviews[1, 24, 37, 41, 42]. How useful and acceptable this antiseptic will prove to be in terms of plaque control on a community basis remains to be seen.

Other antiseptic chemical agents

Apart from chlorhexidine, several other antimicrobial agents have been tested either in vitro or in vivo for anti-plaque activity[1, 24]. These agents include quaternary ammonium compounds and surface-active agents. In one particular investigation[43], in which a large number of agents were screened in the laboratory, the four most promising compounds were found to be chlorhexidine gluconate, dodecylamine, zephiran chloride and victamine C. Several agents have undergone clinical tests for anti-plaque or anti-calculus activity, but none has so far been shown to have an obvious application for prevention of dental caries.

11.3.3 Enzymes

Several enzyme preparations have been used in the past in an attempt to prevent the formation, or cause disruption, of dental plaque and calculus. Early studies included trials of mucinase, polysaccharideases, pancreatic enzymes and various multi-enzyme 'cocktails'[24]. More recently, attention has been concentrated on enzymes

Table 11.2   The effect of dextranase on the incidence of caries in monkeys (from Bowen[48])

| Group | No. of carious lesions | | | No. of carious teeth |
	12 months	24 months	36 months	36 months
Experimental (6 animals)	12	19	27	16
Control (6 animals)	27	32	49	27

which specifically break down the extracellular polysaccharides, such as dextran and mutan, which are produced by some oral streptococci and which make up an important part of plaque matrix.

Dextranase preparations can be obtained from culture supernatants of certain moulds, such as *Penicillium funculosum* and *P. lilacinum*. Such enzymes were shown to disperse accumulations of dextran-forming streptococci in the test-tube, and it seemed logical to test similar preparations for plaque-inhibiting activity in experimental animals. Rather mixed results were reported from experiments carried out on rodents. In one study[44], almost complete protection against caries was achieved by feeding albino hamsters with dextranase produced from culture of *P. funiculosum*, whereas dextranase obtained from *P. lilacinum* had little or no such effect in rats[45].

Several short-term studies on the effects of dextranase mouthwashes on plaque formation in humans have been reported. In two trials, some reduction in plaque accumulation was observed[46, 47]. None of these experiments was continued for long enough to show any effect of the enzyme on the incidence of disease.

Data on the caries-reducing activity of dextranase in the monkey (*Macaca irus*) has also been published[48]. Using a small group of monkeys, dextranase added to the diet produced a significant reduction in the number of carious lesions over a period of 3 years (table 11.2).

Although the caries reduction was impressive, the monkeys in the experimental group also showed a reduced white blood cell count. Thus, further studies on the toxicity of the enzyme preparation, as well as suitable methods of delivery, would be required before it could be administered to humans.

The dextranase enzymes used in the studies reviewed briefly above are effective against the predominantly α-1, 6 soluble glucose polymers by some oral streptococci, rather than the insoluble α-1, 3 linked polymers referred to as 'mutan', which are typical of *Streptococcus mutans*. Guggenheim has isolated a mutanase enzyme from a mould which can hydrolyse the mutan-type of polysaccharide and this has been shown to have a significant caries-reducing effect in rodents consuming a high-sucrose, cariogenic diet[49].

Although various studies on the use of enzymes as potential plaque-control agents have produced some interesting and useful results, it does not appear at present that this is likely to be the most helpful method for widespread use in humans. The dextranase and mutanase enzymes which are aimed at disrupting the carbohydrate components of the plaque matrix would need to be effective against several different linkages for maximum effect, and this would necessitate including several different enzymes in the final product. There are also problems in the potential toxicity of any preparations used, which must be very carefully monitored, and in finding the most appropriate method of delivery to the site of action. Inclusion of dextranase in human diets is unlikely to be feasible, since any cooking procedure would inactivate the enzyme.

11.3.4   Fluoride

Much of the beneficial effect of the fluoride ion in relation to the prevention of caries is thought to be due to its ability to increase the resistance of enamel to acid attack, and this aspect is covered in detail in other chapters. However, for the sake of completeness, it should be mentioned in the context of this chapter that some of the observed cariostatic effect may be due to the influence of fluoride on plaque bacteria and their enzymes (chapter 5). The fluoride ion is well known for its ability to inhibit a variety of enzymes, including some of those involved in acid production by bacteria[50].

It has been suggested by Hamilton[50] that low levels of fluoride may interfere with carbohydrate metabolism by one or more of the following mechanisms: (a) inhibition of enolase and consequently transport of glucose into cells; (b) inhibition of sugar translocation in membranes; (c) interference with cation transport and accumulation in cells; (d) inhibition of cellular phosphatases which dephosphorylate sugar phosphates resulting from transport.

It is also possible that, in addition to inhibition of transport mechanisms and glycolysis, fluoride may have an effect on glycogen synthesis[51, 52]. An inhibitory effect on extracellular polysaccharide production seems less likely from *in vitro* studies[53], although plaque from subjects who have been exposed to relatively high levels of fluoride appears to contain less extracellular polysaccharide than controls with low fluoride exposure[54].

Although fluoride is known to have an inhibitory effect on many bacterial enzymes *in vitro*, the importance of this *in vivo* is not so clear. Most laboratory experiments in the past have been carried out under highly artificial conditions, usually in batch culture systems where the microorganisms may achieve unnaturally high rates of growth. Studies on oral bacteria,

such as *S. mutans*, grown in continuous culture in a chemostat, have shown that the effect of fluoride on acid production varieş according to the conditions employed[55]. When a strain of *S. mutans* was grown under glucose-limited conditions, at a fixed pH of 6.5, it was observed that 15 p.p.m. of fluoride ion could prevent acid production when the organisms were growing slowly (dilution rate $(D) = 0.05\,h^{-1}$, mean generation time $= 14\,h$). In contrast, when the streptococci were allowed to grow ten times faster $(D = 0.5\,h^{-1})$, the rate of acid production was unaffected by as much as 100 p.p.m. of F^-. Fluoride also affected the rate of acid produced when pulses of sugars such as glucose, fructose or sucrose were added to a chemostat culture of *S. mutans*, and similar effects have been noted with mixed cultures of plaque microorganisms[56].

From the data available it is clear that the effect of fluoride on acid production is related to the speed at which bacteria are growing. Not much is known about the actual rate of growth of bacteria within plaque, although it is generaly believed to be slow compared to that of batch grown organisms in laboratory culture media. However, it is likely that different species within plaque grow at different rates and that these rates fluctuate according to the availability of dietary substrates.

As well as inhibiting enzyme activities, fluoride may also influence the colonisation of enamel and pellicle by altering their surface properties, or by exerting a direct bactericidal effect on plaque bacteria[1]. Several investigators have looked for evidence that various fluoride compounds may interfere with plaque formation either *in vitro*, in experimental animals or in humans[57-63]. From most of these studies it seems that fluoride compounds containing bivalent cations do have a plaque-inhibitory effect, while only one study indicated a similar effect with sodium fluoride[58]. Clearly the form in which fluoride is delivered, the concentration and availability of the fluoride ion are all important factors which will influence potential antimicrobial activity.

There is evidence to show that topical application of fluorides can influence the streptococcal populations within plaque, especially the relative numbers of *S. mutans*[64–66]. For example, one study showed that 1.23 per cent APF gel, applied in applicator trays over a period of two weeks, could produce a marked reduction in *S. mutans* levels compared to a placebo gel. A similar effect on relative numbers of *S. sanguis* was not observed[66].

The practical significance of the antimicrobial or anti-enzymic properties of the fluoride ion in relation to the overall caries-reducing effect of this element is not clear at present. No attempt has been made in this brief section to analyse the extensive literature on this topic exhaustively, but more detailed information can be found in recent reviews[67, 68]. However, it does seem probable that the known beneficial effects in terms of reducing enamel solubility may be enhanced by additional antibacterial (or anti-plaque) properties of fluoride.

11.3.5   Methods of delivery of chemotherapeutic agents

In the preceding sections of this chapter, various potential chemical agents for the control of dental plaque and dental caries have been discussed. Any such agent must be administered in such a way that it comes into contact with the target microorganisms at a suitable concentration and for a sufficient length of time, in order to achieve the desired effect.

A wide variety of vehicles have been considered for delivery of chemical agents designed to be effective in controlling caries. These include the following:

> diet
> drinking water
> dentifrices
> prophylaxis pastes (for professional application)
> mouthrinses
> gels and applicator trays
> irrigation devices
> chewing gum
> tablets and lozenges
> powder aerosols

A disadvantage of many of these methods of delivery is that the actual time of exposure of plaque microorganisms to the active ingredient is relatively short, so that frequently repeated applications may be required. Chemotherapeutic agents such as chlorhexidine, which adhere to the tooth surface or plaque and are released over a period of time, have a distinct advantage in this respect.

An interesting new development is the use of devices which are inserted in the appropriate part of the body and slowly release their active chemotherapeutic ingredient over a prolonged period of time. Such controlled-release devices have been used in the eye for treatment of glaucoma and in the uterus for contraceptive purposes. Investigations are now in progress to develop and test similar devices which may be used intra-orally for controlled release of fluoride and, possibly, other cariostatic agents[69].

11.4   Immunisation

The concept that dental caries is an infectious disease caused by specific pathogens, as outlined in chapter 3, has led research workers to explore the possibility that the disease can be prevented by immunisation[72, 73]. Despite some scepticism concerning the likely benefits of immune mechanisms in protection against dental caries[74, 75], a large amount of experimental work has been carried out in recent years (for reviews, see the list of Further Reading at the end of the chapter).

Studies on human populations have indicated that there may be difference in antibody levels between subjects with different amount of caries. In particular, a correlation has been reported between low caries experience and high titres of serum IgG and IgM antibodies against antigens of *S. mutans*[76, 77]. In contrast, there is little evidence to suggest that salivary IgA antibodies play a significant role in protection against caries in man[78, 79].

All the information concerning artificial immunisation against dental caries has so far been obtained from animal experiments, and at the time of writing no human trials have been attempted. The scientific basis of attempting to control dental caries immunologically may be stated simply as follows;

(1) The disease is a specific infection caused by *S. mutans*.

(2) An artificially induced immune response to *S. mutans* antigens may protect against caries.

(3) Protective antibodies may reach caries-susceptible sites either via saliva (local IgA response) or crevicular fluid (systemic IgG and IgM response).

As discussed in chapter 3, it is likely that bacteria other than *S. mutans* may play a role in caries. Thus, even if immunisation against *S. mutans* is highly effective, the possibility remains that other species may continue to cause some disease.

In fact, before the relatively recent explosion of interest in the role of *S. mutans*, investigators explored the possibility of reducing caries by immunising against lactobacilli[80, 81].

As might be expected, the majority of the immunisation studies have been carried out using vaccines prepared from various strains of *S. mutans*, although a limited number of other bacterial species have occasionally been tested. The type of vaccine, dose, route of administration, strain of animal employed and other experimental conditions have varied considerably from study to study. In some cases, whole bacterial cell vaccines have been used, while in others some bacterial product such as crude glucosyl-transferase preparations have been employed. Investigators have attempted to stimulate either systemic or local production of antibodies, or both, by injecting the vaccines at different sites, such as intravenously, intramuscularly or submucosally near the salivary glands. Attempts have also been made to enhance the immune response non-specifically by injecting adjuvants (for example, Freund's adjuvant) together with the antigen. In some cases, serum and salivary antibody levels have been monitored sequentially, while in other studies less attention has been given to one or other of these factors. Apart from differences in the strains and ages of animals used for vaccine studies, details of the experimental procedures adopted have varied amongst different laboratories. Thus gnotobiotic antibiotic-treated and conventional animal systems have been tried, with a variety of dietary regimes (but almost invariably with a high sucrose content).

In view of all the experimental variables outlined above, it is hardly surprising that different success rates have been obtained by different workers. Some of the results reported appear to be contradictory or difficult to interpret, and comparisons between experiments carried out in different laboratories is difficult.

Research in this field has been carried out either in rodents (rats and hamsters) or in monkeys (rhesus, *Macaca mulatta*, and irus, *Macaca fascicularis*). A critical assessment of the published work on caries immunisation up to the end of 1975 has been contributed by Bowen[82], and detailed analyses of more recent investigations are presented in the book edited by McGhee *et al.*[83].

Relatively few investigators have used the hamster for vaccination studies. The published results from this model system are summarised in table 11.3. The earliest of the experiments failed to show a reduction in caries[84], but most of the more recent studies have demonstrated a cariostatic effect. In one study[88], it was shown that local

Table 11.3 Summary of published results on immunisation studies in hamsters*

Antigen	Route	Reduction in caries	Antibodies serum	saliva	Ref.
S.mutans (HS-6)	SC	−	NR	NR	84
S.species (SS-2)	IM	+	+	+	85
GTF	IP	+	+	+	86
S.mutans (6715)	IP	−	NR	NR	87
GTF	SC (salivary)	+	NR	NR	88

* Abbreviations:
  GTF = glucosyltransferase
  SC = subcutaneous
  IM = intramuscular
  IP = intraperitoneal
  NR = not recorded

Table 11.4 Summary of published results on immunisation studies in rats*

Antigen	Route	Reduction in caries	Antibodies serum	saliva	Ref.
S. faecalis	IM	+	+	+	89
GTF	IP	+	+	NR	90
GTF	IP	+	+	NR	91
GTF	IV	−	+	−	92
S. mutans (OMZ 176)	IV	+	+	NR	92
S. mutans (6715)	SC	+	+	NR	93
S. mutans (6715)	SC (salivary)	+	+	+	94
S. mutans (6715)	SC (salivary)	+	+	+	95
GTF	SC (salivary)	+	+	+	96
S. mutans (6715)	SC (salivary)	+	+	+	97
S. mutans (6715)	Oral	+	−	+	98, 99
S. faecalis	IM	+	+	+	100

* For abbreviations see footnote to table 11.3.

immunisation in the salivary gland region with GTF prepared from a strain of *S. mutans* serotype *c* (strain Ingbritt) reduced colonisation of the teeth and the number of carious lesions caused by infection with the homologous strain when compared with sham-injected control animals. There was also some evidence of cross-reactivity and protection against infection with a different serotype (strain 6715, serotype *g*). The type of antibody involved in the protective response in hamsters has not been recorded in several of the published reports.

The rat has been used more extensively in immunisation studies and a summary of the results obtained is given in table 11.4. Although many of these studies have shown a caries-protective effect by a variety of immunisation regimes, some negative results have also been recorded[92, 93]. In one study, variable results were obtained in different experiments[94]. Protection against caries was noted in three out of five experiments, enhancement of caries occurred in one, and no effect was observed in the fifth experiment of this series. Several studies have shown that a protective immune response can be

obtained by immunising the animals locally in the salivary gland region[95-97] or even administering the vaccine orally[98, 99]. Such routes of immunisation generally induce a local salivary IgA response, with or without an accompanying serum (IgG, IgM) response.

Reviewing the results of immunisation experiments using the rodent carries model, Smith and Taubman conclude[101]: Taken together, the immunisation experiments which have been performed in the rat caries model system appear to suggest a correlation between the presence of salivary antibody to *S. mutans* and reductions in caries caused by these bacteria. However, the multifactorial nature of this disease does not permit at present the conclusion that the presence of this antibody is both necessary and sufficient to give rise to the demonstrated effects on pathogenicity.'

Probably the best experimental model for dental caries is the monkey, since the dentitition and pattern of disease is more comparable to that of man. Several immunisation studies have been carried out in monkeys, and the results of these are summarised in table 11.5.

Table 11.5   Summary of published results on immunisation studies in monkeys*

Antigen	Route	Reduction in caries	Antibodies serum	Antibodies saliva	Ref.
S. mutans (Ingbritt)	IV	+	+	NR	102
S. mutans (Ingbritt)	SM	+	+	NR	103
GTF	SM	−	+	NR	103
S. mutans (C)	SC, SM	+	+	+	104–106
S. mutans (6715)	SC (parotid)	+	+	+	107
CAG	Parotid	?	+	+	108
GTF	SC	−	+	+	109
S. mutans (Ingbritt)	SC (parotid)	+	+	−	110
GTF	SC (parotid)	+	+	−	110

* Abbreviations:
   IV = intravenous.
   SM = submucosal.
   SC = subcutaneous.
  CAG = cell-associated glucan.
  GTF = glucosyltransferase.
   NR = not recorded.

Following a successful pilot experiment at the Royal College of Surgeons Research Establishment at Downe[102], in which a small group of irus animals were protected against caries by intravenous injection of whole S. mutans cells, a series of different immunogen preparations were tested[103].

Preparations containing whole cells or disrupted cells conferred protection against dental caries, whereas several glucosyl-transferase enzyme preparations, of varying degress of purity, failed to protect the animals. In fact, there was some indication that the enzyme immunisation may have enhanced the susceptibility of test amimals to the disease, possibly by giving rise to increased numbers of S. mutans in the plaque. The authors of this study also suggested that intra-oral submucosal injection of vaccine might prove to be more effective than conventional subcutaneous injection, presumably by stimulating local antibody production in addition to serum antibodies.

Another group of British workers, working at Guy's Hospital, have reported a series of experiments on immunisations against dental caries in rhesus monkeys (Macaca mulatta), using a heat-killed S. mutans, serotype c vaccine[104, 111]. In one of these studies it was shown that animals which gave a brisk (within one month) serum antibody response to an antigen preparation from the immunising strain developed little or no caries during the two-year experimental period. In contrast. those animals in which the antibody response was slow (5–12 months to attain 1/16 titre) were not protected and rapidly developed caries[104–106]. It is clear, therefore, that several factors, including optimum antibody titres and rate of antibody response, may influence the subsequent developing of caries in immunised animals.

Further studies by this group[112], have indicated that low caries scores obtained in immunised animals could be correlated with a low percentage count of S. mutans in the crevicular fluid and 'crevicular fluid/plaque zone' and an increased serum antibody titre against the organism. A similar relationship was not found between salivary antibodies and S. mutans in saliva or superficial plaque. The authors proposed the hypothesis that the immune components of crevicular fluid may be responsible for protection of smooth surfaces against caries. Thus, it might be argued that a moderate degree of gingivitis should be encouraged in order to increase the flow of crevicular fluid!

In a further study on the immune responses in vaccinated monkeys, evidence of cell-mediated responses, due to T-lymphocytes, in addition to antibody production, has been presented[113, 114]. The authors postulate that T- and B-cell cooperation may also take place. The idea that cell-mediated immunity may play a role in protection against dental caries is perhaps surprising, since access of sensitised lymphocytes to the site of caries initiation must be limited. However, it is essential that all possible mechanisms should be examined in caries vaccine studies. In fact, recent studies indicate that not only lymphocytes but also polymorphonuclear leucotyes may be involved in the 'crevicular domain', helping to confer protection by actively phagocytosing microorganisms, including *S. mutans*[115].

The possible routes by which antibodies and immunologically primed cells may reach caries-susceptible sites are illustrated diagramatically in figure 11.1. The significance of the salivary and crevicular factors may vary at different tooth surfaces. For example, salivary IgA could be of particular relevance in the pits and fissures, whereas crevicular fluid may be more important in the approximal and cervical areas of the tooth.

11.4.1 Mechanisms of action

The protective mechanisms by which the immune response may prevent dental caries are not fully understood, although there is experimental evidence to show that immunisation with vaccines derived from *S. mutans* can be effective in animals. Assuming that antibodies or immunologically sensitised cells reach the tooth–plaque interface by one of the routes described above, the following modes of action may be considered as theoretical possibilities;

(1) Opsonisation and phagocytosis of bacteria.

(2) Lysis of bacteria by antibody and complement.

(3) Interference with colonisation of the tooth, possibly by antiglucosyltransferase activity which prevents production of extracellular glucan.

(4) Inhibition of bacterial metabolism.

At present, most of the available evidence suggests that modes (1) and (3) may occur; there is no experimental support for mode (4).

11.4.2 Passive immunity

In addition to the rapidly increasing number of reports on active immunisation against dental caries, a few investigators have also demonstrated that immunity can be transferred passively. The results of such studies are summarised in table 11.6. In rats, protection has been transferred from dams to their suckling pups via milk. Both locally induced IgA antibody, following intra-mammary or oral immunisation, and systemic IgG antibody appears to be effective[116]. An interesting additional finding from the same research group in Birmingham, Alabama, is that protection can also be achieved by oral administration of bovine milk from cows immunised with *S. mutans*[118].

Passive transfer of immunity to dental caries has also been demonstrated in the monkey model system. In this case, caries reduction was not achieved by transfer of immune serum alone, whereas protection could be shown in animals given separated IgG antibody[117]. However, administration of whole serum together with transfer factor (a soluble extract obtained from pooled lymphocytes) did confer immunity to recipient animals[113].

From these experiments it would appear that both secretory IgA antibody and serum IgG antibody are able to confer a protective effect against dental caries.

11.4.3 Safety aspects and future prospects

For an immunisation programme to stand any chance of success it must be effective, safe and

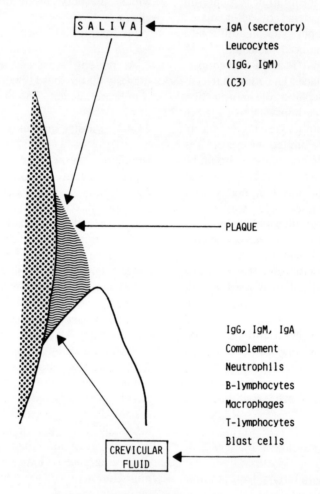

Figure 11.1   Diagram to illustrate routes by which both specific and non-specific immune factors may reach the plaque–tooth interface

acceptable to the general public. Although dental caries is undeniably a most important disease in terms of prevalence, suffering, inconvenience and cost, it is a condition which rarely, if ever, leads to death or serious disability of a patient. Consequently, it is most important that any prospective preventive method, including immunisation, should not carry even a small risk of causing serious damage. This aspect is particularly relevant at the present time (1979), when great public concern is being shown about the balance of risks between a life-threatening con-

Table 11.6   Summary of published results on passive transfer of immunity to dental caries*

Animals	Preparation	Route	Caries reduction	Ref.
Rats	IV-immunised dams (IgG)	Oral (suckling)	+	116
	Intra-mammary immunised dams (IgA)	Oral (suckling)	+	116
	Orally-immunised dams (IgA)	Oral (suckling)	+	116
Rats	Hyperimmune cow's milk	Oral	+	99
Monkeys	Immune serum	IV	−	117, 118
	Immune plasma + transfer factor	SC, IV	+	117, 118
	IgG	IV	+	117, 118
	IgM	IV	−	117, 118
	IgA	IV	−	117, 118

* For abbreviations see footnotes to table 11.5.

dition such as whooping cough (pertussis) and the possibility of serious side-effects from the currently recommended vaccine.

Unfortunately, all known prophylactic immunisation procedures carry some, albeit small, risk of producing unwanted side-effects. One of the main worries about the use of any streptococcal vaccine, including *S. mutans*, is the possibility of including antibodies which cross-react with heart tissue antigens. Some experimental evidence from animal studies supports the idea that such cross-reactions can be produced by immunisation with *S. mutans*, at least in rabbits[119]. Before the widespread use of caries vaccines in humans can be contemplated, it is obvious that their safety must be exhaustively tested.

The greatest risk of side-effects is likely to arise from whole-cell vaccines. Identification and isolation of fractionated 'protective antigens' *S. mutans* could lead to the development of a potentially safer immunogen which would be more acceptable for use in humans*. Studies on this approach are currently in progress in some laboratories.

In addition to finding the most effective and safe vaccine preparation, there is also a need for further studies on the most suitable method of delivery. Such questions as the optimum dose,

* See additional reference 120 for recent new evidence

route of administration, need for adjuvants and other practical considerations remain to be determined. Thus it seems unlikely that widespread human immunisation against dental caries can be contemplated for several years.

The information from studies on rodents and monkeys at the present time may be summarised as follows:

(1)   Immunisation with whole-cell or disintegrated cell vaccines from *S. mutans* can protect experimental animals from caries when challenged orally with the same bacterial strain. Protection has also been observed in animals which harbour *S. mutans* as part of their indigenous oral flora.

(2)   Other immunogens, such as glucosyl transferase preparations, have generally not been effective in conferring protection.

(3)   In some monkey experiments, animals which rapidly produced a high-serum antibody response were protected ('brisk responders'), whereas slow responders were not.

(4)   Reports vary as to the effect of immunisation on the numbers of detectable *S. mutans* in plaque. In some studies, high-serum antibody levels were found to correlate with low numbers of *S. mutans* and reduced caries incidence. In other studies, no obvious effect on colonisation by *S. mutans* was detected.

(5) The caries-protective effect observed in immunised animals may be mediated by serum antibodies via the gingival fluid, or by locally secreted IgA antibodies in saliva, or a combination of the two. Theoretically, different mechanisms may be involved in the protection of different tooth surfaces.

(6) The possibility that cell-mediated immune mechanisms and B- and T-cell cooperation may be significant in caries protection is currently being explored in some laboratories.

(7) Immunisation by passive transfer of both IgA and IgG antibodies has been reported.

(8) It is clear that further elucidation of the mechanisms by which vaccination with *S. mutans* can protect experimental animals, together with more studies on the most effective and safe methods of producing the appropriate immune responses, are required. Only when such information is available will it be proper to consider embarking upon clinical trials in human subjects:

11.5 Summary and Conclusions

In this chapter various methods by which caries may be prevented by measures directed against dental plaque as a whole, or against specific components of plaque, have been considered:

(1) Regular mechanical removal of all plaque deposits by toothbrushing and interdental cleaning aids can prevent caries, but is difficult to achieve on a community basis.

(2) A wide variety of chemical agents have been tested for anti-plaque activity, including antibiotics, antiseptics and enzymes. None of these has yet been shown to be an effective, safe and acceptable method of controlling dental caries in humans.

(3) Prevention of caries by immunisation with *S. mutans* has been demonstrated in experimental animals. Further studies are required before this method can be tested safely in humans.

Further Reading

Bowen, W. H., Genco, R. J. and O'Brien, T. C. (Eds) (1976). Immunological Aspects of Dental Caries: A special supplement of Immunology Abstracts, Information Retrieval Inc., Washington DC and London

Frandsen, A. (Ed.) (1976). *Preventive Dentistry in Practice*, Munksgaard, Copenhagen

Immunological aspects of dental caries (1976). *Journal of Dental Research*, **55** (special issue C)

Loesche, W. J. (1976). Chemotherapy of dental plaque infections. *Oral Science Reviews*, **9** 65–107

McGhee, J. R., Mestecky, J. and Babb, J. L. (Eds) (1978). Secretory immunity and infection, in *Advances in Experimental Medicine and Biology*, vol. 107, Plenum Press, New York and London

Newbrun, E. (1978). *Cariology*, Williams & Wilkins Co., Baltimore

References

1. Loesche, W. J. (1976). Chemotherapy of dental plaque infections. *Oral Sciences Reviews*, **9**, 65–107

2. Frandsen, A. M., Barbano, J. P., Suomi, J. D., Chang, J. J., and Houston, R. (1972). A comparison of the effectiveness of the Charter's, scrub and roll methods of toothbrushing in removing plaque. *Scandinavian Journal of Dental Research*, **80**, 267–71

3. Hanson, F. and Gjermo, P. (1971). The plaque-removing effect of four toothbrushing methods. *Scandinavian Journal of Dental Research*, **79**, 502–6

4. Gillings, B. R. D. (1977). Recent developments in dental plaque disclosants. *Australian Dental Journal*, **22**, 260–6

5. Mandel, I. D. (1974). Indices for measurement of soft accumulations in clinical studies of oral hygiene and periodontal disease. *J. Periodontal Research*, **9**, supplement 14, 7–30

6. Katayama, T., Suzuki, T. and Okada, S. (1975). Clinical observation of Dental plaque maturation. *Journal of Periodontology*, **46**, 610–13

7. Block, P. L., Lobene, R. R. and Derdivanis, J. P. (1972). A two-tone dye test for dental plaque. *Journal of Periodontology*, **43**, 423–6

8. Hill, H. C., Levi, P. A. and Glickman, I. (1973). The effects of waxed and unwaxed dental floss on interdental plaque accumulation and interdental gingival health. *Journal of Periodontology*, **44**, 411–13

9. Wright, G. Z., Banting, D. W., and Feasby, W. H. (1977). Effect of interdental flossing on the incidence of proximal caries in children. *Journal of Dental Research*, **56**, 574–8

10. Lang, N. P., Cumming, B. R., and Löe, H. (1973). Toothbrushing frequency as it relates to plaque development and gingival health. *Journal of Periodontology*, **44**, 396–405

11. Russell, A. L. (1963). International nutrition surveys: a summary of preliminary dental findings. *Journal of Dental Research*, **42**, 233–44

12. Greene, J. C. (1963). Oral hygiene and periodontal disease. *American Journal of Public Health*, **53**, 913–22

13. Sheiham, A. (1970). Dental cleanliness and chronic periodontal disease. *British Dental Journal*, **129**, 413–18

14. Leske, G. S., Ripa, L. W. and Barenie, J. T. (1976). Comparisons of caries and prevalence of children with different daily toothbrushing frequencies. *Community Dentistry and Oral Epidemiology*, **4**, 102–5

15. Tucker, G. J., Andlaw, R. J. and Burchell, C. K. (1976). The relationship between oral hygiene and dental caries incidence in 11-year-old children. *British Dental Journal*, **141**, 75–9

16. Lindhe, J., Axelsson, P. and Tollskog, G. (1975). The effect of proper oral hygiene on gingivitis and dental caries in school-children. *Community Dentistry and Oral Epidemiology*, **3**, 150–5

17. Axelsson, P. and Lindhe, J. (1975). Effect of fluoride on gingivitis and dental caries in a preventive program based on plaque control. *Community Dentistry and Oral Epidemiology*, **3**, 156–60

18. Hamp, S. E., Lindhe, J., Fornell, J., Johansson, L-Å. and Karlsson, R. (1978). Effect of a field program based on systematic plaque control on caries and gingivitis in schoolchildren after 3 years. *Community Dentistry and Oral Epidemiology*, **6**, 17–23

19. Poulsen, S., Agerbaek, N., Melsen, B., Korts, D. C., Glavind, L. and Rölla, G. (1976). The effect of professional tooth-cleansing. *Community Dentistry and Oral Epidemiology*, **4**, 195–9

20. Committee Report (1966). Oral health care for the prevention and control of periodontal disease, in *World Workshop in Periodontics* (Eds Ramfjord, S. P., Kerr, D. A. and Ash, M. M.), University of Ann Arbor, Michigan

21. Applewhite, M. L. (1969). Dental education as it relates to the community. *American Journal of Public Health*, **59**, 1882–6

22. Parsby, J. E. (1976). Communication and behavioural change, in *Preventive Dentistry in Practice* (Ed. Frandsen, A.), Munksgaard, Copenhagen, pp 92–113

23. Sutton, R. and Sheiham A. (1974). The factual basis of dental health education. *Health Education Journal*, **33**, 49–55

24. Parsons, J. C. (1974). Chemotherapy of dental plaque—a review. *Journal of Periodontology*, **45**, 177–86

25. McClure, F. J. and Hewitt, W. L. (1946). The relationship of pencillin to induced rat dental caries and oral *L.acidophilus*. *Journal of Dental Research*, **25**, 441–3

26. Stephan, R. M., Fitzerald, R. J., McClure, F. S., Harris, M. R. and Jordan, H. V. (1952). The comparative effects of penicillin, bactracin, chloromycetin, aureomycin and streptomycin on experimental dental

caries and on certain oral bacteria in the rat. *Journal of Dental Research*, **31**, 421–7

27. Zander, H. A. (1950). The effect of penicillin dentifrice on caries incidence in schoolchildren. *Journal of the American Dental Association*, **40**, 569–74

28. Weld, H. G. and Sandham, H. J. (1976). Effect of long-term therapies with penicillin and sulfadiazine on *Streptococcus mutans* and lactobacilli in dental plaque. *Antimicrobial Agents and Chemotherapy*, **10**, 200–4

29. Loesche, W. J., Green, E., Kenney, E. B. and Nafe, D. (1971). The effect of topical kanamycin sulphate on plaque accumulation. *Journal of the American Dental Association*, **83**, 1063–9

30. Schroeder, H. E., Marthaler, T. M. and Muhlemann, H. R. (1962). Effects of some potential inhibitors on early calculus formation. *Helvetica Odontologica Acta*, **6**, 6–9

31. Löe, H. and Schiøtt, C. R. (1970). The effect of mouthrinses and topical application of chlorhexidine on the development of dental plaque and gingivitis in man. *Journal of Perodontal Research*, **5**, 79–83

32. Löe, H., von der Fehr, F. R. and Schiøtt, C. R. (1972). Inhibition of experimental caries by plaque prevention. The effect of chlorhexidine mouthrinses. *Scandinavian Journal of Dental Research*, **80**, 1–9

33. Schiøtt, C. R. and Löe, H. (1972). The sensitivity of oral streptococci to chlorhexidine. *Journal of Peiodontal Research*, **7**, 192–4

34. Emilson, C. G., Krasse, B. and Westergren, G. (1976). Effect of a fluoride-containing chlorhexidine gel on bacteria in human plaque. *Scandinavian Journal of Dental Research*, **84**, 56–62

35. Emilson, C. G. and Fornell, J. (1976). Effect of toothbrushing with chlorhexidine gel on salivary microflora, oral hygiene, and caries. *Scandinavian Journal of Dental Research*, **84**, 308–19

36. Emilson, C. G. (1977). Susceptibility of various microorgannisms to chlorhexidine. *Scandinavian Journal of Dental Research*, **85**, 255–65

37. Rölla, G. and Melsen, B. (1975). On the mechanism of the plaque inhibition by chlorhexidine. *Journal of Dental Research*, **54**, B57–62

38. Regolati, B., König, K. G. and Mühlemann, H. R. (1969). Effects of topically applied disinfectants on caries in fissures and smooth surfaces of rat molars. *Helvetica Odontologica Acta*, **13**, 28–31

39. Kornman, K. S., Clark, W. B., Kreitzman, S. N. and Alvarez, C. (1973). Caries control in the albino rat with chlorhexidine gluconate (Hibitane). *Archives of Oral Biology*, **18**, 165–70

40. Fitzgerald, R. J. (1972). Inhibition of experimental dental caries by antibiotics. *Antimicrobial Agents and Chemotherapy*, **1**, 296–302

41. Gjermo, P. (1974). Chlorhexidine in dental practice. *Journal of Clinical Periodontology*, **1**, 143–52

42. Nagle, P. J. and Turnbull, R. S. (1978). Chlorhexidine: an ideal plaque inhibiting agent? *Journal of the Canadian Dental Association*, **44**, 73–7

43. Turesky, S., Glickman, I. and Sandberg, R. (1972). In vitro chemical inhibition of plaque formation. *Journal of Periodontology*, **43**, 263–9

44. Fitzgerald, R. J., Keyes, P. H., Stoudt, T. H. and Spinell, D. M. (1968). The effects of dextranase preparation on plaque and caries in hamsters, a preliminary report. *Journal of the American Dental Association*, **76**, 301–4

45. Guggenheim, B., König, K. G., Mühlemann, H. R. and Regolati, B. (1969). Effect of dextranases on caries in rats harboring an indigenous cariogenic bacterial flora. *Archives of Oral Biology*, **14**, 555–8

46. Lobene, R. R. (1971). A clinical study of the effect of dextranase on human dental

plaque. *Journal of the American Dental Association*, **82**, 132–5

47. Keyes, P. H., Hicks, M. A., Goldman, B. M., McCabe, R. M. and Fitzgerald R. J. (1971). Dispersion of dextranous bacterial plaques on human teeth with dextranase. *Journal of the Americal Dental Association*, **82**, 136–41

48. Bowen, W. H. (1971). The effect of dextranase on caries activity in monkeys (*Macaca irus*). *British Dental Journal*, **131**, 445–9

49. Guggenheim, B., Regolati, B. and Mühlemann, H. R. (1972). Caries and plaque inhibition by mutanase in rats. *Caries Research* **6**, 253–4

50. Hamilton, I. R. (1977). Effects of fluoride on enzymatic regulation of bacterial carbohydrate metabolism. *Caries Research*, **11**, supplement 1, 262–78

51. Weiss, S., King, W. J., Kestenbaum, R. C., and Donohue, J. J. (1965). Influences of various factors on polysaccharide syntheses *in Streptococcus mitis*. *Annals of the New York Academy of Sciences*, **131**, 839–50

52. Hamilton, I. R. (1969). Studies with fluoride-sensitive and fluoride-resistance strains of *Streptococcus salivarius*. I. Inhibition of both intracellular polyglucose synthesis and degradation by fluoride. *Canadian Journal of Microbiology*, **15**, 1013–19

53. Schachtele, C. F. (1971). Discussion of paper by Hamilton, I. R. *Caries Research*, **11**, supplement 1, 278–87

54. Broukal, Z. and Zajicek, O. (1974). Amount and distribution of extracellular polysaccharides in dental microbial plaque. *Caries Research*, **8**, 97–104

55. Hunter, J. R., Baird, J. K. and Ellwood, D. C. (1973). Effect of fluoride on the transport of sugars into chemostat-grown *Streptococcus mutans*. *Journal of Dental Research*, **52**, 954

56. Ellwood, D. C. (1977). Discussion of paper by Kleinberg, I., Chatterjee, R.,

Reddy, J. and Craw, D. *Caries Research*, **11**, supplement 1, 317–20

57. König, K. C. (1959). Dental caries and plaque accumulation in rats treated with stannous fluoride and penicillin. *Helvetica Odontologica Acta*, **3**, 39–44

58. Birkeland, J. M. (1972). Effect of fluoride on the amount of dental plaque in children. *Scandinavia Journal of Dental Research*, **80**, 82–4

59. Dolan, M. M., Kavanagh, B. J. and Yankell, S. L. (1972). Artificial plaque prevention with organic fluorides. *Journal of Periodontology*, **43**, 561–3

60. Balmelli, O. P., Regolati, B. and Mühlemann, H. R. (1974). Inhibition of streptococcal deposits on rat molars by amine fluoride. *Helvetica Odontologica Acta*, **18**, supplement 8, 45–53

61. Tinanoff, N., Brady, J. M. and Gross, A. (1976). The effect of NaF and SnF_2 mouth rinses on bacterial colonization of tooth enamel: TEM and SEM studies. *Caries Research*, **10**, 415–26

62. Suzuki, T., Sobue, S. and Suginaka, H. (1976). Mechanisms of antiplaque action of diamine silver fluoride. *Journal of Osaka University Dental School*, **16**, 87–95

63. Gross, A. and Tinanoff, N. (1977). Effect of SnF_2 mouthrinse on initial bacterial colonization of tooth enamel. *Journal of Dental Research*, **56**, 1179–83

64. Woods, R. (1971). The short-term effect of topical fluoride applications on the concentration of *Streptococcus mutans* in dental plaque. *Australian Dental Journal*, **16**, 152–5

65. Loesche, W. J., Murray, R. J., and Mellberg, J. R. (1973). The effect of topical fluoride on percentage of *Streptococcus mutans* and *Streptococcus sanguis* in interproximal plaque samples. *Caries Research*, **7**, 283–96

66. Loesche, W. J. Syed, S. A., Murray, R. J. and Mellberg, J. R. (1975). Effect of topical acidulated phosphate fluoride on

percentage of *Streptococcus mutans* and *Streptococcus sanguis* in plaque II. Pooled occlusal and pooled approximal samples. *Caries Research*, **9**, 139–55

67. Brown, W. E. and König, K. G. (Eds) (1977). Cariostatic mechanisms of fluoride. *Caries Research*, **11**, supplement 1

68. Newbrun, E. (Ed.) (1972). *Fluorides and Dental Caries*, Charles C. Thomas, Springfield

69. Mirth, D. B. and Bowen, W. H. (1976). Chemotherapy: antimicrobials and methods of delivery, in *Microbial Aspects of Dental Caries* (Eds Stiles, H. M., Loesche, W. J. and O'Brien, T. C.), Information Retrieval Inc., Washington DC and London, pp. 249–62

70. Axelsson, P. and Lindhe, J. (1974). The effect of a preventive programme on dental plaque, gingivitis and caries in schoolchildren. Results after one and two years. *Journal of Clinical Periodontology*, **1**, 126–38

71. Luoma, H. (unpublished data)

72. Colman, G. (1978). The prospect of immunization against dental caries. *Dental Update*, **8**, 137–40

73. Lehner, T., Challacombe, S. J. and Caldwell, J. (1978). Immunization with *Streptococcus mutans* against dental caries in rhesus monkeys, in *New Trends and Developments in Vaccines* (Eds Voller, A. and Friedman, H.), MTP

74. Sims, W. (1970). The concept of immunity in dental caries. I. General considerations. *Oral Surgery, Oral Medicine, Oral Pathology*, **30**, 670–7

75. Sims, W. (1972). The concept of immunity in dental caries. II. Specific immune responses. *Oral Surgery, Oral Medicine, Oral Pathology*, **34**, 69–86

76. Challacombe, S. J. (1974). Serum complement-fixing antibodies in human dental caries. *Caries Research*, **8**, 84–95

77. Challacombe, S. J. and Lehner, T. (1976). Serum and salivary antibodies to cariogenic bacteria in man. *Journal of Dental Research*, **55**, C139–48

78. Challacombe, S. J. (1978). Salivary IgA antibodies to antigens from *Streptococcus mutans* in human dental caries, in *Secretory Immunity and Infection* see ref. 83, pp. 355–67

79. Huis in't Veld, J., Bannet, D., Van Palenstein Helderman, W., Carmargo, P. S. and Backer Dirks, O. (1978). Antibodies against *Streptococcus mutans* and glucosyltransferases in caries-free and caries-active military recruits, in *Secretory Immunity and Infection*, see ref. 83, pp. 369–81

80. Rosebury, T., Foley, G., Greenberg, S. and Pollack, F. (1934). Studies of lactobacilli in relation to caries in rats. II. Attempt to immunize rats on caries-producing diets against lactobacilli. *Journal of Dental Research*, **14**, 231–2

81. Williams, N. B. (1944). Immunization of human beings with oral lactobacilli. *Journal of Dental Research*, **23**, 403–11

82. Bowen, W. H. (1976). Relevance of caries vaccine investigations in rodents, primates and humans: critical assessment, in *Immunological Aspects of Dental Caries* (Eds Bowen, W. H., Genco, R. J. and O'Brien, T. C.), Information Retrieval Inc., Washington DC and London, pp. 11–20

83. McGhee, J. R., Mestecky, J. and Babb, J. L. (Eds), (1978). *Secretory Immunity and Infection. Advances in Experimental Medicine and Biology*, vol. 107, Plenum Press, New York and London

84. Fitzgerald, R. J. and Keyes, P. H. (1962). Attempted immunization of albino hamsters against induced dental caries. *International Association for Dental Research*, abstract No. 146

85. Gaffar, A., Coleman, G. J. Marcussen, H. and Kestembaum, R. C. (1970). Effects of inoculating a levan-forming cariogenic streptococcus on experimental caries in hamsters. *Archives of Oral Biology*, **15**, 1393–6

86. Gaffar, A., Marcussen, H. W., Schlissel, J. H. and Volpe, A. R. (1971). Effect of specific immunization with an enzyme on experimental dental caries in hamsters. *International Association for Dental Research*, abstract No. 349

87. Gaffar, A. (1976). Effects of specific immunization on dental caries in hamsters. *Journal of Dental Research*, **55**, C221–3

88. Smith, D. T., Taubman, M. A. and Ebersole, J. L. (1978). Cross-protective aspects of glucosyltransferase antigens in the hamster caries model, in *Secretory Immunity and Infection*, see ref. 83, pp. 271–9

89. Wagner, M. (1967). Specific immunization against *Streptococcus faecalis* induced dental caries in the gnotobiotic rat. *Bacteriological Proceedings*, **67**, 99

90. Bahn, A. N., Pinter, J. K., Quillan, P. D. and Hayashi, J. A. (1969). Immunization with enzymes against caries in the rat. *International Association for Dental Research*, abstract No. 64

91. Hayashi, J. A., Shklair, I. L. and Bahn, A. N. (1972). Immunization with dextran-sucrases and glycosidic hydrolases. *Journal of Dental Research*, **51**, 436–42

92. Guggenheim, B., Mühlemann, H. R., Regolati, B. and Schmid, R. (1970). The effect of immunization against strepto-cocci or glucosyltransferases on plaque formation and dental caries in rats, in *Dental Plaque* (Ed. McHugh, W. D.), Livingstone, Edinburgh and London, pp. 287–96

93. Tanzer, J. M., Hageage, G. J. and Larson, R. H. (1970). Inability to immunologically protect rats against smooth surface caries. *Journal of Dental Research*, **49**, 165

94. Tanzer, J. M., Hageage, G. J. and Larsen, R. H. (1973). Variable experiences in immunization of rats against *Streptococcus mutans*-associated dental caries. *Archives of Oral Biology*, **18**, 1425–39

95. Taubman, M. A. and Smith, D. J. (1974). Effects of local immunization with *Streptococcus mutans* on induction of immunoglobulin A antibody and experimental dental caries in rats. *Infection and Immunity*, **9**, 1079–91

96. Taubman, M. A. and Smith D. J. (1977). Effect of local immunization with gluco-syltransferase fractions from *Streptococcus mutans* on dental caries in rats and hamsters. *Journal of Immunology*, **118**, 710–20

97. McGhee, J. R., Michalek, S. M., Webb, J., Navia, J. M., Rahman, A. F. R. and Legler, D. W. (1975). Effective immunity to dental caries: protection of gnotobiotic rats by local immunization with *Streptococcus mutans*. *Journal of Immunology*, **114**, 300–5

98. Michalek, S. M., McGhee, J. R., Mestecky, J., Arnold, R. R. and Bozzo, L. (1976). Ingestion of *Streptococcus mutans* induces secretory IgA and caries immunity. *Science*, **192**, 1238–40

99. Michalek, S. M., McGhee, J. R., Arnold, R. R. and Mestecky, J. (1978). Effective immunity to dental caries: selective induction of secretory immunity by oral administration of *Streptococcus mutans* in rodents, in *Secretory Immunity and Infection*, see ref. 83, pp. 261–9

100. Peri, B. A. and Wagner, M. (1977). Immune response and dental caries incidence in *S. faecalis*-monoassociated Harvard caries-resistant and caries-susceptible rats. *Infection and Immunity*, **16**, 805–11

101. Smith, D. J. and Taubman, M. A. (1976). Immunization experiments using the rodent caries model. *Journal of Dental Research*, **55**, C193–205

102. Bowen, W. H. (1969). A vaccine against dental caries: a pilot experiment in monkeys (*Macaca irus*). *British Dental Journal*, **126**, 159–63

103. Bowen, W. H., Cohen, B., Cole, M. F. and Colman, G. (1975). Immunization against dental caries. *British Dental Journal*, **139**, 45–58

104. Lehner, T., Challacombe, S. J. and Caldwell, J. (1975). An immunological investigation into the prevention of caries in deciduous teeth of rhesus monkeys. *Archives of Oral Biology*, **20**, 305–10

105. Lehner, T., Challacombe, S. J. and Caldwell, J. (1975). Immunological and bacteriological basis for vaccination against dental caries in rhesus monkeys. *Nature*, **254**, 517–20

106. Lehner, T., Caldwell, J. and Challacombe, S. J. (1977). Effects of immunization on dental caries in the first permanent molars in rhesus monkeys. *Archives of Oral Biology*, **22**, 393–7

107. Evans, R. J., Emmings, F. G. and Genco, R. J. (1975). Prevention of *Streptococcus mutans* infection of tooth surfaces by salivary antibody in irus monkeys (*Macaca fascicularis*). *Infection and Immunity*, **12**, 293–302

108. Genco, R. J., Emmings, F. G., Evans, R. T. and Apicella, M. (1976). Purification, characterization and immunogenicity of cell-associated glucan from *Streptococcus mutans. Journal of Dental Research*, **55**, C115–20

109. Russell, M. W., Challacombe, S. J. and Lehner, T. (1976). Serum glucosyltransferase-inhibiting antibodies and dental caries in rhesus monkeys immunized against *Streptococcus mutans. Immunology*, **30**, 619–27

110. Schick, H. J., Klimek, F. J. Wimann, E. and Zwisler, O. (1978). Preliminary results in the immunization of irus monkeys against dental caries, in *Secretory Immunity and Infection*, see ref. 83, pp. 261–9

111. Lehner, T., Challacombe, S. J. and Caldwell, J. (1975). An experimental model for immunological studies of dental caries in the rhesus monkey. *Archives of Oral Biology*, **20**, 299–304

112. Caldwell, J., Challacombe, S. J. and Lehner T. (1977). A sequential bacteriological and serological investigation of rhesus monkeys immunized against dental caries with *Streptococcus mutans. Journal of Medical Microbiology*, **10**, 213–24

113. Lehner, T., Challacombe, S. J., Wilton, J. M. A. and Ivanyi, L. (1976). Immunopotentiation by dental microbial plaque and its relationship to oral disease in man. *Archives of Oral Biology*, **21**, 749–53

114. Lehner, T., Challacombe, S. J., Wilton, J. M. A. and Caldwell, J. (1976). Cellular and humoral immune responses in vaccination against dental caries in monkeys. *Nature*, **264**, 69–72

115. Sculley, C. and Lehner, T. (1979). Bacterial and strain specificities in opsonization, phagocytosis and killing of *Streptococcus mutans. Clinical and Experimental Immunology*, **35**, 128

116. Michalek, S. M. and McGhee, J. R. (1977). Effective immunity to dental caries: passive transfer to rats of antibodies to *Streptococcus mutans* elicits protection. *Infection and Immunity*, **17**, 644–50

117. Lehner, T., Russell, M. W., Challacombe, S. J., Sculley, C. M. and Hawkes, J. E. (1978). Passive immunization with serum and immunoglobulins against dental caries in rhesus monkeys. *Lancet*, 1 April, 693–5

118. Lehner, T., Russell, M. W., Wilton, J. M. A., Challacombe, S. J., Scully, C. M. and Hawkes, J. E. (1978). Passive immunization with antisera to *Streptococcus mutans* in the prevention of caries in rhesus monkeys, in *Secretory Immunity and Infection*, see ref. 83, pp. 303–15

119. Van de Rijn, I., Bleiweis, A. S. and Zabriskie, J. B. (1976). Antigens in *Streptococcus mutans* cross reactive with human heart muscle. *Journal of Dental Research*, **55**, C59–64

120. Lehner, T., Russell, M. W. and Caldwell, J. (1980). Immunisation with a purified protein from *Streptococcus mutans* against dental caries in Rhesus monkeys. *Lancet*, **i**, May 10, 995–6

Chapter 12

Prevention of Caries by Increasing the Resistance of the Tooth

This chapter deals with the prevention of dental caries by increasing the resistance of the tooth. Increasing the resistance of the tooth to carious dissolution will be dealt with under three specific headings. The topical application of fluoride agents is a well-recognised caries-preventive procedure. The development of these agents, clinical trials, and their mechanisms of action will be discussed in the first section. In the second, the development and use of fissure sealants will be discussed. The use of sealants on occlusal surfaces of posterior teeth can act as a physical barrier on caries-susceptible surfaces which are least benefited by fluoride. The topic of remineralisation will be discussed in the third section. Remineralisation has already been dealt with in connection with the formation of the histological zones in the small lesion of enamel caries (chapter 6). However, in this section, remineralisation will be discussed in more general terms in order to obtain a broader perspective.

12.1   Topical Fluorides

12.1.1   Mechanisms by which fluoride reduces caries

The aim of topical fluoride therapy is the deposition of fluoride into the surface layer of tooth enamel to form fluorapatite, so as to decrease the caries susceptibility of the tissue:

$$Ca_{10}(OH_2)(PO_4)_6 + 2F \rightarrow$$

hydroxyapatite

$$\rightarrow Ca_{10}F_2(PO_4)_6 + 2OH^-$$

fluorapatite

Mechanisms whereby fluoride reduces caries are complex, but may be summarised under the following headings:

By rendering enamel more resistant to acid dissolution

Under the influence of fluoride: (1) larger crystals are formed, with fewer imperfections—this stabilises the lattice and presents a smaller surface area per unit volume for dissolution; (2) enamel has a lower carbonate content, thus giving reduced solubility; (3) reprecipitation of calcium phosphates occurs and fluoride favours their crystallisation as apatite.

It is claimed that the initial rate of dissolution of hydroxyapatite is the same as fluorapatite[1]. However, the subsequent formation of secondary precipitates, such as calcium fluoride, on the surface of the enamel crystals reduces the rate of diffusion of hydrogen ions and of undissociated acid to the crystals, thus reducing their rate of solution.

By inhibiting bacterial enzyme systems which convert sugars into acids in plaque

For this to occur, fluoride must be present as free ionic fluoride and not be bound up in plaque[2].

By inhibiting storage of intracellular polysaccharides

In this way the accumulation of carbohydrate within the cell is prevented. This could otherwise be used to form acids between meals.

At high concentration, fluoride is toxic to bacteria

Certain species may therefore be eliminated for short periods after topical fluoride therapy. However, this is obviously only a temporary benefit of topical fluoride therapy.

By reducing the tendency of the enamel surface to adsorb proteins

Several *in vitro* reports have shown that plaque does not build up so readily on enamel surfaces treated with fluoride. This may be because fluoride reduces the surface energy of the teeth[3], and the tendency of the enamel surface to adsorb proteins[4].

Clinical trials have failed to demonstrate any plaque-reducing effect. However, a pilot study on humans demonstrated a significant reduction in plaque in fluoride-treated quadrants relative to controls after topical application of a fluoride gel[5].

Modification in size and shape of teeth

Animal experiments have suggested that fluoride intake during tooth development may reduce the size of teeth and produce more rounded cusps and shallower fissures. Such observations have been recorded in humans from high-fluoride areas in the UK[6]. However, the scientific basis for these observations is poor.

Remineralisation

Fluoride favours precipitation of calcium and phosphate ions in the form of apatite rather than as soluble calcium phosphates[7]. Experiments on remineralisation of carious human enamel *in vitro* have shown that the presence of low concentrations of fluoride enhances greatly the reprecipitation of mineral ions into the damaged enamel[8].

12.1.2 Fluoride agents

Sodium fluoride

Bibby[9], in 1942, was the first to use fluoride solutions on teeth in the dental office as a caries-preventive measure. He reported that applications of 0.1 per cent sodium fluoride, three times a year, produced a 33 per cent reduction in caries experience in children from 10 to 13 years of age. In this study, on 78 children, the solution was applied to half of the mouth, the untreated half acting as a control.

Sodium fluoride was selected on the basis that it was a soluble salt and was employed in the artificial fluoridation of water supplies. After this, research was directed towards finding the optimum concentration and the most effective technique. This led to the classical studies reported by Knutson[10], in 1948, in which a 2 per cent solution was used.

Technique

(1)   Tooth crowns were cleaned using a rubber cup and prophylaxis paste.
(2)   A 2 per cent solution was applied to teeth in an isolated and dried quadrant, or to half the mouth.
(3)   Teeth were allowed to remain moist with the solution for 3–4 minutes.
(4)   Application was repeated on the other quadrants.
(5)   Second, third and fourth applications, not preceded by prophylaxis, were given at intervals of about one week.
(6)   Treatments were recommended at 3, 7, 11 and 13 years of age, to coincide with eruption of new teeth.

Reductions in caries were reported as 30–40 per cent among children living in low-fluoride areas.

Further studies by other workers confirmed the preventive properties of topically applied sodium fluoride. According to other workers[11], certain aspects of its potential usefulness needed further investigation, although these questions also apply to other agents. But:

(1)   More long-term studies must be carried out to determined precisely how long after treatment a topical agent continues to exert a beneficial effect.
(2)   Some investigations suggest that a fall-off in effectiveness may occur in less than three years[12].
(3)   Optimum frequency of application remains to be determined.

Advantages of Sodium Fluoride

(1)   It is stable chemically when stored in plastic or polythene containers.
(2)   It has an acceptable taste.
(3)   The solution is non-irritating to the gingiva.
(4)   It does not cause discoloration to teeth.

Disadvantage   With the Knutson[10] technique,

the patient must make four visits within a relatively short time.

Stannous fluoride

Because of the time-consuming regimen described by Knutson[10], further laboratory studies were undertaken to find a more effective agent.

Of the compounds tested, stannous fluoride (SnF_2) was shown by Muhler, Boyd and Huysen[13], in 1950, to be more effective in reducing the rate of dissolution of enamel by acid *in vitro*. A study compared[14] the efficacy of 2 per cent SnF_2 and 2 per cent NaF when applied according to Knutson's technique[10]. Stannous fluoride proved to be more affective than sodium fluoride, reductions being 59 per cent and 30 per cent, respectively. Subsequent studies[15, 17] reported that annual applications of 8 per cent stannous fluoride produced significant caries reduction. This single regimen was more desirable than the much longer technique advocated by Knutson[10].

Technique

(1)   Rubber cup prophylaxis; tooth surfaces cleaned and polished with pumice for 5–10 seconds each (the pumice carried between contact points using unwaxed dental floss).

(2)   Either a quadrant or half the mouth is isolated and dried.

(3)   A freshly-prepared 8 per cent solution of SnF_2 is applied continuously to the teeth with cotton applicators, so that the enamel surfaces are kept moist with it for 4 minutes. Reapplication is usually required every 15–30 seconds.

In highly susceptible patients, the topical application should be repeated at least once every six months; for those not particularly caries-prone; a single treatment can be given once a year. One study[18] showed that a second application of 8 per cent SnF_2, given within a few days, provided no additional preventive effect.

Much of the work dealing with SnF_2 as a topical fluoride agent has been conducted by Muhler and his associates[13] at the University of Indiana, USA. They have reported on many occasions that annual or six-monthly applications of an 8 per cent solution of SnF_2 produces a significant decrease in the development of new carious lesions, and their trials indicate benefits exceeding the 30–40 per cent reductions generally accepted for 2 per cent NaF. Levels of prevention ranging from 47 to 78 per cent on new DMF surfaces have been recorded.

Other investigators have found SnF_2 effective, although usually to a lesser extent. One study[19] reported a 26 per cent lower increment in DMF teeth after two annual applications of 8 per cent SnF_2 solution. In another[20], a single application produced a reduction of about 17 per cent in development of new carious teeth after one year, whereas another[21] showed that six monthly treatments led to a 23 per cent reduction in new lesions.

However, in conflict with many favourable reports, a few more recent studies using SnF_2 have shown extremely disappointing results. In one study[22] it was found that in the case of children it failed to yield any reductions after one year. Negative results were also obtained in a two-year study in Sweden[23] in a group of children after two annual applications of a 10 per cent SnF_2 solution. Another trial[24] similarly found no preventive effect in children who received a topical application of 8 per cent SnF_2 annually for two years, after either the first or second year.

Disadvantages of SnF_2

(1)   It is not stable in aqueous solution, undergoes fairly rapid hydrolysis and oxidation, and forms stannous hydroxide and the stannic ion. This reaction reduces its effectiveness, and consequently a fresh solution must be used each time.

(2)   Because an 8 per cent solution of SnF_2 is astringent and disagreeable in taste, its application is unpleasant[11]. Unfortunately, the addition of flavouring agents is contra-indicated.

(3)   The solution sometimes causes a reversible tissue irritation, shown by gingival blanching. This reaction usually occurs in patients with poor gingival health.

(4) Pigmentation and staining of teeth after SnF_2 has been reported by many. It usually appears in association with carious lesions, hypocalcified areas of enamel, and around the margins of restorations. One study[25] estimated that 95 per cent of children had pigmented teeth after SnF_2 application, whereas another[22] reported staining in 60 per cent.

(5) Because SnF_2 does produce staining it is difficult to measure caries in test and control groups. Enamel lesions can be masked clinically, photographically and by radiography. This may lead to errors in diagnosis and be responsible for many so-called 'reversals' reported in SnF_2 studies[26].

Acidulated phosphate fluoride (APF)

Brudevold and co-workers[27], in 1963, reported laboratory studies showing that an APF solution produced an increased uptake of fluoride by enamel, compared with either stannous fluoride or neutral sodium fluoride.

The success of a topical fluoride agent depends largely on the extent to which it is capable of depositing fluoride in the enamel as fluorapatite. An ideal one would react with enamel to form maximal amounts of fluorapatite quickly. Water fluoridation forms fluorapatite in the enamel, in terms of months or years, whereas a topical solution must react in minutes.

The crystalline structure of enamel is made more stable by acquisition of fluoride according to the following reaction:

$$Ca_{10}(PO_4)_6(OH)_2 + 2F^- \rightleftharpoons Ca_{10}(PO_4)_6F_2 + 2OH^-$$

enamel hydroxyapatite + fluoride   fluorapatite + hydroxyl

Fluoride competes with, and displaces, the hydroxyl groups of the hydroxyapatite molecule to form fluorapatite. There are two ways of speeding up this reaction: (1) raising the concentration of fluoride in solution, and (2) lowering the pH, thus making the solution more acid. However, both methods may produce undesirable side-effects:

(a) increasing fluoride concentration may cause the following:

$$Ca_{10}(PO_4)_6(OH)_2 + 20F^- \rightleftharpoons 10CaF_2 + 6PO_4^- + 2OH^-$$

enamel hydroxyapatite + high   calcium fluoride + phosphate
concentration of fluoride   + hydroxyl

Calcium fluoride has a different crystal structure from apatite and its formation is associated with decomposition of the mineral phase of enamel.

(b) Lowering the pH. It is accepted that enamel in the presence of acid may break down according to the following reaction:

$$Ca_{10}(PO_4)_6(OH)_2 + 8H^+ \rightleftharpoons 10Ca^{++} + 6HPO_4^- + H_2O$$

enamel hydroxyapatite + acid   calcium + phosphate + water

Thus, increased fluoride could be deposited into enamel only if both calcium fluoride formation, and demineralisation, could be suppressed. Brudevold noticed that both of these unfavourable reactions resulted in phosphate as a breakdown product. He reasoned that since the reactions are reversible, introduction of phosphate into the solution containing high fluoride at low pH would suppress the undesirable effects because of a shift in equilibrium of the reactions from left to right, yielding intact hydroxyapatite as the principal reaction product.

Therefore, if enamel is brought into contact with high concentrations of fluoride at low pH, in the presence of phosphate, rapid fluoride deposition should occur with no significant enamel breakdown.

Initial clinical studies on topically applied acidulated phosphate fluoride solutions have given excellent results. After two years of annual applications children showed a 67 per cent smaller increment in DMF teeth, and a 70 per cent reduction in DMF surfaces compared with untreated controls[28]. When a 2 per cent solution of sodium fluoride was applied to half the mouth, and a 2 per cent sodium fluoride solution acidified with orthophosphoric acid (APF) to the other half, it was found that the half treated with the acid phosphate had about 50 per cent fewer new carious lesions than that treated with neutral sodium fluoride, the difference being highly significant[29].

The preventive effects shown in more recent studies have tended to be smaller than those obtained initially, but are nevertheless encouraging.

One study[22] reported that after two annual applications of APF, children had 44 per cent fewer new DMF teeth and 52 per cent fewer new DMF surfaces compared with untreated controls. The results of another study[30] showed a 49 per cent reduction in DMF teeth after two years in children who received the topical application at six-monthly intervals.

Technique   The technique with APF solution is similar to that with other fluoride agents. The crowns of teeth are cleaned with prophylaxis paste using a rubber cup, and unwaxed dental floss is employed to carry the paste between interstitial contact regions. The solution is then applied to a dried and isolated quadrant, or half the mouth, enamel surfaces remaining moist for four minutes.

Advantages of APF

(1)   It is chemically stable when stored in plastic or polythene containers.

(2)   It has a tolerable taste (and can be flavoured without upsetting the fluoride content).

(3)   It will not stain enamel surfaces or pellicle.

(4)   It is not astringent to gingival tissues.

(5)   Clinical trials have shown it to be an effective caries preventive agent.

(6)   Laboratory studies have established that enamel takes up significantly more fluoride from APF than from other fluoride agents.

APF Gels   Relatively few studies have been carried out on these gels. Application in wax trays produced a 24 per cent reduction in DMF surfaces after three years, compared with controls[31]. A further study[32] found, after one year, 28 per cent fewer new DMF surfaces among children 8–12 years of age after a single treatment with APF gel in foam-rubber trays, while in another [33], a 41 per cent reduction was reported over two years. Use of an APF solution over a similar time-span yielded non-significant reductions.

In one major study[34], test groups received either APF gel, APF solution, neutral sodium fluoride or stannous fluoride. After three years, significant reductions were found only in the case of APF gel. Supervised self-application of fluoride gels in polyvinyl mouthpieces was tested [35] at Cheektowaga, USA. Children used it for 6 minutes each school day for two years. At the end of 21 months, reductions of 75 per cent and 80 per cent in new DMF surfaces among two groups were recorded.

The clinical advantage of using gels is that the whole mouth can be treated at once rather than separate quadrants by solution technique, but since gels are viscous, poorly fitting trays or mouthpieces may apply them only to freely exposed buccal, lingual and occlusal surfaces. Moreover, to be effective against smooth-surface caries, the gel must penetrate the interstitial regions.

Yet because gels are thixotropic to some extent they are able to flow under pressure. Thus, with a well-fitting tray, they have a better chance of entering interstitial sites. This applies especially to the new generation of thixotropic fluoride gels now available commercially. However, since gels must be used in trays, the design of these is of extreme importance: variations in results of trials could well be related to this factor.

In addition to the clinical advantage of treating the whole mouth at once, gels have another important advantage. Substantial amounts of fluoride are deposited into enamel from topical treatments but most of it soon leaches away into the oral environment[36–37].

Laboratory experiments indicate that this loss is essentially complete within 24 hours. If fluoride ions can be 'trapped' at the enamel surface for longer periods, this could result in a greater uptake by enamel.

Several workers have shown an increase in enamel fluoride *in vitro*, after application of coating materials to the enamel[38]. Fluoride gels also exhibit a somewhat similar mechanism, a thin layer remaining on enamel surfaces acting as a fluoride ion reservoir. A significant increase in fluoride content of surface enamel has been shown 4 and 60 days after a gel application[39]. In another study, higher levels of fluoride were deposited from an APF gel than from an APF solution[40]. In addition, APF gel was more effective in preventing artificial caries *in vitro* than either an APF solution or other topical fluoride agents[41].

Therefore, it is evident that fluoride gels have great potential as caries-preventive agents, provided that the problems are borne in mind.

12.1.3 Fluoride methods compared

A study in the USA gave an idea (table 12.1) of how much can be achieved by spending a given amount of money on different methods of fluoridation, and also compared the number of cavities which could be treated for the same sum.

Table 12.1 Comparative results per $100 000 spent

	Cavities prevented
1. Water fluoridation	666 660
2. Self-applied fluorides	233 330
3. Topical fluorides	60 000
4. Fluoride dentifrices	25 600
5. Dental restorations	16 666 cavities restored

Water fluoridation has the lowest cost per cavity by a clear margin. However, topical fluorides can be seen to be effective, not only in children but also in young adults. Teeth should preferably be treated as soon after eruption as possible, since these benefit most from topical fluoride therapy[43, 44].

It would be reasonable to expect some benefit in adults of all ages, although clinical trials in this area are limited and conflicting.

Benefits might be more in prevention of secondary caries around existing restorations, rather than in prevention of initial lesions as in children and young adults.

Recent evidence has also shown that topical fluorides can give additional caries prevention even in areas receiving fluoridated drinking water[45].

12.1.4 Fluoride mouthrinses

Fluoride mouthrinsing is one of several topical fluoride techniques available which may be particularly suited to community dental health programmes. The results of early trials were disappointing[46]. It was not until a decade ago that renewed interest was shown by workers in Sweden. In one study[47], the use of monthly 0.2 per cent sodium or potassium fluoride rinses demonstrated substantial reductions in anterior approximal caries. Later it was found that the addition of manganese ions enhanced the effect of potassium fluoride[48].

In a comprehensive multi-group trial[49], the unsupervised daily use of an 0.05 per cent sodium fluoride mouthrinse over a two-year period was shown to reduce the incidence of caries in 10–12-year-old children by about half. This reduction was significantly greater than that obtained by supervised fortnightly rinsing with an 0.2 per cent sodium fluoride solution in the same trial. In this latter group, only a 21 per cent caries reduction was found, indicating the importance of frequent exposure in the use of topical fluorides. A 44 per cent reduction in DMFS increament was produced in a 20-month trial in the USA[50] with weekly rinsing with a solution of 0.2 per cent sodium fluoride.

In a further multi-group trial[51] the effect of fluoride toothpastes and fluoride mouthrinses was evaluated on caries incidence in Swedish schoolchildren. Two sodium fluoride solutions were used, 0.5 per cent and 0.05 per cent. Ten millilitres of the 0.5 per cent solution was used for each rinse, containing about 23 mg F^-. The 0.5 per cent rinse was prepared by dissolving 10 ml of 0.6 per cent NaF in 100 ml of tap water. This solution contained 27 mg F^-. Three study groups were used to test the fluoride rinses. There was a

23 per cent reduction in DMFS score in the fluoride group compared with the control. When the caries increments were considered for various tooth surfaces it was found that occlusal caries was not affected by the fluoride rinse.

The largest reduction in caries was on buccal and approximal surfaces. The children who rinsed only when they attended the school clinic used the mouthwash three to four times a year on average. The third group used a 0.05 per cent NaF solution. However, they used 110 ml of this solution and had to use all of this volume. Therefore, the total fluoride content was slightly higher for this group than for the two other groups. The children rinsed about three times a year. Using a 0.05 per cent solution three times a year, no reduction in caries was obtained. It was concluded that daily rinsing with such a weak solution would probably be necessary before a reduction in caries was obtained with a 0.05 per cent solution.

Two years after the above trial had ended[52], re-examination of children who had taken part in the fortnightly rinsing with 0.5 per cent NaF took place. One hundred and forty children were available for re-examination. A difference was found between control and test groups, but this difference was not statistically significant. Thus, no prolonged caries prophylactic effect could be found two years after the end of a programme based on fortnightly rinsing with 0.5 per cent sodium fluoride solution. It appears that the beneficial effect of supervised mouthrinsing with fluoride solution can only be maintained if mouthrinsing is continued. This study by Koch in Sweden on mouthrinsing is one of the largest so far reported and is the only one in which the caries increment was determined when the fluoride rinsing programme had ended.

Sodium fluoride

In a more recent study in the UK[53], more than 400 15-year-old subjects completed a three-year double-blind trial testing the daily supervised use of a mouthrinse containing 0.05 per cent sodium fluoride. The control rinse was similar, except for the omission of fluoride. There was a 36 per cent reduction (3.7 DMFS) over the three-year period. The highest percentage reductions were found on anterior approximal and free smooth surfaces. No adverse effects on oral soft tissues were found, and ingestion of fluoride from the rinses was low. With respect to cost-effectiveness, it was considered that one supervisor could organise a daily mouthrinsing programme for 800 subjects at a cost of $8.00 (£4.00) per child per year. These results were in agreement with other fluoride mouthrinsing studies[51], in that caries reductions were greatest on free smooth surfaces and anterior approximal surfaces.

Although it had previously been suggested that fortnightly rinsing with an 0.5 per cent sodium fluoride solution had an unfavourable effect upon gingival health[54], this was not observed in the above British trial[53]. This lack of adverse effect on gingival health has also been demonstrated in other studies. A further double-blind British study carried out over two years with supervised 0.2 per cent sodium fluoride rinsing for one minute[55], produced its greatest caries reduction on posterior approximal surfaces. With respect to the posterior teeth only, a 48 per cent reduction was found. This study therefore differs from others with respect to the surfaces showing the greatest reductions.

In addition to sodium fluoride, acidulated phosphate fluoride (APF) has also been used in mouthrinse studies in recent years. One such study compared three groups of 8–11-year-old children over a three-year period[56]. One group received daily 5 ml sodium fluoride rinses containing 0.02 per cent fluoride, whereas the second group used an acidulated phosphate fluoride rinse, also containing the equivalent of 0.2 per cent fluoride. The third group received a neutral placebo. The solutions were kept in the mouth for one minute and then swallowed. At the end of the study, reductions in DMFS of 27 per cent and 30 per cent were found in the neutral sodium fluoride and APF groups, respectively. Enamel biopsies showed that the APF solution was superior to sodium fluoride in depositing fluoride in intact enamel.

All rinsing studies referred to so far have been carried out in non-fluoride areas. The effect of rinsing in a 20-month study using a rinse containing 0.1 per cent stannous fluoride was conducted on 900 children, 8–13 years of age, who resided in an area where the water had been fluoridated to a level of 1 p.p.m.[57]. The children rinsed three times for 10, 20 and 30 seconds, every other school day. The children in study and control groups had a similar caries experience at the start of the study. Of the two dental examiners employed, both found a small reduction in caries increment at the end of the trial. This is an interesting result, because some benefit was apparently obtained by rinsing in addition to that derived from the consumption of fluoridated drinking water.

Thus, many studies have shown that fluoride incorporated into a mouthrinse is effective in reducing the incidence of dental caries over a period from one to three years. This has been observed in fluoridated and non-fluoridated areas. However, the observation by Koch[52] is important in that no difference between study and control groups was observed two years after cessation of mouthrinsing. It appears, therefore, that the beneficial effect of mouthrinsing with fluoride solutions can only be maintained if continued. Further studies are necessary to investigate whether benefits are maintained if the rinsing regimen is gradually phased down to (for example) monthly rinses. Alternatively, it may be sufficient to change to another fluoride regimen, such as annual topically applied fluorides, to maintain the benefits gained by fluoride rinsing.

This summary demonstrates that fluoride mouthrinsing may provide an answer to the problems of insufficient professional manpower and excessive costs that currently hinder topical fluoride programmes.

12.1.5 Fluoride dentifrices

Because a large segment of the population uses a dentifrice in conjunction with toothbrushing, the incorporation of fluoride into dentifrices is a logical and practical approach to the problem of delivering topical fluorides to a large number of people. Many studies on fluoride-containing dentifrices have been carried out. It can be concluded that several formulations containing stannous fluoride, sodium fluoride or sodium monofluorophosphate have anti-cariogenic properties, and reduce caries by 15–30 per cent.

The abrasives and other ingredients of dentifrices must be compatible with the dentifrice's fluoride system. Abrasives such as calcium pyrophosphate, insoluble sodium metaphosphate and acrylic particles have shown compatibility with their respective fluorides and have been reviewed in detail elsewhere[58]. Because dentifrices are proprietary products and are readily available, the levels of fluoride have to be kept low—in the region of 0.1 per cent—to avoid the danger of ingestion of possibly toxic quantities by children.

Hargreaves and Chester[59] carried out trials in which they investigated the effect of increasing the concentration of monofluorophosphate (MFP) to 2 per cent. The caries reductions found over a three-year period did not differ markedly from those in studies using lower concentrations of MFP. The greatest effect was found on smooth surfaces. One year after termination of the study, 221 children were re-examined. It was reported that a statistically significant difference in DMF increment between test and placebo groups still remained[60].

Although the caries reduction produced by using fluoride-containing dentifrices is low—an average of 20 per cent reduction in DMFS—it is nevertheless significant. Because this technique does not depend upon professional or supervised care, it represents a very useful and important part of a caries-preventive programme.

12.1.6 Fluoride-containing prophylaxis pastes

Early on in the development of topical fluoride programmes, it was recommended that, before application of the fluoride agent, teeth should be cleaned with a polishing paste. A rubber cup prophylaxis has therefore been an integral part of the topical fluoride therapy. It would be an attractive proposition if, by incorporating a fluoride compound into a polishing paste, a prophylaxis and topical fluoride application could be carried out in one procedure. However, because the fluoride ion is highly reactive, it readily forms complexes with the other constituents of the polishing paste and therefore tends to become inactivated.

The collective findings with an 8–9 per cent stannous fluoride–lava pumice prophylaxis paste, indicate that its use alone on a semi-annual basis will produce a modest caries-preventive effect. The cariostatic effect, however, is not comparable to that produced by a topical application of fluoride preceded by a prophylaxis with a non-fluoride paste. Thus, the recommendation for using a fluoride-containing prophylaxis paste is a controversial subject. The more recent development of zirconium silicate–stannous fluoride and silicone dioxide–acidulated phosphate fluoride prophylaxis pastes may lead to more successful results. No clinical trials have been reported which confirm the promising laboratory results with fluoride-containing polishing pastes.

Prophylaxis with a fluoride-containing polishing paste should not replace the topical application of fluorides. To date there is not adequate data to recommend any professionally applied fluoride-polishing paste as the sole fluoride agent in a topical fluoride programme. A thorough prophylaxis will remove a thin, but significant, layer of surface enamel of the order of 2–4 μm. This layer is rich in fluoride and highly mineralised. Therefore, if a prophylaxis is not to be followed by a topical application of a concentrated fluoride solution or gel, a fluoride-containing polishing paste should be used for cleaning the teeth initially to replace the fluoride which is removed.

12.1.7 Fluoride varnishes

In recent years, varnishes containing fluoride have been produced in an attempt to maintain the fluoride ion in intimate contact with the enamel surface for longer periods than conventional topical fluoride applications. After initial studies on extracted teeth, favourable results have been obtained in clinical trials. In one study[61], a 30 per cent reduction in caries increment between the study and control groups was found over a 15-month period. The varnish yielded 2.26 per cent available fluoride and was stated to be remarkably water-tolerant so that it could cover moist teeth.

In a recent *in vitro* study[62], a high concentration of fluoride was found in the outermost layer of enamel after treatment with the varnish. In a recent clinical trial, 376 5-year-old children were treated with a fluoride varnish using a half-mouth technique[63]. At the end of the second year only 20 per cent of the control first permanent molars were carious compared with 13 per cent on the test side. Further long-term clinical studies need to be carried out before this method can be recommended as an effective caries-preventive agent. Today, fluoride varnishes should be regarded as experimental agents.

12.2 Fissure Sealants in Caries Prevention

12.2.1 Development of techniques

Numerous studies have shown that the fluoridation of public water supplies and the use of fluoride preparations can reduce caries significantly. Whereas the approximal sites show the greatest reductions, the occlusal surfaces of posterior teeth are least benefited[64]. A number of techniques have been proposed in an attempt to prevent occlusal caries. In a study of prophylactic odontotomy[65] the occlusal fissures are filled, but this was not widely accepted since it necessitated the preparation of cavities in sound teeth. The use of chemical agents to seal pits and fissures, such as ammoniacal silver nitrate,[66] zinc chloride and potassium ferrocyanide[67], met with little success, as did the use of copper cement[68].

The eventual development of new synthetic resins led to the possibility of sealing occlusal fissures with adhesive materials which required no cavity preparation. Early work with the epoxy resins was unsuccessful, since the bond strength of these adhesives to the enamel surface was poor due to the presence of water in the tissue. The introduction of the cyanoacrylate group of adhesives seemed likely to overcome this difficulty by utilising a small amount of water for polymerisation. Initial application was found in medicine for the non-suture closure of arterial incisions[69]. However, methyl-2-cyanoacrylate was found to be unsatisfactory, since it was degraded in the tissues with some histotoxicity due to degradation by-products of formaldehyde and methyl cyanoacetate[70]. In spite of this, it was methyl-2-cyanoacrylate which was chosen as a fissure sealant. Reports showed that this material containing a filler could adhere to enamel surfaces *in vitro*[71] and *in vivo*[72] for relatively long periods. Adhesion was promoted by initial etching of the enamel surface with phosphoric acid solution[71, 73].

Early trials using the material gave encouraging results[72,74], although it was necessary for re-application every six months. A further trial, carried out in Britain[75], showed an almost total failure of the material as a fissure sealant after a six-month period. However, since slightly modified techniques were used with respect to acid treatment of the enamel surface prior to application of the resin, as well as alteration of the liquid–powder ratio of the resin, it is difficult to compare the results.

Two trials using a higher homologue, ethyl-2-cyanoacrylate and polymethyl methacrylate[76,77] showed significant reductions in occlusal caries. However, a third trial using the identical material, and also carried out in Japan[78], gave poor results.

A polyurethane sealant containing fluoride (Epoxylite 9070, Lee Pharmaceuticals, California, USA) has also been developed[79]. Report of this material as a fissure sealant has proved unsatisfactory in laboratory studies[80], and after a two-year trial period[81]. However, this flexible coating was designed to provide a high fluoride level in surface enamel due to release of fluoride ions, rather than as a permanent seal to occlusal fissures. In this respect, it might be regarded as a sophisticated topical fluoride application.

The other chemical sealant which has been used with apparent success is based on the class of monomers known as bis-GMA resins[82], the reaction product of bisphenol A and glycidyl methacrylate. With the addition of ceramic fillers, this has been used to produce a new generation of anterior filling materials, namely the composites. The basic material was first used as a fissure sealant in a three-year trial[83], in which it was applied only at the commencement. The material was chemically polymerised using benzyl peroxide as the catalyst and results showed a 30 per cent protection after three years.

Two materials of this type have been employed by several workers in laboratory[80] and clinical trials[81]. Although the two resin systems are essentially similar, the method of polymerisation differed. One material (Epoxylite 9075, Lee Pharmaceuticals, California, USA) employed a chemical catalyst/accelerator system and used a silane coupling agent to maintain adhesion[84]. Results of a two-year clinical trial with this material produced a significant reduction in occlusal caries[81]. Full retention was reported as being 51 per cent, with a 64 per cent reduction in caries compared with controls. In addition, partial retention of sealant was a further 15 per cent.

The second development of the bis-GMA resin[85] led to the incorporation of an ultraviolet light-sensitive catalyst, benzoin methyl ether (Nuva-Seal, L.D. Caulk Co., Milford, Delaware, USA). After application, the material is polymerised by exposure to long-wave ultraviolet light. Results of clinical trials after two years have shown a highly significant reduction in occlusal caries[85,86]. A recent trial in Britain using the identical material also showed a highly significant reduction in occlusal caries two years after a single application[81]. The results of this trial showed 80 per cent full retention of sealant after two years, with a further 15.3 per cent showing partial retention of the material.

More recently, the effectiveness of Nuva-Seal was reported in a five-year trial in Kalispell, Montana[87]. The children who took part in the trial were of two age-groups: 5–8-year-olds and 10–14-years-olds. The sealant was applied using portable equipment in a school environment. After one year of the trial (table 12.2), results on 900 pairs of homologous teeth showed an 81 per cent reduction in caries and an 88 per cent total retention of sealant[88]. After the second year of the trial (table 12.2), the sealant was reported as showing a 67 per cent reduction in caries relative to controls. Seventy-three per cent of test teeth showed full retention of the sealant. Failure of the sealant was recorded if the treated tooth was either carious, restored or extracted. If a two-surface (class II) restoration was found in the tooth, although it may have been inserted as a result of approximal caries, it nevertheless was counted as a sealant failure in this trial. The final report of the trial, five years after placement of the sealant, showed 56 per cent of treated sites retained sealant[89]. This resulted in a 92 per cent prevention of dental caries in sites with retention of material.

In the UK, several clinical trials using a number of fissure sealants have been carried out by Rock. The results after two years involving four commercial sealants were presented in 1974[90]. Each sealant was applied to two teeth in the mouths of 100 children between 11 and 13 years of age. The teeth sealed were in diagonally opposite quadrants, and teeth on the opposite side of each arch served as matched contralateral controls. The results after two years with Nuva-Seal are shown in table 12.3. The material was fully intact on 80 per cent of teeth, and had produced an 89 per cent reduction in occlusal caries relative to controls. In addition, a further 15.3 per cent of teeth were classed as showing partial retention. Of the 170 teeth used in this aspect of the trial, only 5 teeth (2.9 per cent) in the test group showed evidence of occlusal caries two years after the initial application of the sealant. However, 49 of the control teeth (28.8 per cent) were carious (table 12.4). One feature of relevance is that the numbers of teeth remaining fully sealed after two years were very similar to the numbers retaining sealant six months after application. This indicates that if the sealant is to

Table 12.2   Nuva-Seal (from Horowitz[87])

Time since application (years)	Complete retention (%)	Caries reduction (%)
1	88	81
2	73	67

Table 12.3   Nuva-Seal retention (from Rock[90])

Time since application (months)	Full retention (%)	Partial retention (%)	Sealant lost (%)
6	91.1	7.2	1.7
12	86.2	10.3	3.5
24	80.0	15.3	4.7

Table 12.4   Nuva-Seal: incidence of occlusal caries (from Rock[90])

Time since application (years)	No. of teeth in study	Caries Test teeth	Control teeth
2	170	5 (2.9%)	49 (28.8%)

be lost, it is lost early on, probably as a result of an incorrect application technique or polymerisation failure, rather than failure of the sealant/enamel bond.

In another Nuva-Seal study[91], 205 children between 5 and 17 years of age participated initially. Between them, 427 pairs of teeth were included in the study, one of each pair being sealed. At six months, 39 per cent of all teeth were graded as having the sealant completely intact, with a further 44.2 per cent classed as showing partial retention. However, the total retention figure of 83.2 per cent may be the significant one regarding prevention of caries as partial loss of sealant usually occurs on cuspal slopes. This may not reduce the efficacy of the seal.

A further two-year study using Nuva-Seal was carried out in the Aberdare region of South

Wales[92]. The age range of the 106 patients was 6–13 years, presenting a complete spectrum of the mixed dentition. Of the 275 teeth sealed in the study, 86.2 per cent were found to be fully sealed after two years, with 6.2 per cent showing partial retention, while 7.6 per cent showed loss of sealant (table 12.5). Regarding caries incidence, 9.1 per cent of test teeth were classed as being carious, whereas 36 per cent of controls became carious over the two-year period (table 12.6).

Table 12.5   Nuva-Seal retention (from Douglas and Tranter[92])

No. of teeth	Time since application (months)	Full retention (%)	Partial retention (%)	Sealant lost (%)
275	24	86.2	6.2	7.6

Table 12.6   Nuva-Seal: incidence of occlusal caries (Douglas and Tranter[92])

No. of teeth	Carious test teeth	Carious control teeth
275	25 (9.1%)	99 (36.0%)

12.2.2   Mechanism of sealant retention

The use of an acid solution to etch the enamel surface is an essential prerequisite for the successful bonding of resin to the hard tissue. The acid usually employed is phosphoric acid with an exposure time of 60 s. Buonocore[73] used 85 per cent phosphoric acid solution to etch or 'condition' enamel prior to the use of acrylic restorative materials, in order to improve the edge adaptation. Since then, many workers have used a solution of 50 per cent phosphoric acid, buffered with 7 per cent zinc oxide by weight, as an etching agent prior to bounding of sealants or composite resins to enamel.

Silverstone[80] has shown that the acid solution produces changes to the enamel surface in two distinct ways. In the first, a shallow layer of enamel, approximately 10 μm in depth, is re-

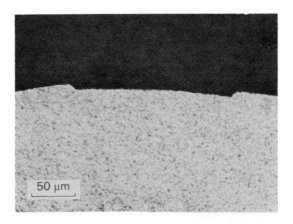

Figure 12.1   Longitudinal ground section showing a region of enamel exposed to 30 per cent phosphoric acid for 60 s examined in water between crossed polars. A layer of enamel measuring 8 μm has been removed from the window region by etching

moved by etching (figure 12.1). In this manner plaque, surface and sub-surface cuticles are effectively removed from the site to be bonded. In addition, chemically inert crystals in surface enamel are also removed, so favouring attempts at chemical union between hard tissue and resin. In the second, after removal of the surface layer by etching, the remaining enamel surface is rendered porous by the acid solution (figure 12.2). It is into this porous region that the resin is able to penetrate and so bond with the enamel. The depth of enamel rendered porous can be measured accurately in polarised light[80]. Examination of the enamel/resin junction with electron microscopy shows that an excellent bond occurs between enamel and resin irrespective of the material used (figure 12.3). The most important parameter is to obtain a satisfactory initial etch. Demineralisation of enamel to reveal the fitting resin surface demonstrates the extent of penetration of the resin into etched enamel. Tags of up to 50 μm in length are identified routinely (figure 12.4) and present a formidable area for retention.

12.2.3   Range of etchants and solutions

Many studies have been carried out with a 50 per cent solution of phosphoric acid buffered with 7

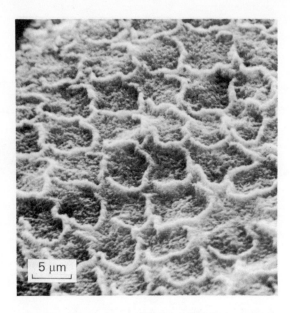

Figure 12.2   Scanning electron micrograph of an enamel surface which has been etched with phosphoric acid for 60 s. The etch pattern is one in which prism centres have been removed preferentially—termed a type 1 etching pattern

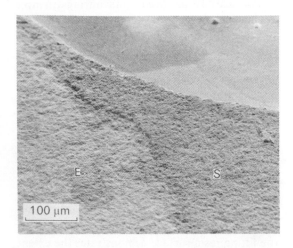

Figure 12.3   Examination of the enamel/sealant junction with the scanning electron microscope shows no evidence of separation of the sealant (S) from the enamel (E), in spite of section preparation and examination procedures

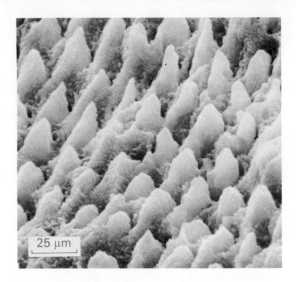

Figure 12.4   Scanning electron micrograph of a sample of fissure sealant after demineralisation of the adjacent enamel. The inner fitting surface of the resin shows tags which are approximately 30 μm in length

per cent zinc oxide by weight[93,94]. However, in a recent study[80] a number of different acid solutions, as well as phorphoric acid in the concentration range 20–70 per cent, were investigated for their effects on enamel surfaces *in vitro*. Phosphoric acid was found to be the most successful agent for etching enamel surfaces prior to application of a resin. The degree of etching increased with decreasing acid concentration (figure 12.5).

The most retentive conditions for a sealant were found to be in the range 30–40 per cent, with a 30 per cent (w/w) unbuffered solution of phosphoric acid being the most effective single agent.

In a further study[95] phosphoric acid solutions in the concentration range 5–80 per cent (w/w) were investigated for their effects on human enamel surfaces, with special reference to the variation in degree of etching over single tooth surfaces. When using acid concentrations of 5–15 per cent and 70–80 per cent, only minimal surface changes were found. The most evenly distributed etching patterns were found with solutions of 30–40 per cent phosphoric acid used with 60 s exposure periods. A 30 per cent unbuffered solution of phosphoric acid produced the most consistent and evenly distributed etch over a single enamel surface.

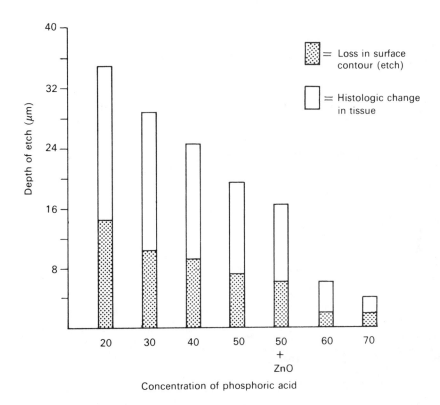

Figure 12.5 Histogram showing the depth of enamel affected by a 60-s exposure to various concentrations of phosphoric acid. This consists of both the loss in depth due to etching and the region showing histological change due to the creation of porous regions (From Silverstone, L. M., 1974, 8, 2–26; courtesy of *Caries Research*)

12.2.4 Types of etching pattern

In a recent report by Silverstone and co-workers[96] three basic etching patterns were found when human dental enamel was exposed to phosphoric acid. In the first, called type 1 etching pattern, there was a generalised roughening of the enamel surface, but with a distinct pattern showing hollowing of prism centres with relatively intact peripheral regions (figure 12.2). The average diameter of the hollowed regions was 3μm. This was found to be the most common of the three patterns observed.

In the second, or type 2 etching pattern, prism peripheries appeared to be removed, or heavily damaged (figure 12.6). Therefore, the prism cores were left projecting towards the original enamel surface. This damage of the peripheral regions of the prisms was seen to extend along the

length of the prism, thus aiding in delineating individual prisms. When viewed from the original surface, separate bundles or columns of material were seen, the gaps separating them corresponding to the peripheral regions of the prisms. Thus, this type 2 etching pattern is the reverse of the honeycomb pattern of type 1 damage, and both patterns are produced by exposure to a similar solution of phosphoric acid for an identical exposure time.

Some etched regions showed neither type 1 nor type 2 etching patterns exclusively. These areas appeared as a generalised surface roughening, referred to as a type 3 etching pattern (figure 12.7). The whole region in the type 3 etching pattern was one in which the surface topography could not be related to a prism pattern. All three patterns of etching were found to occur on the one enamel surface produced by identical con-

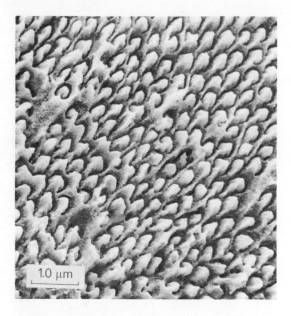

Figure 12.6 Scanning electron micrograph of an enamel surface which has been exposed to 40 per cent phosphoric acid for 60 s. In this case the etching pattern is one in which there has been a preferential removal of prism peripheries—termed a type 2 etching pattern

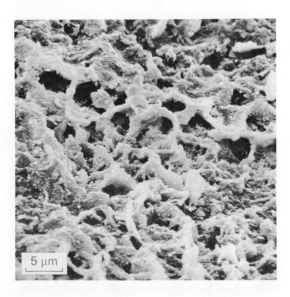

Figure 12.7 Scanning electron micrograph of an enamel surface treated with 30 per cent phosphoric acid for 60 s. The etching pattern shows a generalised surface roughening with no apparent evidence of a prism pattern—termed a type 3 etching pattern

ditions of acid attack. This highlights the variation in structure that can occur in enamel, not only from tooth to tooth or surface to surface, but also from site to site on a single tooth surface.

12.2.5 Caries susceptibility of acid-etched enamel

No evidence of caries or demineralisation of test teeth has been reported which could be related to the original etching of the enamel. Acid etching is an essential stage in the bonding mechanism and it appears to be confined to the cuspal slopes, rather than to the base of the fissure, and this is the region where the bond occurs[80]. In addition, a number of studies have shown that etched enamel, not covered by resin, will be remineralised on contact with the oral fluid[97]. Quantitative studies on enamel solubility rates have shown recently that the solubility rate of acid-etched enamel returns to that of adjacent sound enamel after 24 h exposure to oral fluid[98]. In addition, fissure-sealed enamel surfaces artificially abraded *in vitro*, show a lower solubility rate than adjacent sound enamel[98]. These results were interpreted as being due to the retention of tags of sealant, which penetrated for up to 50 μm into the enamel surface. Thus, fissure-sealed enamel surfaces which have been worn down might well be less susceptible to caries than adjacent sound enamel.

In a community dependent upon an average civilised diet, the high prevalence of dental caries cannot be controlled by reparative techniques alone. Caries prevention programmes must be run in addition to restorative procedures if the disease is to be controlled. From all available evidence, fissure sealants are likely to play an important role in caries prevention to augment fluoride and other techniques, since they are intended to protect caries-susceptible surfaces that are least benefited by fluoride. The occlusal surface accounts for nearly half the caries of a school life-time in English children[99]. Since it is the surface least protected by fluoride and most accessible to the clinical operator, the use of fissure sealants can have a highly significant caries-preventive effect. Some of the materials currently available, together with others under development, offer an exciting preventive technique to be employed in conjunction with other caries control measures.

12.3   Remineralisation Phenomena

12.3.1   Rationale

It is now 60 years since it was first concluded that enamel, artificially softened by acid, becomes partially rehardened after immersion in saliva[100]. More recently[101] it has been shown beyond doubt that a considerable degree of rehardening of acid-softened enamel may be achieved by exposure to saliva. Even more rehardening takes place if a remineralising solution, containing calcium and phosphate ions at an appropriate concentration and in a certain ratio, is used. It is clear that in deficient enamel, new mineral will precipitate from solution. In such experiments flat facets are prepared on human caries-free enamel surfaces by grinding and polishing. These facets are then tested for hardness by means of a Knoop diamond indenter. The same surfaces are softened by exposure to acid which results in a reduction in hardness of the enamel surface. Finally, the softened surfaces are exposed to a rehardening medium prepared from calcium phosphate solution. In this way the enamel may recover over 90 per cent of its lost hardness[101].

In experimental studies on the 'remineralisation' of enamel caries[102, 103], carious lesions, and artificial caries-like lesions, were exposed to either saliva or a synthetic calcifying fluid *in vitro*. After exposure, there was a significant reduction in pore volume throughout the lesions, resulting in the histological appearance of a much earlier stage in lesion formation than that existing prior to experiment (figures 12.8(a) and 12.8(b)). This occurred with both natural and artificial lesions and was found when either saliva or the calcifying fluid were employed. However, the synthetic

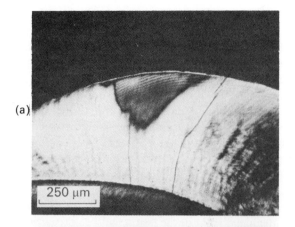

(a)

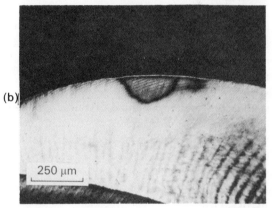

(b)

Figure 12.8 (a) Longitudinal ground section from the control half of a carious lesion examined in water with the polarising microscope. (b) Longitudinal ground section taken from the test half of the same lesion as in (a), also examined in water with polarised light. This half of the lesion had the surface exposed to a synthetic calcifying fluid and shows a significant degree of remineralisation. The test lesion is smaller than its control and exhibits a considerable reduction in pore volume

calcifying fluid, which contained no organic material, was more effective in producing these changes than was saliva[103]. When examined in quinoline with polarised light, the most obvious change in the modified lesion was a significant broadening of the dark zone as a consequence of its extension back towards the enamel surface, into the region identified in chapter 6 as the body of the lesion (figure 6.5). In addition, lesions which showed no evidence of a dark zone in quinoline were also exposed to the synthetic calcifying fluid. After the experiment, many of the lesions demonstrated dark zones positioned at the 'correct' histological site between the translucent zone and the body of the lesion when examined in quinoline. The imbibition behaviour of 'new' dark zones, and those which increased in width after experiment, was consistent with that of the dark zone proper. Thus, part of the body of the lesion (zone 3) had reverted to the histological characteristics of the dark zone (zone 2)[103].

Prior to these findings, the dark zone at the advancing front of the lesion had been regarded as a breakdown stage successional to the translucent zone and preceding the body of the lesion. It has always been difficult to explain why in the first zone of enamel caries, the translucent zone, relatively large pores are found, whereas in the succeeding stage of breakdown, the dark zone, a smaller pore system is found in addition to the large pores. The micropores in the dark zone were explained as being due to demineralisation, or 'opening up', of specific sites in the tissue which were not attacked in the first zone of breakdown. If some of the relatively large pores of the body of the lesion could, in effect, become the minute ones of the dark zone, then this could indicate that the micropore system of the dark zone may not be formed by a simple process of continuing demineralisation. Thus, the zone may not be a stage in the sequential breakdown of the tissue as was previously thought. The micropores may be formed by 'remineralisation', whereby either the size or the accessibility of the large pores was reduced by the deposition of material. The results from *in vitro* studies suggest that mineral deposition could account for the 'closing down' of the original pores created as a result of demineralisation, such as are found in the translucent zone, although *in vivo* organic material might also contribute.

If this is the case, then this lends further support to the concept that the carious process in enamel is a dynamic one with phases of demineralisation alternating with phases of remineralisation, rather than a more simple process

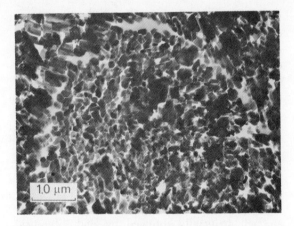

Figure 12.9   Transmission electron micrograph through the control half of a section of a carious lesion cut perpendicularly to the prisms. A channel can be seen surrounding the prism which is filled with the embedding material. This is characteristic of carious enamel

of continuing dissolution. In this way, the variation in distribution and width of the dark zone over the advancing front of the enamel lesion may be explained as functions of the efficacy of the 'remineralisation' process. Of significance in this respect are the observations[104] that lesions of 'arrested' caries have wide, well-marked, dark zones.

Through the comparison of ultra-thin sections of remineralised lesions with those of untreated lesions, electron microscopy has revealed that remineralised enamel is less porous and possesses dense collections of foreign crystals, especially at prism junctions (figures 12.9 and 12.10). These crystals, which may be identified throughout the tissue near the centre of lesions, are larger and have a more plate-like habit than the hydroxyapatite crystals of sound enamel. Carious enamel also shows enlarged crystals at prism junctions, but in this case the crystals do not achieve the size or density of those identified in remineralised enamel. The relatively intact surface zone which persists over a lesion as sub-surface demineralisation progresses often shows signs, at microscopically observable points, of minor damage. These points of damage disappear after remineralisation[105], which may also be accounted

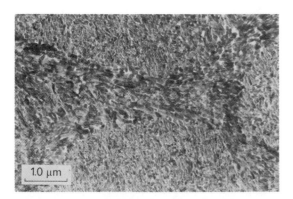

Figure 12.10 Transmission electron micrograph through the test half of the same lesion seen in figure 12.9 after exposure to a calcifying fluid *in vitro*. The tail of a prism can be seen in the centre, with heads of adjacent prisms above, below and to one side. There is no evidence of junctional gaps between the prisms, as is evident in the control half of the same lesion. The tail region of the prism is densely packed with crystals

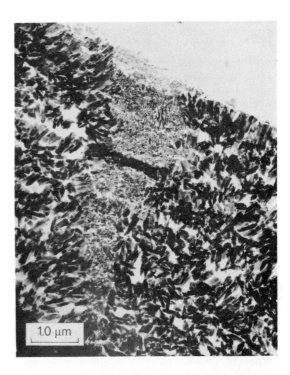

Figure 12.11 Transmission electron micrograph of an ultra-thin section of surface enamel from an erupted human tooth which had been exposed to a calcifying fluid for four days *in vitro*. A narrow, cleft-like, defect has become filled with rounded crystals, much smaller than the surrounding apatite crystals. Over the outer surface of the tooth a deposit of granular mineral has occurred. These features were not seen in the control half of the same surface

for by the precipitation on to, and into defects within, the enamel surface of small crystals and granular deposits, as seen by electron microscopy. Similar precipitates also form on the surfaces of sound enamel exposed to remineralising solutions[106] (figure 12.11). These crystals and granules are different, in size and habit, from those deposited in deeper tissue but, as yet, the identity of all these crystals remains uncertain. Nevertheless, there is evidence, based on measured increases in intrinsic birefringence, that regrowth of apatite occurs[106].

Thus, remineralising experiments, based both upon hardness measurements and changes in histology, leave no doubt that it is possible for calcium salts to precipitate on enamel surfaces and within tissue softened artificially or by caries. Other parameters of the remineralising process have also been defined. By hardness measurement it has been shown that there is a limit to the degree of softening beyond which rehardening is poor. The rate of rehardening is dependent upon pH and the degree of saturation of the mineralising solutions[107]. In saturated solutions, spontaneous precipitation is faster than crystal growth within the microspaces of softened enamel. Below this maximum level, conditions seem more favourable for crystal growth within the tissue, but the continued lowering of the concentrations of ionic calcium and phosphate, or the lowering of pH, can slowly deactivate the remineralising capacity of the solution.

The presence of sodium and chloride ions increases the stability and range of pH over which the solutions are active in rehardening buffer-softened enamel[108]. Certain ions appear to have an inhibiting effect[109]. However, the inhibition produced by poisons such as copper(II) ions can be reversed by washing out with calcium chloride, as is also true in the mineralisation of rachitic cartilage[110]. It has been suggested that copper(II) ions inhibit the nucleation but not the growth of apatite crystals[111]. In enamel, it is possible that inhibition and reactivation of remineralisation indicate that rehardening is not simply a matter of the infilling of microspaces. Rather, crystals form in the microspaces on surfaces with active groups necessary to trigger crystallisation before spontaneous precipitation takes place in the bulk of the calcifying solution.

Histological studies have shown that conditioning of sound enamel surfaces by exposure to remineralising solutions resulted in an increased resistance to artificial caries[106] associated with a decreased surface solubility. As shown by both rehardening[101] and histological studies[103, 105], saliva can be used to remineralise enamel *in vitro,* although it is not as efficient as the synthetic solutions. Moreover, remineralisation of softened enamel can be achieved by exposure, *in vivo,* to oral fluids. However, from the point of view of dental caries prevention, probably the most important observations of all relate to the influence of the fluoride ion on remineralisation[101, 103]. Not only does the presence of fluoride accelerate rehardening by a factor of four, but also it results in producing a greater degree of remineralisation of a lesion in a shorter exposure time compared to using a calcifying fluid with no fluoride[8].

12.3.2   Biological role of saliva in remineralisation

Dental caries is a rare disease in animals other than man, and it is therefore unlikely that the character and composition of saliva has arisen as a specific evolutionary response to this disease. Nevertheless, it is important to try and understand the role of saliva, from the remineralisation point of view, in order to define the most likely forms of prophylaxis against the disease.

Human saliva varies in composition from individual to individual, from gland to gland in the same individual and from time to time in the same gland; for example, stimulated saliva differs from resting saliva. Organic components are several proteins, including glycoproteins and enzymes, carbohydrates, both protein-bound and dialysable, lipids and a number of compounds of low molecular weight, such as urea, amino acids and organic acids[112]. The major inorganic components are calcium, phosphate, sodium, potassium, magnesium, chloride, and hydrogen carbonate ions and dissolved carbon dioxide. As well as fluoride, trace amounts of iron, copper, cobalt, bromide and iodide are present[113]. The average amount[114] of calcium present is 5.8 mg/100 ml (2.2–11.3 mg%) and of phosphorus 16.8 mg/100 ml (6.1–71.0 mg%). Almost half the calcium is complexed in either organic or inorganic form, whereas 90 per cent of the phosphorus is inorganic, 10 per cent of this being in the form of complexes.

In spite of the complexing, appreciable amounts of calcium and phosphorus (as PO_4) are present in ionic form. Calculations of the activity products from the ionic activities of calcium and phosphate reveal that both resting and stimulated saliva are always saturated or supersaturated with respect to hydroxyapatite[113]. As regards other forms of calcium phosphate found in the mouth, resting saliva is undersaturated, and stimulated saliva saturated, with respect to both brushite ($CaHPO_4, 2H_2O$) and octacalcium phosphate ($Ca_8H_2(PO_4)_6, 5H_2O$).

With this composition it is not surprising that at times in most people, and frequently in some, solid calcium phosphate is deposited on the teeth in the form of calculus. A number of different phosphates may be present in calculus including hydroxyapatite, octacalcium phosphate, whitlockite and brushite. It is possible that by nucleating, organic material on the tooth surfaces accelerates the mineralising process. In some animals, such as rats, there appears to be a positive gain in the degree of enamel mineralisation after the tooth has erupted into the mouth and has therefore been exposed to saliva[115]. However, it is not certain if there is more than a minimal increase in mineral, as the tooth erupts into the mouth, in most animals including man, although the possibility of the existence of a critical maturation phase at this time has been discussed[116, 117].

True mastication evolved with the emergence of the mammalian vertebrates and involved appropriate modifications of both jaws and teeth, the latter becoming more generally varied in crown form, the grinding molars being particularly complex. The enamel covering the teeth became thicker and, with its prismatic structure, mechanically more efficient[118]. Related to this, and most important to this discussion, was the reduction in number of tooth generations to a maximum of two, the permanent teeth functioning for most of the life of the individual animal. It is therefore understandable that the surfaces, especially between teeth, became choice habitats for microorganisms, for here are available sheltered microenvironments, sources of food and essential minerals, such as calcium and phosphate, from either saliva or the tooth surfaces themseves. In turn, the organisms might have had a role in helping to cleanse, or at least loosen, wedged debris from the teeth and even if, as a consequence of fermented organic acids, some of the tooth surfaces were demineralised, the integrity could be restored when access to saliva was regained. In this way it is possible to see the biological interrelation between the composition of saliva and the maintenance of tooth surfaces. Of great interest in this respect is the observation[119] on the repeated exposure of human enamel to acid buffers containing calcium and phosphate ions. Surfaces exposed to a series of successively more undersaturated buffers became increasingly more resistant to demineralisation than control surfaces. This could be a model of the effect on enamel of the combined activities of saliva and acid-producing bacteria.

However, in such considerations as these, it is possible to think only in terms of enamel as constituting tooth surfaces. This is because modern man tends to eat soft, cooked foods so that it is quite usual, even in old age, for the tooth crowns to remain covered with enamel. But this is unnatural since most animals (including primitive man indulging in heavy mastication) rapidly grind crowns into flattened surfaces, exposing dentine in the process. Exposed dentine reacts by occluding the odontoblast tubules, which originally housed cell processes, with mineral. Dentine may also acquire mineral from saliva[120] and this is undoubtedly an important function since, in order that the combined enamel–dentine surfaces might not become too irregular,

the dentine should be as hard as possible. Thus, the maintenance role of saliva really applies as much to dentine as to enamel and, even in modern man, dentine exposed to saliva by trauma or caries may become sufficiently hard ('arrested' dentine caries) for it to need no restorative treatment.

12.3.3   The present situation and possibilities for the future

It may properly be asked why, with a built-in system of protection, does a tooth decay? The answer is complex but, briefly, there are two important factors. First, absence of natural heavy mastication and consequent attrition leaves persistent grooves and fissures on the occlusal surfaces as well as curved, rather than flattened, contacting surfaces between teeth. In both types of situation, food—fermenting under the action of microorganisms—can only be cleaned away with great difficulty. The second factor is the inclusion of large quantities of sucrose in the diet which is not only rapidly fermented but also leads to the establishment of dense masses of microorganisms, the dental plaque. Thus, saliva never reaches the surfaces at risk and it is the contents of the plaque which determine what happens at the tooth surface. The plaque itself acquires mineral from saliva, but whether remineralisation can occur depends very much on the prevailing, often acidogenic, conditions at the tooth surfaces. From the very high incidence of the disease it is obvious that the natural restorative process cannot match the rate of dissolution.

It is not beyond the bounds of possibility that some boost to the restorative role of the saliva–plaque complex can be provided. The addition of calcium sucrose phosphate to the diets of test animals does not seem to have a notable caries-reducing effect[121] and does not justify earlier optimism. However, the addition of calcium glycerophosphate to the diet of monkeys has produced a reduction in caries[122]. In the test animals, concentrations of calcium in plaque were increased, and these could contribute to the buffering capacity and reduce the ability to dissolve enamel. Perhaps remineralisation is also encouraged.

From the various experiments which have been discussed here, it is apparent that if demineralisation of enamel exceeds certain limits, complete remineralisation is not possible even with prolonged exposure to the more efficient, synthetic remineralising solutions. Once established, dental caries is likely to persist and the principal aim must therefore be to prevent the disease from starting in the first place. Prolonged searches have therefore been made for substances which are known not only to contribute to the protection of the tooth surfaces but also to stand a reasonable chance of actually penetrating the plaque and reaching surfaces at risk. In this respect, the marked reducing effect on caries of the fluoride ion has attracted most attention, yet, even now, the exact way in which it acts to reduce caries is in doubt. There are several possibilities. First, flouride released from the tooth surface may act as an enzyme poison and so reduce acid production by organisms[123]. Secondly, fluorapatite is less soluble than hydroxyapatite, so that if fluoride is incorporated into tooth mineral in this way, either during development or possibly later in the mouth, its overall solubility will be reduced. Thirdly, the presence of fluoride ions improves nucleation of apatite and results in crystals of better form. The last two possibilities are both important from the point of view of remineralisation.

Unfortunately, a full understanding of remineralisation is still hindered by the lack of knowledge of the re-formed mineral. Because of the variability of habit of each of the forms of calcium phosphate, it is not possible to identify the different crystals morphologically. Moreover, not only is it difficult to distinguish hydroxyapatite from octacalcium phosphate by means of electron diffraction, but both octacalcium phosphate and dicalcium phosphate are fairly easily hydrolysed to hydroxyapatite. Even X-ray diffraction studies fail to distinguish between intact demineralised and remineralised enamel.

Hydroxypatite should form, in experimental systems at least, at and above pH 6.8^{124}, and electron probe studies show that remineralised enamel has the same Ca:P ratio (about 2.1) as normal enamel[125]. Recent measurements on various parameters of the model remineralising system show that fluoride not only increases the rate of deposition of calcium phosphate, but also becomes incorporated into the mineral, probably as fluorapatite or fluorohydroxyapatite. This in itself would be a direct contribution to the known, reduced acid solubility of remineralised enamel.

Among these various possibilities must lie the explanation of the small, but positive, beneficial effect of ingesting fluoridated water after the teeth have formed and have erupted into the mouth although, of course, the principal benefit accrues from incorporation during the formation of teeth. And it may be concluded that a beneficial effect on enamel could be achieved by conditioning surfaces with remineralising solutions *in vivo* as has been done *in vitro*. The most serious difficulty is the time required for such conditioning which, with present knowledge, would be too great even for prophylactic treatment in a dental office. In view of this, it is not surprising that intense interest continues in the possibilities of incorporating, in some beneficial way, fluoride into the tooth surface by means of the topical application of relatively strong solutions.

The literature concerning topical applications of fluoride to tooth surfaces is exhaustive and has been summarised at the beginning of this chapter.

The topical use of fluoride in acid solutions[126] has been suggested on the grounds that, in this way, fluoride is more readily taken up by apatite and more effectively reduces solubility. However, some of the tooth mineral must dissolve, resulting in the formation of calcium fluoride and more soluble phosphates, the latter possibly accounting for the failure to reduce caries in early trials with acidulated fluoride. It has been proposed that much of this demineralisation would be prevented by the use of phosphoric acid[126]. A relatively brief exposure to sodium fluoride and phosphoric acid together reduced enamel solubility significantly, and fluoride appeared to be incorporated primarily as fluorapatite, calcium fluoride being absent or present in small quantities only. These experiments were followed by successful clinical trials[127] in which a substantial reduction in caries was induced in a group of children treated once a year with acid phosphate-flouride (APF); there also appeared to be a marked improvement over a parallel group in which 8 per cent stannous fluoride had been used.

Current experimental work suggests that both APF and stannous fluoride treatments reduce enamel solubility, although possibly by different mechanisms[128]. Initial leaching by APF may be followed by fluoride-stimulated remineralisation as acid concentrations in the plaque are reduced. Tin(II) ions tend to inhibit remineralisation, but the complex formed with tin(II) after fluoride treatment is extremely resistant to acid attack.

A note of caution has been sounded already[123]. The fact that high fluoride concentrations lower solubility *in vitro* does not prove the mechanism by which fluoride works *in vivo,* either via water supplies or topical application. Nevertheless, it is hoped that this brief and selective review will illustrate the likely interrelations between fluoride action and remineralising processes.

Therefore, it can be concluded that there exists in the mouth a natural biological remineralising process in which the integrity of surfaces of the tooth is maintained by means of precipitation of new mineral from saliva. The use of synthetic remineralising solutions is more efficient than saliva, but once mineral loss from enamel exceeds certain limits remineralisation is poor. For this reason it is unlikely that carious enamel which has cavitated can be repaired. With a fuller knowledge of the biology of dental plaque it is conceivable that remineralising processes could be boosted against the initial establishment of caries. It is possible that the main cariostatic action of fluoride is in producing remineralisation[8].

As understanding of the complex physical and chemical reactions at tooth surfaces improves, there must be real hope that a truly effective prophylaxis against dental caries will be evolved in the not too distant future.

References

1. Gray, J. A., Frances, M. D. and Griebstein, W. J. (1962). Chemistry of enamel dissolution, in *Chemistry and Prevention of Dental Caries* (Ed. Sognnaes, R. F), Charles C. Thomas, Springfield, Ill., pp. 164–79

2. Jenkins, G. N. (1967). The mechanism of action of fluoride in reducing caries incidence. *International Dental Journal,* **17,** 552–63

3. Glantz, P. (1969). Reduction in the surface energy in teeth by fluoride. *Odontologia Revy,* **20,** 17

4. Ericson, T. and Ericsson, Y. (1967). Effect of partial fluorine substitution on the phosphate exchange and protein adsorption of hydroxylapatite. *Helvitica Odontologica Acta,* **11,** 10–14

5. Pearlman, B. A. and Joyston-Bechal, S. J. (1973). A pilot study on the use of fluoride as a plaque preventive agent. *Journal of Dental Research,* **52,** 953

6. Forrest, J. R. (1956). Caries incidence v enamel defects in areas with different levels of fluoride in the drinking water. *British Dental Journal,* **100,** 195–200.

7. McCann, H. G., and Brudevold, F. (1966). The mechanism of the caries inhibitory effect of fluoride, in *Environmental Variables in Oral Disease* (Eds. Kreshover, S. S. and McClure, F. D.), American Association for the Advancement of Science, Washington, DC, pp. 121–3

8. Silverstone, L. M. (1977). Remineralization phenomena. In *Cariostatic Mechanisms of Fluoride* (Eds Brown, W. E. and Konig, K. G.), *Caries Research,* **11** (suppl. 1), 59–84

9. Bibby, B. G. (1942). Preliminary report on the use of sodium fluoride applications in caries prophylaxis. *Journal of Dental Research*, **21**, 661

10. Knutson, J. W. (1948). Sodium fluoride solutions: technique for application to the teeth. *Journal of the American Dental Association*, **36**, 37–9

11. Horowitz, H. S. and Heifetz, S. B. (1970). The current status of topical fluoride in preventive dentistry. *Journal of the American Dental Association*, **81**, 166–77

12. Syrrist, A. and Karlsen, K. (1954). A five year report on the effect of topical applications of sodium fluoride on dental caries experience. *British Dental Journal*, **97**, 1–6

13. Muhler, J. C., Boyd, T. M. and Huysen, G. (1950). Effect of fluorides and other compounds on the solubility of enamel, dentine and tricalcium phosphate in dilute acids. *Journal of Dental Research*, **29**, 182–196

14. Howell, C. L., Gish, C. W., Smiley, R. D. and Muhler, J. D. (1955). Effect of topically applied stannous fluoride on dental caries experience in children. *Journal of the American Dental Association*, **50**, 14–17

15. Slack, G. L. (1956). The effect of topical application of stannous fluoride on the incidence of dental caries in six year old children. *British Dental Journal*, **101**, 7–11

16. Nevitt, G. A., Witter, D. H. and Bowman, W. D. (1958). Topical applications of sodium fluoride v stannous fluoride. *Public Health Reports*, **73**, 847–850.

17. Gish, C. W., Howell, C. L. and Muhler, J. C. (1959). A new approach to the topical application of fluoride in children with results at the end of 4 years. *Journal of Dentistry for Children*, **26**, 300–3

18. Mercer, V. H. and Muhler, J. C. (1972). Comparison of single topical applications of sodium fluoride and stannous fluoride. *Journal of Dental Research*, **51**, 1325–30

19. Peterson, J. K. and Williamson, L. (1962). Effectiveness of topical application of eight per cent stannous fluoride. *Public Health Reports*, **77**, 39–40

20. Law, F. R., Jeffreys, M. H. and Sheary, H. C. (1961). Topical application of fluoride solutions in dental caries control. *Public Health Reports*, **76**, 287–90

21. Harris, R. (1963). Observations on the effect of 8 % sodium fluoride on dental caries in children. *Australian Dental Journal*, **8**, 335–40

22. Wellock, W. D., Maitland, A. and Brudevold, F. (1965). Caries increments, tooth discoloration, and state of oral hygiene in children given single annual applications of acid phosphate-fluoride and stannous fluoride. *Archives of Oral Biology*, **10**, 453–60

23. Torell, P. and Ericsson, Y. (1965). Two year clinical tests with different methods of local caries preventive fluorine application in Swedish school children. *Acta Odontologica Scandinavica*, **4**, 287–322

24. Horowitz, H. S. and Lucye, H. S. (1966). A clinical study of stannous fluoride in a prophylaxis paste and as a solution. *Journal of Oral Therapy*, **3**, 17–25

25. Backer Dirks, O. (1967). The relation between the fluoridation of water and dental caries experience. *International Dental Journal*, **17**, 582

26. Forrester, D. J. and Auger, M. F. (1971). A review of currently available topical fluoride agents. *Journal of Dentistry for Children*, **38**, 272–8

27. Brudevold, F., Savory, A., Gardner, D. E., Spinelli, M. and Speirs, R. (1963). A study of acidulated fluoride solutions. *Archives of Oral Biology*, **8**, 167–77

28. Wellock, W. D. and Brudevold, F. (1963). A study of acidulated fluoride solutions. II. The caries inhibition effect of single annual topical applications of an acidic fluoride and phosphate solution, a two year experience. *Archives of Oral Biology*, **8**, 179–82

29. Pameijer, J. H. N., Brudevold, F. and Hunt, E. E. (1963). A study of acidulated fluoride solutions. III. The cariostatic effect of repeated topical sodium fluoride applications with and without phosphate. A pilot study. *Archives of Oral Biology*, **8**, 183–5

30. Cartwright, H. V., Lindahl, R. L. and Bawden, J. W. (1968). Clinical findings on the effectiveness of stannous fluoride and acid phosphate-fluoride as caries reducing agents in children. *Journal of Dentistry for Children*, **35**, 36–40

31. Horowitz, H. S. (1969). Effect on dental caries of topically applied acidulated phosphate-fluoride: results after two years. *Journal of the American Dental Association*, **78**, 568–72

32. Bryan, E. G. and Williams, J. E. (1970). The cariostatic effectiveness of a phosphate-fluoride gel administered annually to school children: final results. *Journal of Public Health Dentistry*, **30**, 13–16

33. Ingraham, R. Q. and Williams, J. E. (1970). An evaluation of the utility of application and cariostatic effectiveness of phosphate-fluorides in solution and gel states. *Journal of Tennessee Dental Association*, **50**, 5–12

34. Cons, N. C., Janerich, D. T. and Senning, R. S. (1970). Albany topical fluoride study. *Journal of the American Dental Association*, **80**, 777–81

35. Englander, H. R., Heyes, P. H. and Gestwicki, M. (1967). Clinical anticaries effect of repeated topical sodium fluoride applications by mouth pieces. *Journal of the American Dental Association*, **75**, 638–44

36. Mellberg, J. R., Laasko, P. V. and Nicholson, C. (1966). The acquisition and loss of fluoride by topically fluoridated human tooth enamel. *Archives of Oral Biology*, **11**, 1213–20

37. Brudevold, F., McCann, H. G., Nilsson, R., Richardson, B. and Coklica, V. (1967). The chemistry of caries inhibition: problems and challenges in topical treatments. *Journal of Dental Research*, **46**, 37–45

38. Mellberg, J. R. and Nicholson, C. R. (1968). *In vitro* evaluation of an acidulated fluoride-phosphate prophylaxis paste. *Archives of Oral Biology*, **13**, 1223–34

39. Hotz, P. (1972). Fluoride level in surface enamel after application of fluoride gels. *Helvitica Odontologica Acta*, **16**, 32–4

40. Clarkson, B. H. (1972). The *in vitro* uptake of fluoride from five topical fluoride agents and its effect on artificial lesion formation. *Journal of Dental Research*, **51**, 1262

41. Clarkson, B. H. and Silverstone, L. M. (1974). The effect on enamel of several different topical fluoride agents *in vitro*. *Journal of the International Association of Dentistry for Children*, **5**, 27–32

42. Gish, C. W. (1968). *American Dental Association Newsletter*, **21**, 23

43. Averill, H. M., Averill, J. E. and Ritz, A. G. (1967). A two year comparison of three topical fluoride agents. *Journal of the American Dental Association*, **74**, 996–1001

44. Horowitz, H. S. and Heifetz, S. B. (1969). Evaluation of topical applications of stannous fluoride to teeth of children born and reared in a fluoridated community: final report. *Journal of Dentistry for Children*, **36**, 355–61

45. Englander, H. R., Sherrill, L. T., Miller, B. G., Carlos, J. R., Mellberg, J. R. and Senning, R. S. (1971). Incremental rates of dental caries after repeated topical sodium fluoride applications in children with lifelong consumption of fluoridated water. *Journal of the American Dental Association*, **82**, 354–9

46. Bibby, B. G., Zander, H. A., McKelleget, M. and Labunsky, B. (1946). Preliminary reports on the effect on dental caries of the use of sodium fluoride in a prophylactic

cleaning mixture and in a mouthwash. *Journal of Dental Research,* **25**, 207–11

47. Torell, P. and Siberg, A. (1962). Mouthwash with sodium fluoride and potassium fluoride. *Odontologica Revy,* **13**, 62–71

48. Gerdin, P. O. and Torell, P. (1969). Mouth rinses with potassium fluoride solutions containing manganese. *Caries Research,* **3**, 99–107

49. Torell, P. and Ericsson, Y. (1965). Two-year clinical tests with different methods of local carries-preventive fluorine application in Swedish school-children. *Acta Odontologica Scandinavica,* **23**, 287–322

50. Horowitz, H. S., Creighton, W. E. and McClendon, B. J. (1971). The effect on human dental caries of weekly oral rinsing with a sodium fluoride mouthwash. *Archives of Oral Biology,* **16**, 609–16

51. Koch, G. (1967). Effect of sodium fluoride in dentifrice and mouthwash on incidence of dental caries in schoolchildren. *Odontologica Revy,* **18** (suppl. 2)

52. Koch, G. (1969). Caries increment in school children during and two years after end of supervised rinsing of the mouth with sodium fluoride solution. *Odontologica Revy,* **20**, 323

53. Rugg-Gunn, A. J. Holloway, P. J. and Davies, T. G. H. (1973). Caries prevention by daily fluoride mouthrinsing. *British Dental Journal,* **135**, 353–60

54. Koch, G. and Lindhe, J. J. (1967). The effect of supervised oral hygiene on the gingive of children. The effect of sodium fluoride. *Journal of Periodontical Research,* **2**, 53–64

55. Brandt, R. S., Slack, G. L. and Waller, D. (1972). The use of a sodium fluoride mouthwash in reducing the dental caries increment in eleven year old English schoolchildren. *Proceedings of the British Paedodontic Society,* **2**, 23–5

56. Aasenden. R., DePaola, P. F. and Brudevold, F. (1972). Effects of daily rinsing and ingestion of fluoride solutions upon dental caries and enamel fluoride. *Archives of Oral Biology,* **17**, 1705–14

57. Radole, A. W., Gish, C. W., Peterson, J. K., King, J. D. and Segreto, V. A. (1973). Clinical evaluation of stannous fluoride as an anticaries mouthrinse. *Journal of the American Dental Association,* **86**, 404–8

58. Heifetz, S. G. and Horowitz, H. S. (1972). Fluoride dentrifices, in *Fluorides and Dental Caries* (Ed Newbrun, E.), Charles C. Thomas, Springfield, Ill., p. 22

59. Hargreaves, J. A. and Chester, C. G. (1973). Clinical trails amongst Scottish children of an anti-caries dentifrice composed of 2% Sodium monofluorophosphate. *Community Dentistry and Oral Epidemiology,* **1**, 47–57

60. Hargreaves, J. A., Chester, C. G. and Wagg, B. J. (1975). Assessment of children in active and placebo groups 1 year after termination of clinical trial of a 2% sodium monofluorophosphate dentrifice. *Caries Research,* **9**, 291 (abstract)

61. Heuser, H. and Schmidt, F. F. M. (1968). Zahrikanesprophylaxe durch Treperumprëgniening des Zahrschnelyes mit Fluedlack. *Stoma,* **21**, 91–100

62. Koch, G. and Petersson, L. A. (1972). Fluoride content of enamel surface treated with a varnish containing sodium fluoride. *Odontological Revy,* **23**, 437–46

63. Murray, J. J., Winter, G. B. and Hurst, C. P. (1977). Duraphàt fluoride varnish a 2-year clinical trial in 5-year-old children. *British Dental Journal,* **143**, 11–5

64. Backer Dirks, O., Houwink, B. and Kwant, G. W. (1961). The results of $6\frac{1}{2}$ years of artificial fluoridation of drinking water in the Netherlands. *Archives of Oral Biology,* **5**, 284–300

65. Hyatt, T. P. (1928). A statistical study of the location of dental caries shows the practical value of prophylactic odontotomy. *Dental Digest,* **34**, 235

66. Klein, H. and Knutson, (J. W). Studies in dental caries: effect of ammoniacal silver nitrate on caries in the first permanent

molar. *Journal of the American Dental Association,* **29**, 1420–6

67. Ast, D. B., Busherl, A. and Chase, H. C. (1950). A clinical study of caries prophylaxis with zinc fluoride and potassium ferrocyanide. *Journal of the American Dental Association,* **41**, 437–42

68. Miller, J. (1950). Clinical investigations in preventive dentistry. *British Dental Journal,* **91**, 92–8

69. Nathan, H. S., Nachlas, M. M., Solomon, R. D., Hapern, B. D. and Seligman, A. M. (1960). Non-suture closure of arterial incisions using a rapidly polymerizing adhesive. *Annals of Surgery,* **152**, 648–59

70. Cameron, J. L., Woodward, S. C., Pulaski, E. J., Sleeman, K. H., Brandes, G., Kulkarni, R. K. and Leonard, F. (1965). The degradation of cyanoacrylate tissue adhesive I. *Surgery,*, **58**, 424–30

71. Gwinnett, A. J. and Buonocore, M. G. (1965). Adhesives and caries prevention: a preliminary report. *British Dental Journal,* **119**, 77–80

72. Cueto, E. L. and Buonocore, M. G. (1967). Sealing of pits and fissures with an adhesive resin: its use in caries protection. *Journal of the American Dental Association,* **73**, 121–8

73. Buonocore, M. G. (1955). Simple method of increasing the adhesion of acrylic filling materials to enamel surfaces. *Journal of Dental Research,* **34**, 849–53

74. Ripa, L. W. and Cole, W. W. (1970). Occlusal sealing and caries prevention: results 12 months after a single application of adhesive resin. *Journal of Dental Research,* **49**, 171–3

75. Parkhouse, R. C. and Winter, G. B. (1971). A fissure sealant containing methyl 2-cyanoacrylate as a caries preventive agent: a clinical evaluation. *British Dental Journal,* **130**, 16–9

76. Ninomiya, F., Suchara, Y., Yano, K., Ueka, S., Kobayashi, C. and Sugihara, I. (1968). A clinical evaluation of the efficacy of ethylcyanomethacrylate monomer and methylethacrylate polymer as a filling material for the prevention of tooth caries (in Japanese) *Journal of Kyushu Dental Society,* **22**, 239–43

77. Akeuchi, M., Shimizu, T., Kizu, T., Eto, M., Nakagawa, M., Ohsawa, T. and Oishi, T. (1971). Sealing of the pit and fissure with resin adhesive. IV. Results of five year field work and a method of evaluation of field work for caries prevention. *Bulletin of the Tokyo Dental College,* **12**, 295–316

78. Nakagaki, Y., Takayama, Y., Sakakibara, Y. and Matsuoka, S. (1971). Clinical study on single application with cyanoacrylate sealant (in Japanese). *Japanese Journal of Dental Health,* **20**, 276–9

79. Lee, H. L. and Swartz, M. L. (1971). Sealing of developmental pits and fissures: 1, *In vitro* study. *Journal of Dental Research,* **50**, 133–40

80. Silverstone, L. M. (1974). Fissure sealants: laboratory studies. *Caries Research,* **8**, 2–26

81. Rock, W. P. (1974). Fissure sealants: further results of clinical trials. *British Dental Journal,* **136**, 317–21

82. Bowen, R. L. (1963). Properties of a silica–reinforced polymer for dental restorations. *Journal of the American Dental Association,* **66**, 57–64

83. Roydhouse, R. H. (1968). Prevention of occlusal fissure caries by use of a sealant. A pilot study. *Journal of Dentistry for Children,* **35**, 253–62

84. Lee, H. L., Stoffey, D., Orlowski, J., Swartz, M. L., Ocumpaugh, D. and Neville, K. (1972). Sealing of developmental pits and fissures. III. Effects of fluoride on adhesion of rigid and flexible sealers. *Journal of Dental Research,* **51**, 191–201

85. Buonocore, M. G. (1970). Adhesive sealing of pits and fissures for caries prevention with use of ultraviolet light. *Journal of the American Dental Association,* **80**, 324–8

86. Buonocore, M. G. (1971). Caries prevention in pits and fissures sealed with an adhesive resin polymerized by ultraviolet light: a two year study of a single adhesive application. *Journal of the American Dental Association*, **82**, 1090–3

87. Horowitz, H. S., Heifetz, S. B. and McCune, R. J. (1974). The effectiveness of an adhesive sealant in preventing occlusal caries: findings after two years in Kalispell, Montana. *Journal of the American Dental Association*, **89**, 885

88. McCune, R. J., Horowitz, H. S. and Heifetz, S. B. (1973). Pit and fissure sealants: one year results from a study in Kalispell, Montana. *Journal of the American Dental Association*, **87**, 1177

89. Horowitz, H. S., Heifetz, S. B. and Poulsen, S. (1977). Retention and effectiveness of a single application of an adhesive sealant in preventing occlusal caries: final report after five years of a study in Kalispell, Montana. *Journal of the American Dental Association*, **95**, 1133–9

90. Rock, W. P. (1974). Fissure sealants: further results of clinical trials. *British Dental Journal*, **136**, 317–21

91. Burt, B., Berman, D. S., Gelbier, S. and Silverstone, L. M. (1975). Retention of a fissure sealant six months after application. *British Dental Journal*, **138**, 98–100

92. Douglas, W. H. and Tranter, T. C. (1975). A clinical trial of a fissure sealant–Results after 2 years. *Proceedings of the British Paedodontic Society*, **5**, 17–28

93. Gwinnett, A. J. (1967). A study of enamel adhesives. *Archives of Oral Biology*, **12**, 1615–20

94. Buonocore, M. G., Matsui, A. and Gwinnett, A. J. (1968). Penetration of resin dental materials into enamel surfaces with reference to bonding. *Archives of Oral Biology*, **13**, 61–70

95. Silverstone, L. M. (1975). The acid etch technique: *In vitro* studies with special reference to the enamel surface and the enamel-resin interface, in *Proceedings of an International Symposium on the Acid Etch Technique* (Eds), Silverstone, L. M. and Dogon, I. L. North Central Publishing Co., Minnesota, pp. 13–39

96. Silverstone, L. M., Saxton, C. A., Dogon, I. L. and Fejerskov, O. (1975). Variation in the pattern of acid etching of human dental enamel examined by scanning electron microscopy. *Caries Research*, **9**, 373–87

97. Albert, M. and Grenoble, D. E. (1971). An in vivo study of enamel remineralisation after acid etching. *Journal of the Southern Californian Dental Association*, **39**, 747–51

98. Silverstone, L. M. (1977). Fissure sealants: the susceptibility to dissolution of acid-etched and subsequently abraded enamel *in vitro*. *Caries Research*, **11**, 46–51

99. Oswald, J. (1973). Fluoridation–the alternative. The pattern of dental caries. *Proceedings of the 80th Health Congress of the Royal Society of Health*, London. Royal Society Health Journal, **93**, 257–60

100. Head, J. (1912). A study of saliva and its action on tooth enamel in reference to its hardening and softening. *Journal of the American Medical Association*, **59**, 2118–22

101. Koulourides, T., Cueto, H. and Pigman, W. (1961). Rehardening of softened enamel surfaces of human teeth by solutions of calcium phosphate. *Nature (Lond.)*, **189**, 226–7

102. Silverstone, L. M. and Poole, D. F. G. (1968). The effect of saliva and calcifying solutions upon the histological appearance of enamel caries. *Caries Research*, **2**, 87–96

103. Silverstone, L. M. (1977). Remineralization phenomena. *Caries Research*, **11** (suppl. 1), 59–84

104. Crabb, H. S. M. (1966). Enamel caries: observations on the histology and pattern of progress of the approximal lesion.

British Dental Journal, **121**, 115–29, 167–74

105. Silverstone, L. M. (1973). Structure of carious enamel, including the early lesion, in *Oral Sciences Reviews No. 3: Dental Enamel* (Eds. Melcher, A. H. and Aarb, G.), Munksgaard, Copenhagen, pp. 100–60

106. Silverstone, L. M. (1971). The effect of topical application of calcifying fluids on human dental enamel *in vitro*. *Journal of the International Association of Dentistry for Children*, **2**, 39–54

107. Koulourides, T. (1968). Experimental changes of enamel mineral density. In *Art and Science of Dental Caries Research* (Ed. Harris, R. S.), University Press, Chicago, pp. 355–78

108. Silverstone, L. M. (1972). Remineralization of human enamel *in vitro*. *Proceedings of the Royal Society of Medicine*, **65**, 906–8

109. Feagin, F., Walker, A. A. and Pigman, W. (1969). Evaluation of the calcifying characteristics of biological fluids and inhibitors of calcification. *Calcified Tissue Research*, **4**, 231–44

110. Sobel, A. e. (1950). The local factor in calcification. Metabolic Interrelations, *Transactions 2nd Macy Conference*, **2**, 113–43

111. Sherman, B. S. and Sobel, A. E. (1965). Differentiation between crystal growth in mineralizing tissues and macromolecules. *Archives of Oral Biology*, **10**, 323–42

112. Caldwell, R. C. (1968). Organic components of human salivary secretions. In *Art and Science of Dental Caries Research* (Ed. Harris, R. S.), University Press, Chicago, pp. 43–53

113. McCann, H. G. (1968). Inorganic components of salivary secretions. In *Art and Science of Dental Caries Research* (Ed. Harris, R. S.), University Press, Chicago, pp. 55–78

114. Becks, H. and Wainwright, W. W. (1946). Human saliva. XVII. Relationship of total calcium and inorganic phosphorus to rate of flow of resting saliva. *Journal of Dental Research*, **25**, 275–83

115. Speirs, R. L. (1967). Factors influencing 'maturation' of developmental hypomineralized areas in the enamel of rat molars. *Caries Research*, **1**, 15–31

116. Darling, A. I. (1965). Discussion in *Caries-Resistant Teeth* (Ciba Foundation Symposium), Churchill, London, pp. 141–8

117. Backer Dirks, O. (1966). Posteruptive changes in dental enamel. *Journal of Dental Research*, **45**, 503–11

118. Poole, D. F. G. (1967). Phylogeny of tooth tissues: enameloid and enamel in recent vertebrates with a note on the history of cementum. In *Structural and Chemical Organization of Teeth* (Ed. Miles, A. E. W.), Academic Press, New York, chap. 3, pp. 111–49

119. Koulourides, T. and Dimitriadis, A. (1970). Increase in resistance of human enamel to softening by exposure to acid buffers containing calcium and phosphate. *Archives of Oral Biology*, **15**, 1079–87

120. Starkey, W. E. (1971). Dimensional changes associated with enamel maturation in rabbits. *Archives of Oral Biology*, **16**, 479–93

121. Grenby, T. H. (1971). Tests of calcium sucrose phosphate as a preventive agent against dental caries in rats and *in vitro*. *Journal of Dental Research*, **50**, 1213

122. Bowen, W. H. (1972). The cariostatic effect of calcium glycerophosphate in monkeys. *Caries Research*, **6**, 43–51

123. Jenkins, G. N. (1968). *In vitro* studies using chemicals. In *Art and Science of Dental Caries Research* (Ed. Harris, R. S.), University Press, Chicago, pp. 331–54

124. Neuman, W. F. and Neuman, M. W. (1958). *The Chemical Dynamics of Bone Mineral*, University Press, Chicago

125. Wei, S. H. U. (1970). Electron microprobe analyses of the remineralization of en-

amel. *Journal of Dental Research*, **49**, 621–5

126. Brudevold, F., Savory, A., Gardner, D. E., Spinelli, M. and Speirs, R. (1963). A study of acidulated fluoride solutions. I. *In vitro* effects on enamel. *Archives of Oral Biology*, **8**, 167–77

127. Wellock, W. D., Maitland, A. and Brudevold. F. (1965). Caries increments, tooth discolouration, and state of oral hygiene in children given single annual applications of acid phosphate-fluoride and stannous fluoride. *Archives of Oral Biology*, **10**, 453–60

128. Koulourides, T. and Housch, T. (1972). Influence of strong versus weak acid priming of enamel on the efficacy of SnF_2 applications. *Proceedings 50th General Session of the International Association for Dental Research*, Abstract No. 624

Index